MW01118081

DERMATOLOGY - LABORATORY AND CLINICAL RESEARCH

ENCYCLOPEDIA OF DERMATOLOGY

(6 VOLUME SET)

VOLUME 6

DERMATOLOGY - LABORATORY AND CLINICAL RESEARCH

Additional books in this series can be found on Nova's website under the Series tab.

Additional e-books in this series can be found on Nova's website under the e-book tab.

DERMATOLOGY - LABORATORY AND CLINICAL RESEARCH

ENCYCLOPEDIA OF DERMATOLOGY

(6 VOLUME SET)

VOLUME 6

MEGHAN PRATT
EDITOR

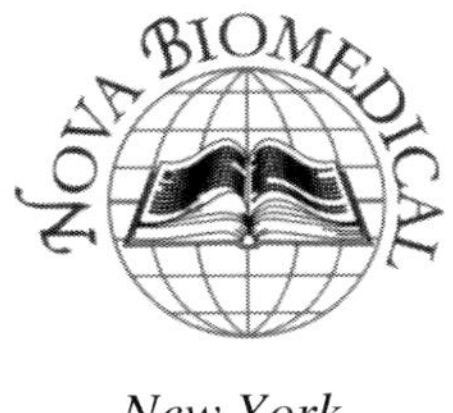

New York

Additional color graphics may be available in the e-book version of this book.

Library of Congress Cataloging-in-Publication Data

ISBN: 978-1-63483-326-4

Library of Congress Control Number: 2015954518

Published by Nova Science Publishers, Inc. † New York

CONTENTS

Preface **xiii**

Volume 1

Chapter 1 Cellular and Histological Changes in Dermis Aging **1**
C. M. Bernal-Mañas, C . Ferrer, E. Beltrán-Frutos, V. Seco-Rovira and L. M. Pastor

Chapter 2 Non-Invasive Methods in the Study of the Dermal Structure and Composition **43**
Jalil Bensaci and Georgios N. Stamatas

Chapter 3 Dermal and Epidermal Interaction: A Critical Role for Skin Homeostasis **63**
Carla Abdo Brohem and Márcio Lorencini

Chapter 4 Melanogenesis and Natural Hypopigmentation Agents **83**
H. M. Chiang, H. W. Chen, Y. H. Huang, S. Y. Chan, C. C. Chen, W. C. Wu and K. C. Wen

Chapter 5 Fungal Melanins: Biosynthesis and Biological Functions **159**
Rodrigo Almeida-Paes, Joshua Daniel Nosanchuk and Rosely Maria Zancope-Oliveira

Chapter 6 The Coat Color Genes Regulate Eumelanin and Pheomelanin Synthesis in Melanocytes **191**
Tomohisa Hirobe

Chapter 7 The Role of Melanin Production in *Gaeumannomyces Graminis* Infection of Cereal Plants **221**
Hanafy Fouly, Shelby Henning, Osman Radwan, Henry Wilkinson and Bruce Martin

Chapter 8 Skin Anatomy and Physiology Research Developments in Melanocytes **249**
Naoki Oiso and Akira Kawada

Chapter 9	Optical Spectroscopy and Structural Properties of Synthetic and Natural Eumelanin *Giuseppe Perna and Vito Capozzi*	**271**
Chapter 10	Melanic Pigmentation in Ectothermic Vertebrates: Occurrence and Function *Classius de Oliveira and Lilian Franco-Belussi*	**293**
	Volume 2	
Chapter 11	Fairness in a Natural Way -- Novel Polyherbal Ingredients Inhibiting Melanin Synthesis and Transfer *S. Gokulshankar, M. S. Ranjith, Babu, M. A. Deepa, B. K. Mohanty and G. Prabhakaran*	**307**
Chapter 12	The Melanocortin-1 Receptor: A Key Melanoma Risk Determinant and a Critical Regulator of the UV DNA Damage Repair Response *Stuart G. Jarrett, Alexandra Amaro-Ortiz, Jason Tucker and John D'Orazio*	**323**
Chapter 13	MC1R, EDNRB and Kit Signaling in Pigmentation Regulation and related Disorders *Javier Pino and Lidia Kos*	**365**
Chapter 14	Multiple Genes and Diverse Hierarchical Pathways Affect Human Pigmentation *C. Ganesh, Anita Damodaran, Martin R. Green, Sheila Rocha, Nicole Pauloski and Shilpa Vora*	**389**
Chapter 15	Acquired Skin Pigmentation *Hideo Nakayama*	**413**
Chapter 16	The Pro-Opiomelanocortin (POMC) and Melanocortin System in Regulation of Human Skin Pigmentation *Han-En Tsai, Elsa C Chan, Gregory J. Dusting and Guei-Sheung Liu*	**441**
Chapter 17	Overview on the Melanocyte Precursor Migration from the Neural Crest *Toyoko Akiyama and Ai Shinomiya*	**455**
Chapter 18	Radiation Treatment and Alopecia – Past and Present Concerns *Paula Boaventura, Dina Pereira, José Teixeira-Gomes and Paula Soares*	**473**
Chapter 19	Psychosocial Aspects in Alopecia Areata: Studies on Stress Involvement in Adults and Children *Liana Manolache*	**489**
Chapter 20	The Power of the Gene: The Origin and Impact of Genetic Disorders Alopecia: Causes, Diagnosis And Treatment *Naoki Oiso and Akira Kawada*	**505**

Chapter 21 Alopecia Areata: Treatment Options **521**
Emina Kasumagić-Halilovic and Nermina Ovcina-Kurtovic

Chapter 22 The Genetic Basis of Alopecia Areata **535**
F. Megiorni, M. Carlesimo, A. Pizzuti and A. Rossi

Chapter 23 Ocular Rosacea: Recent Advances in Pathogenesis and Therapy **545**
Alejandro Rodriguez-Garcia

Chapter 24 Invasive Candidiasis Epidemiology, Diagnosis and Treatment **571**
Mayra Cuéllar Cruz, Guillermo Quindós and Everardo López Romero

Volume 3

Chapter 25 Candida Parapsilosis Complex **617**
D. V. Moris, M. S. C. Melhem, M. A. Martins and R. P. Mendes

Chapter 26 Oral Candidiasis: Conventional and Alternative Treatment Options **655**
C. E. Vergani, P. V. Sanitá, E. G. O. Mima, A. C. Pavarina and A. L. Machado

Chapter 27 Candida Spp. in Oral Cavity of Children with Immunodeficiencies **687**
Dorota Olczak-Kowalczyk, Maria Roszkowska-Blaim, Małgorzata Pańczyk-Tomaszewska, Maria Dąbkowska, Ewa Swoboda-Kopeć, Beta Pyrżak, Ewa Krasuska-Sławińska and Renata Górska

Chapter 28 Oxidative Stress and the Development of Antifungal Agents for the Treatment of Candidiasis **717**
Maxwel Adriano Abegg and Mara Silveira Benfato

Chapter 29 Inhalation and Topical Steroid Therapy and Oral Candidiasis: A Brief Overview **735**
Arjuna N. B. Ellepola, H. M. H. N. Bandara and Hugh D Smyth

Chapter 30 Fluorescent Staining for the Diagnosis of Oral Erythematous Candidiasis **749**
Yoichi Nakagawa

Chapter 31 Cyanosis: Causes, Symptoms and Treatment **761**
K. R. Ramanathan

Chapter 32 Perinatal Cyanosis: Neuropsychological Functioning **767**
Ashlee R. Loughan, Robert Perna and Hana Perkey

Chapter 33 Laryngomalacia: A Cause of Cyanosis in Pediatric Age **789**
Marco Berlucchi, Diego Barbieri, Daniela Tonni, Silvana Molinaro, Patrizia Bardini and Nader Nassif

Chapter 34 The Visual Recognition of Cyanosis and the Influence of Lighting and Color Vision **805**
Stephen J. Dain

Chapter 35 Keratinocytes in Psoriasis: Key Players in the Disease Process **815**
Inas Helwa, Meg Gullotto and Wendy B. Bollag

Chapter 36 Types, Triggers and Treatment Strategies of Psoriasis **871**
Spyridoula Doukaki and Maria Rita Bongiorno

Volume 4

Chapter 37 A New Strategy for the Treatment of Psoriasis — Keratin 17 (K17)-Targeting Therapy **911**
JiXin Gao and Gang Wang

Chapter 38 Narrow-Band Ultraviolet Light B (UVB) and Psoralen Plus UVA Effect in the Circulating Levels of Biological Markers in Psoriasis **937**
Susana Coimbra and Alice Santos-Silva

Chapter 39 Psoriasis Vulgaris Investigated by Electron Paramagnetic Resonance **959**
Kouichi Nakagawa and Daisuke Sawamura

Chapter 40 Psoriasis and Comorbidities **981**
Nayra Merino de Paz, Marina Rodríguez-Martín and Patricia Contreras Ferrer

Chapter 41 Nutrition and the Treatment of Psoriasis **999**
Emily de Golian, Maryam Afshar and Nancy Anderson

Chapter 42 Psoriasis and Cardiovascular Disease - Update **1009**
Manisha R. Panchal, Helen Coope, Anton B Alexandroff and John McKenna

Chapter 43 Bullous Pemphigoid: An Overview **1017**
Alexandre Carlos Gripp, Aline Bressan, Cândida Naira Lima e Lima-Santana and Daniele do Nascimento Pereira

Chapter 44 Bullous Pemphigoid Due to Anti-TNFαlpha **1025**
Vincenzo Bettoli, Stefania Zauli, Michela Ricci and Annarosa Virgili

Chapter 45 Desquamative Gingivitis as an Oral Manifestation of Mucous Membrane Pemphigoid: Diagnosis and Treatment **1031**
Hiroyasu Endo, Terry D. Rees, Hideo Niwa, Kayo Kuyama, Hirotsugu Yamamoto and Takanori Ito

Chapter 46 Associations between Bullous Pemphigoid and Internal Malignancies: A Literature Review **1045**
Yuta Kurashige, Norihiro Ikoma, Tomotaka Mabuchi, Akira Ozawa and Kenichi Iwashita

Chapter 47 New Therapeutic Advances in the Management of Acne **1051**
Vincenzo Bettoli, Stefania Zauli and Annarosa Virgili

Chapter 48 A Large-Scale European Observational Study to Describe the Management of Acne in Clinical Practice **1069**
S. Seité and B. Dreno

Chapter 49 Skin Aging **1079**
Samira Yarak and Carolina A. Pontes da Silva

Chapter 50 A Procedure for the Assessment of Skin Aging **1093**
Natsuko Kakudo, Satoshi Kushida, Nobuko Saito, Kenji Suzuki and Kenji Kusumoto

Chapter 51 Aged Skin and Strenuous Exercise: Can the Skin Handle the Heat? **1099**
Stuart A. Best and Martin W. Thompson

Chapter 52 New Insights on the Regulation of Extracellular Matrix Proteins During Skin Aging **1121**
Connie B. Lin and Michael D. Southall

Chapter 53 Improved Cell Metabolism and Strengthening of the Extracellular Matrix by Nicotinamide, and Copper for Anti-Skin Aging **1141**
Neena Philips, Philips Samuel, Halyna Siomyk, Harit Parakandi, Hui Jia, Sesha Gopal and Hossam Shahin

Chapter 54 Skin Morphology of Caucasian Women during Aging **1157**
H. Zahouani, R. Vargiolu, C. Guinot, E. Tschachler and F. Morizot

Chapter 55 Molecular Understanding of the Development of "Age Spots" **1179**
Connie B. Lin and Miri Seiberg

Chapter 56 Skin Rejuvenation – Ultrastructural Study **1197**
Tokuya Omi and Shigeru Sato

Volume 5

Chapter 57 The Role of Sun Exposure in Skin Aging **1215**
Raja Dahmane, Ruza Pandel, Polonca Trebse and Borut Poljsak

Chapter 58 Photoprotection Practices **1245**
Jacqueline Selph, Ritva Vyas and Meg Gerstenblith

Chapter 59 Risk Factors for Sun Exposure During Spring Break among College Students **1265**
Marvin E. Langston, Stephanie G. Lashway and Leslie K. Dennis

Chapter 60 Sun Exposure and Protection Habits and Vitamin D Levels in Children and Adolescents With a History of Malignancy **1283**
Yael Levy-Shraga and Dalit Modan-Moses

Chapter 61 The Surgeon General's Call to Action to Prevent Skin Cancer: Facts for Consumers **1301**
Surgeon General of the United States

Chapter 62 The Surgeon General's Call to Action to Prevent Skin Cancer **1305**
Meg Watson, Erin Garnett, Gery P. Guy and Dawn M. Holman

Chapter 63 False and Misleading Health Information Provided to Teens by the Indoor Tanning Industry: Investigative Report **1415**
U.S. House of Representatives Committee on Energy and Commerce-Minority Staff

Chapter 64 Metabolomic Assessment of Sunscreen Efficacy **1429**
Manpreeet Randhawa and Michael D. Southall

Chapter 65 The History and Evolution of Sunscreen **1445**
Mary Laschinger and Anna H. Chacon

Chapter 66 Psychology Behind the Use of Sunscreens, Tanning and Skin Cancer Prevention **1457**
Shailee Patel, Tulsie Patel and Katlein França

Chapter 67 The Role of Antioxidants in Sunscreens: The Case of Melatonin **1467**
Ana Flo Sierra, Víctor Flo Sierra, Ana Cristina Calpena Campmany and Beatriz Clares Naveros

Volume 6

Chapter 68 UV Filters, Their Degradation Reactions and Eco-Toxicological Effects **1505**
Albano Joel M. Santos and Joaquim C. G. Esteves da Silva

Chapter 69 Assessment of Sunscreen Safety by Skin Permeation Studies: An Update **1523**
Lucia Montenegro

Chapter 70 UV Protection by Woolen Fabric Dyed with Natural Dyestuff **1541**
Ana Sutlović, Anita Tarbuk, Ana Marija Grancarić and Đurđica Parac-Osterman

Chapter 71 Light Conversion for UV Protection by Textile Finishing and Care **1571**
Tihana Dekanić, Anita Tarbuk, Tanja Pušić, Ana Marija Grancarić and Ivo Soljačić

Chapter 72 The Potential of Mycosporine-Like Amino Acids as UV-Sunscreens **1601**
Rajesh P. Rastogi, Ravi R Sonani, Datta Madamwar and Aran Incharoensakdi

Chapter 73 Guidelines for School Programs to Prevent Skin Cancer **1619**
Karen Glanz, Mona Saraiya and Howell Wechsler

Chapter 74 Shade Planning for America's Schools **1651**
Centers for Disease Control and Prevention

Chapter 75 Sun Safety for America's Youth Toolkit **1703**
Centers for Disease Control and Prevention

Chapter 76 Burn Diagnosis, Management, and Research **1739**
Amy L. Strong, Kavitha Ranganathan, Eric T. Chang, Michael Sorkin, Shailesh Agarwal and Benjamin Levi

Chapter 77 Pediatric Burn in Bangladesh: A Tertiary Level Hospital Experience **1775**
Kishore Kumar Das, M Quamruzzaman and Syed Shamsuddin Ahmed

Chapter 78 Mulligan's Mobilisations with Movement: A Manual Therapy Approach to the reatment and Management of Hand Burn Injuries **1789**
Natalia Montes Carrasco, Maria Jesús Trancón Bergas, Carmen Oreja Sánchez, Maria Virginia Vicente Blanco and Javier Nieto Blasco

Chapter 79 Epidemiological Characteristics of Burn Injuries **1803**
Bishara Atiyeh and Michel Costagliola

Chapter 80 Current and Future Directions of Burn Resuscitation and Wound Management **1813**
Jeanne Lee, Leslie Kobayashi and Raul Coimbra

Index **1823**

PREFACE

This encyclopedia presents important research on dermatological advances. This six set volume includes discussions on the structure and composition of the dermis layer of the skin; the biosynthesis, functions and health benefits of melanin; the genetics, as well as the geographic variation and disorders, of skin pigmentation; the causes, diagnosis and treatment of alopecia, rosacea, candidiasis, cyanosis, psoriasis, and bullous pemphigoid; new research on skin aging; risk factors, protection practices and health effects of sun exposure; skin cancer prevention; the use of sunscreen; skin cancer prevention guidance for schools and youth; and the epidemiology, management and impact on muscle and joint functions of burns.

In: Encyclopedia of Dermatology (6 Volume Set)
Editor: Meghan Pratt

ISBN: 978-1-63483-326-4

Chapter 68

UV FILTERS, THEIR DEGRADATION REACTIONS AND ECO-TOXICOLOGICAL EFFECTS

Albano Joel M. Santos and Joaquim C. G. Esteves da Silva*

Centro de Investigação em Química da Universidade do Porto (CIQ-UP),
Departamento de Química e Bioquímica, Faculdade de Ciências,
Universidade do Porto, Porto, Portugal

ABSTRACT

Sunscreens or sunscreen agents are more notoriously known as ultraviolet (UV) filters, and they are the prime components of many personal care products and pharmaceuticals. Most UV filters are organic compounds that absorb UV radiation, therefore protecting us from solar radiation and its nefarious effects on human skin and health. The protective character of UV filters regarding UV radiation, would presuppose a stable nature towards alterations in general. However, the compounds are well known to undergo degradation, and in many cases quite substantially, either by influence of UV radiation itself (by photolysis or photo-isomerization) or through contact with water disinfecting agents, such as chlorine. These degradation reactions might be quite troublesome, since they generate degradation by-products that either do not present the appropriate UV-protective capabilities, as is the case with photo-isomers, or possess toxicological profiles potentially damaging for both the human health and the environment, as is the case with free-radicals or even disinfection by-products (DBP's).

INTRODUCTION

Ultraviolet (UV) radiation constitutes about 6.2% of the total solar radiation that is able to reach the Earth's surface, given the filtration and mitigation capabilities of the protective ozone layer. Out of this specific portion of the solar radiation, mostly is attributed to UVA radiation (320-400 nm) while a very small portion is attributed to UVB radiation (290-320 nm).

* Corresponding author: Joaquim C.G. Esteves da Silva; jcsilva@fc.up.pt

The highly energetic UVC radiation (100-290 nm) is completely blocked by the ozone layer and therefore does not reach the surface of the planet [1]. Despite the beneficial character of UV radiation (it enhances the production of vitamin D, improving the human resistance towards different pathologies; increases the calcium absorption by the organism; etc.), it is also known to enhance the occurrence of skin cancer, as well as other serious but less prominent issues like inflammations, sunburns, and allergic reactions [1]. It is in this context that sunscreens or sunscreen agents play a fundamental role, by preventing or attenuating the damaging effects of UV radiation on the human skin and health [1].

Sunscreen products include complex formulations of different compounds, of which UV filters are of the utmost importance, since these are the compounds that indeed protect us from UV radiation. As Salvador and Chisvert [2] refer, a sunscreen is defined as any product containing UV filters in its formulation, in order to protect the skin from the negative effects of UV radiation, significantly decreasing its impact on human health [2]. The mechanism of protection, however, is based on two processes that are intimately linked to the two existing types of filters in question: essentially absorption of UV radiation in the case of the vastly more numerous organic UV filters; and reflection or scattering in the case of the few existing inorganic UV filters [3].

UV filters generally display either simple or multiple aromatic structures, often conjugated with carbon-carbon double bonds or carbonyl groups, which attributes them the ability to absorb or scatter UV radiation. These compounds will absorb UV radiation, therefore evolving towards a superior energetic state but returning thereafter to the original state by emitting energy through vibrational transitions or photochemical reactions [4]. As it was already mentioned, UV filters are classified as either organic (UV-absorbent) or inorganic (UV-scattering) compounds. The most prominent classes of UV filters are the benzophenones, salicylates, cinnamates, triazines, *p*-aminobenzoic acid derivatives, dibenzoyl methane derivatives and camphor derivatives, and there are globally about 55 filters approved, regulated and controlled worldwide, out of which merely two are inorganic (zinc oxide and titanium dioxide) [1, 4, 5].

Table 1 includes all the UV filters currently approved in the EU, as well as all their relevant physical-chemical properties [3, 6].

As for the nature of UV filters, these compounds present the features common to most priority organic pollutants (POP's), such as the presence of aromatic rings in association with long and unsaturated aliphatic chains. Most of the filters consist of geometrical isomers (*E* and *Z* forms), although the commercial formulations include solely the *E* isomer. As is visible in Table 1, these compounds exhibit commonly increased lipophilicity, enabling their association with particles rich in organic matter content, such as soils and sediments, as well as high resistance towards biotic degradation, which enhances their accumulation, concentration and persistence in the environment and the food chain [3, 6, 7].

UV Filter Degradation Reactions

Regarding their purpose of application, protection of human skin from the effects of UV radiation, there is the assumption that UV filters are quite stable to general degradation.

Table 1. Physical-chemical properties of the UV filters currently approved and regulated in and by the EU (adapted from [3] and [6])

Structure	INCI name	Acronym	Molecular weight	Log K_{OW}§	Log BCF **;§§	Log K_{OC} ††;§§	Solubility /g/L‡‡	λ_{max} /nm
Benzophenones	Benzophenone-3	BZ3	228.24	3.79	1.38	3.10	0.21	290
	Benzophenone-4	BZ4	308.31	0.88	-	-	0.65	240†; 288
PABA and derivatives	*p*-Aminobenzoic acid	PAB	137.14	0.83	-	-	915	282
	PEG-25 PABA	P25	277.41	-	-	-	-	310*
	Ethylhexyl dimethyl PABA	EDP	277.40	6.15	3.74	3.38	2.1×10^{-3}	310
Salicylates	Homosalate	HS	262.35	6.16	-	-	0.02	-
	Ethylhexyl salicylate	ES	250.34	5.77	-	-	0.028	240*
Cinnamates	Ethylhexyl methoxycinnamate	EMC	290.40	5.80	5.80	4.10	0.15	306†
	Isopentyl *p*-methoxycinnamate	IMC	248.32	4.06	-	-	0.06	-
Camphor derivatives	Camphor benzalkonium methosulfate	CBM	409.55	0.28	-	-	-	288*
	Terephtalydene dicamphor sulfonic acid	TDS	562.69	1.35	-	-	0.014	340*
	Benzylidene camphor sulfonic acid	BCS	320.40	2.74	-	-	0.038	297*
	Polyacrylamidomethyl benzylidene camphor[d]	PBC		-	-	-	-	-
	4-Methylbenzylidene camphor	MBC	254.37	4.95	3.51	3.89	5.1×10^{-3}	300†
	3-Benzylidene camphor	3BC	240.34	4.49			9.9×10^{-3}	292*
Triazines	Ethylhexyltriazone	ET	826.10	15.53	-	-	-	310†
	Diethylhexyl butamido triazone	DBT	765.98	11.90	-	-	4.6×10^{-7}	-
	Bis-Ethylhexyloxyphenol methoxyphenyl triazine	EMT	627.81	13.89	-	-	4.9×10^{-8}	340†
Benzotriazoles	Drometrizole trisiloxane	DRT	225.25	9.79	-	-	1.3×10^{-5}	344; 303
	Methylene bis-benzotriazolyl tetramethylbutylphenol	MBT	658.87	14.35	-	-	3.0×10^{-8}	340†
Benzimidazole derivatives	Phenyl benzimidazole sulfonic acid	PBS	274.30	0.01	0.50	2.46	0.26	300†
	Disodium phenyl dibenzimidazole tetrasulfonate	DPD	674.60	-	-	-	-	250
Dibenzoylmethane derivatives	Butyl methoxydibenzoyl methane	BDM	310.39	2.41	4.51	3.23	0.037	358*
	Diethylamino hydroxybenzoyl hexyl benzoate	DHH	397.51	6.93	-	-	9.5×10^{-4}	360†
Others	Octocrylene	OCR	361.49	7.35	-	-	2.0×10^{-4}	300†
	Polysilicone 15	P15		-	-	-	-	313‡

Data is originated from SciFinder, American Chemical Society, 2008.

UV filters shadowed in green colour, represent the most popular and frequently used compounds in commercial formulations of sunscreen products.

* Rastogi, S.C., Jensen, G.H. (1998), Identification of UV filters in sunscreen products by high-performance liquid chromatography–diode-array detection, *J. Chromatogr. A* 828 (1-2), 311-316.

† De Orsi, D., Giannini, G., Gagliardi, L., Porrà, R., Berri, S., Bolasco, A., Carpani, I., Tonelli, D. (2006), Simple extraction and HPLC determination of UV-A and UV-B filters in sunscreen products, *Chromatographia* 64 (9-10), 509-515.

‡ Philippe Maillan Formulation, R&D Cosmetics, DSM Nutritional Products; Measurement of UV Protection in Hair.

§ Octanol-water partition coefficient (K_{OW}); it regards the ratio between the concentration of a substance in octanol and in water, in equilibrium and at a determined temperature.

** Bio-concentration factor (BCF); it regards the concentration of a substance in an organism and in the water body around it.

†† Organic carbon distribution coefficient (K_{OC}); it regards the ratio between the mass of a substance adsorbed into the soil (by unity of mass of organic carbon in the soil) and the concentration of the same substance in equilibrium in solution.

‡‡ In water and at 25°C.

§§ Giokas, D.L., Salvador, A., Chisvert, A. (2007), UV filters: from sunscreens to the human body and the environment, *Trends in Analytical Chemistry* 26 (5), 360-374.

However, such assumptions are not exactly accurate, in fact, it is well reported and established that UV filters experience degradation from two essential sources: photo-degradation, upon exposure to UV radiation; and degradation induced by disinfecting agents such as chlorine, when in contact with these in aqueous solution [3, 4]. Figure 1 presents the paths of degradation and their consequential by-products.

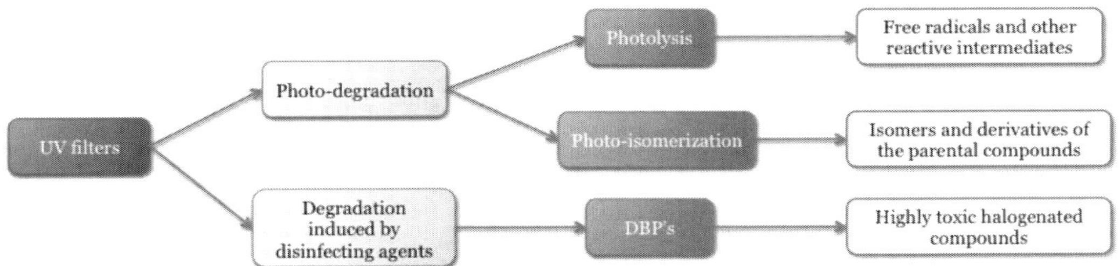

Figure 1. Degradation processes experienced by UV filters.

Photo-Degradation of UV Filters

Photolysis

The direct dissociation of a molecule upon the absorption of a determined amount of energy from a given type of radiation is ever more likely when that amount is equivalent or higher than the bonding energy of that same molecule. When this molecule reaches a higher or excited energy state, it dissociates, and the process is regarded as photolysis [14].

Photolysis is usually a rather complex set of reactions that lead to the formation of reactive species or fragments, and it can be experienced either by direct or indirect paths. Direct photolysis occurs upon the absorption of radiation by specific portions of the UV filters' structure itself, denominated chromophores. Indirect photolysis occurs upon the absorption of radiation by other structures or compounds rather than the UV filter, named photosensitizers, therefore initiating a series of reactions that will induce the transformation or degradation of the filters [3, 8, 9, 14]. Organic compounds will also experience degradation when in contact with reactive species, such as singlet oxygen, hydroxyl radicals, photo-excited organic matter and others [8, 9].

This type of photochemical reactions is one of the most important abiotic processes that control the fate and behaviour of UV filters when in the environment, in particular the aquatic compartments, and in general their prominence is far more significant than the biotic processes of degradation [3, 8], which will be approached in more detail further ahead.

There are numerous studies that have dealt with the subject of photo-degradation, with emphasis on photolysis. The general notion that must be underlined is that as the filters are exposed to UV radiation, they gradually lose their UV-protective features or capabilities [10, 11], which is also accompanied by the formation of several toxic and harmful by-products, as it has been demonstrated with EMC [12]. Sayre [13] stressed the complexity of the photo-degradation issue, since UV filters are used as part of a formulation of several different filters in commercial sunscreen products, and not in singular. In other words, the photochemical profile and behaviour of a matrix of multiple filters is fundamentally different than that displayed by a single UV filter, since the photo-degradation reactions of many filters are known to enhance or even induce the degradation reactions of others, even those supposedly more stable [13]. Serpone has also carried out some interesting studies on the photo-degradation or photo-stability of certain UV filters [10, 11]. His approach [11], delved on the photo-degradation of different UV filters and its extension in aerobic aqueous medium. The study was carried on the basis of the record of any and every alteration to the UV radiation absorbance as a function of irradiation time, with any loss of absorbance being subsequently directly correlated with loss of UV-protective capabilities. Results have shown that, in the case of the filter PAB, for instance, UV radiation absorbance capacity decreased about 35% just within the first hour of irradiation, whereas in the case of a very similar filter, EDP, the UV absorbance decrease was almost complete just after 20 minutes of irradiation. As for TDS, it was defined as the most photo-unstable UV filter of the study, with 90% UV radiation absorbance decrease after just 10 minutes of irradiation, while BZ3 was considered the most photo-stable, with a UV absorbance decrease of 20% and throughout two hours of irradiation.

Photo-degradation studies have always focused on its relation towards photo-protection alterations [10], ability of the filter mixture to enhance photolysis [10, 13], or the toxicological potential of by-products [12], but seldom has it focused on degradation in the environmental context [15]. Sakkas [15] approached simultaneously the disinfection by-product (DBP) formation as well as the photo-degradation by-products. Results have shown that photochemical reaction rates depend, not only on the environmental conditions, but also on the presence of other relevant compounds in solution, in particular dissolved organic matter (DOM). In the case of the filter EDP, degradation decreased significantly with the increase of DOM levels in solution, which is easily explained by the fact that DOM actively competes with any other present organic compound for the incident photons, in regards to photo-degradation. The authors were also able to identify several photo-degradation by-products, namely from dealkylation and hydroxylation, and in all the different sources of water samples studied (distilled water; swimming-pool water; and sea water).

Photo-Isomerization

Contrary to photolysis, photo-isomerization reactions yield new species closely related to the parental structures, but potentially more toxic and harmful than the original compounds. Regarding UV filters in particular, this translates essentially into the production of photo-isomers that may be related but no longer possess the required UV-protective features of the parental molecules, which is prominently evident in several classes of filters: cinnamates; salicylates; camphor derivatives; and dibenzoylmethane derivatives [10, 16-18].

The photo-isomerization of UV filters is both a fast and reversible process, when in aqueous solution, giving origin to a mixture of *E* and *Z* isomers in equilibrium. In the environment, UV filters will always be found in either of these two isomeric forms, given the existence of carbon-carbon exocyclic double bonds in their structure. However, commercial formulations of these compounds contain solely the *E* form of the compounds, despite their immediate photo-isomerization into the *Z* form upon exposure to UV radiation [19].

Another notable disadvantage of these reactions is, as approached earlier, apart from the loss of UV-protective capabilities, the production of potentially more troublesome by-products. For instance, the isomeric forms of UV filters might be chiral and therefore enantiomers, with similar physical-chemical properties, but the compounds will display very distinct environmental fate, behaviour and eco-toxicological profile. Contrary to the biological processes of degradation, that might be stereo-selective or enantio-selective [20], these abiotic processes are apparently not enantio-selective [19]. In light of this, the stereo-isomer composition of UV filters in natural waters seems indeed paramount in order to understand the compounds' fate and behaviour in the environment, but seldom has the theme been the subject of serious and focused investigation [3].

Díaz-Cruz [3] reviews the only existing study focused specifically on the subject: Buser [21] studied the chirality of MBC, showing that the stereo-isomer composition of the filter depended in fact on biological degradation occurring in waste water treatment plants, other water bodies like rivers or lakes, as well as plant or animal life.

There are numerous other studies on the photo-degradation or photo-stability of UV filters in general. One of the most important and popular UV filters, EMC, has been the subject of several interesting studies [10, 22-25]. In a study already mentioned, Sakkas [15] investigated the photochemical behaviour of the filter EDP in different water samples (sea water; swimming pool water; and distilled water) and under natural or artificial solar radiation. Results demonstrate that the filter degrades photo-chemically, originating several by-products; influence of dissolved organic matter (DOM) was also evaluated, showing that its presence decreases the photo-degradation reaction rates, since it competes with the filters for the incident photons; several by-products were also successfully identified. Huong [24] studied the photo-isomerization of EMC under artificial solar radiation and in several different solvents. Results showed significant loss in UV-absorbance capacity after irradiation, occurrence of chemical environmentally-dependent photo-isomerization *E* ➔ *Z* as well as irreversible degradation of the filter structure; *Z* isomer displays considerable lower UV-absorbance capacity; and photo-degradation by-products were also detected and successfully identified. Pattanaargson [22] also approached the photo-isomerization of EMC in different solvents and under natural solar radiation. The relevant results were as follows: photo-isomerization *E* ➔ *Z* resulted in significant loss of UV-absorbance capacity; *E-Z* equilibrium in solution does occur but it depends on solvent polarity. Pattanaargson and Limphong [23] approached the photo-stability of EMC on a chromatographic basis, in order to determine the obtained photo-degradation by-products. The authors have successfully determined one photo-degradation by-product, identified as the *Z* form of the filter, referring that after one day of irradiation, approximately half of the amount of the original *E* form of the filter had been transformed into the by-product. No irreversible compound structure degradation of the filter was detected. Maier [26] carried out a spectroscopically-focused study on the spectral alterations undergone by a set of sunscreen products upon exposure to artificial solar radiation, and its reflection on the UV-absorbance capacity. Results have shown the following: loss in UVB-absorbance capacity never exceeded 5% and considering all the irradiation times; UVA-absorbance capacity loss was generally much more significant and frequent; all products displayed increased spectroscopic photo-instability at increasing wavelengths. Gaspar and Maia Campos [27] evaluated the *in vitro* photo-stability of different combinations of UV filters in sunscreen products, under artificial solar radiation. Results have demonstrated that the interaction between filters within a formulation influences their photo-stability; and formulations containing the filter OCR increased their UVA-absorbance capacity. Huong [28] carried out another study similar to the one mentioned before for EMC [24], but focused now on BDM [28]. As far as the results are concerned, BDM demonstrated photo-instability in non-polar solvents, with significant alterations in its absorption spectra;

these alterations, despite significant, were found to be reversible after protection and storage of the irradiated solutions in the dark, but also found to be inhibited depending on the solvent conditions; the general behaviour of BDM was considered analogous to that of EMC, and it displayed quite significant and irreversible degradation of the filter structure in aqueous solution; several photo-degradation by-products were detected and successfully identified; photo-degradation in general was found to be significantly influenced and dependent on the medium and experimental conditions.

Many other similar studies exist, like Mturi's and Martincigh's [29] that dealt with the photo-stability of BDM in different solvents; or Hojerová's study [30], that ascertained the protective efficiency of several sunscreen products containing different UV filter formulations, and concluded that the sunscreen products' UV-protective efficiency is quite distinct from one another, even between commercial products with the same labeled sun protection factor (SPF); Rodil [25] also evaluated the photo-stability of several UV filters, as well as the eco-toxicological profile of their photo-degradation by-products in aquatic microorganisms; Perugini [31] carried out a very interesting study on the effect of nanoparticle encapsulation of the filter EMC on its photo-stability; and Scalia [32] evaluated the effect of the natural antioxidant quercetin, on the photo-stability of a combination of two of the most popular UV filters used worldwide, EMC and BDM.

Degradation Induced by Disinfecting Agents

The water disinfection process has the fundamental purpose of destroying aquatic microbiological organisms, which represent the ultimate contagion source of disease. This is contrary to the concept of sterilization, which involves complete destruction of every microorganism, something that may not always be achievable or even necessary or beneficial [33].

For more than a century, chlorine has been the most popular disinfecting agent used worldwide, successfully controlling and even eliminating water-borne infectious diseases altogether [8]. Despite this, there are several other types of less popular disinfecting agents, like ozone or even UV radiation, both used in high-scale swimming-pool water disinfection, but also bromide-based water disinfecting agents, used in lower-scale swimming pools [33]. Although the removal of relevant pathogens and microorganisms is rather effective, the removal of DOM is not. Removal of organic pollutants is rather complex and varies significantly [3].

The disinfection process transforms the organic compounds in the water, giving origin to the so-called disinfection by-products (DBP's), or in this particular case, chlorinated DBP's. Over the years, chlorinated DBP's have been directly associated with several and serious potential toxicological effects, which forced authorities to consider the problem of production of these compounds in the context of drinking water disinfection process [3, 8]. Reports indicate that exposure to chlorinated DBP's might be directly associated with the occurrence of several cancers in human vital organs, so Gopal [33] approached predictive models for production and kinetics of DBP formation, their health effects, removal techniques, and guideline implementation.

Given the use of other aforementioned water disinfecting agents, apart from the vastly more popular chlorine, based on either bromide or iodine, important focus is now being given to brominated and iodinated DBP's. These compounds are reported to be significantly toxic, not only in the range of carcinogenicity, but also genotoxicity and cytotoxicity. Such compounds include iodo-acids, like iodo-acetic acid, bromonitromethanes, iodinated-trihalomethanes, 3-Chloro-4-(dichloromethyl)-5-hydroxy-2(5H)-furanone (best known by its historical name, Mutagen X or MX), halogenated-aldehydes, halogenated-amides, bromate, and many others [35]. Also a particular reason for concern is yet another by-product of chlorine disinfection, the production of chloramines, which are originated from the reaction of chlorine with ammonia. Research has indicated that chloramines potentiate the iodo-acids and iodinated-trihalomethane production and accumulation within the water compartments [8].

Researchers have previously approached the general pathways of introduction and movement of synthetic organic pollutants, into and throughout the environment, with emphasis on the aquatic compartments [6, 8]. Generally speaking, the mode of introduction of these compounds into the environmental compartments will very much depend on their pattern of use or application [8]. When in the environment, however, these are transformed, chemically, photo-chemically or biologically. Usually, these processes will lead to the compounds' structure breakdown and subsequent elimination, but at the same time degradation by-products may also be produced, often more persistent and toxic than the original structures [6, 8]. Figure 2 represents the pathways involved in the generic fate and behaviour of UV filters and corresponding by-products in the environment [6].

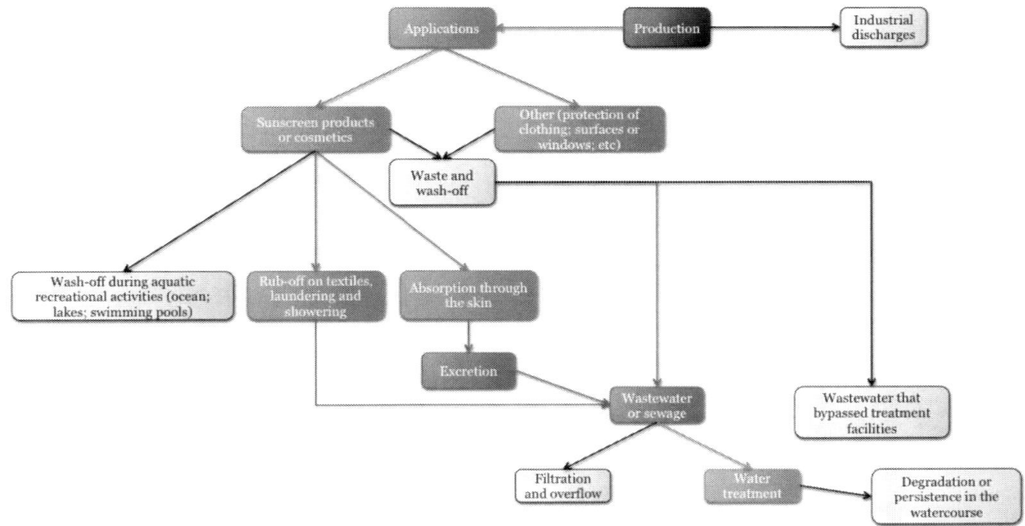

Figure 2. Relevant pathways of introduction of UV filters and their degradation by-products, into the environment (inspired by and adapted from [6]; boxes filled in light grey correspond to potential processes of release into the environment).

An evaluation on the occurrence of DBP's was carried out in Turkish superficial waters with low levels of dissolved organic carbon [36]. Results have shown that, given the susceptibility of the DBP precursors to associate with soils and sediments, events like ground-level run-off or leaching from soils as well as re-suspension into the watercourse from sediments, increased their levels in the superficial aquatic compartments. Upon treatment with chlorine disinfecting agents, it led to the production and increase of DBP's in drinking water.

There isn't any data available on the determination of UV filters DBP's in water treatment facilities [3]. Nonetheless, given the combined action of solar radiation and the presence of disinfecting species in solution, UV filters will be readily halogenated, giving origin to halogenated species of the parental compounds as well as many other DBP's as a result of the degradation of the original structure. Up to this moment, there are only four studies focused on the UV filter degradation reactions in aqueous solution on the presence of chlorine disinfecting agents [1, 37-39], along with a comprehensive review on both the UV filter photo-degradation by-products in aqueous solution, and the UV filters' DBP formation studies until 2012 [40].

Regarding the study of these compounds, very little is still known about the degradation reactions induced by disinfecting agents, and what is indeed known is focused solely on a very limited number of the most popular UV filters [1, 37-39]. More focus should be given towards the disinfection process and its implications on the degradation of UV filters.

Eco-Toxicological Effects of UV Filters and Their Degradation by-Products

The physical-chemical properties of UV filters, presented in Table 1, such as water solubility, vapour pressure and polarity, are crucial in order to determine their behaviour in the environment. As already mentioned, data points to their substantial tendency to concentration and accumulation within the environment and food chain, which, associated with their also reported significant potential for eco-toxicity, is quite problematic [3, 6, 8, 15, 41, 42].

Díaz-Cruz and Barceló [43] have reviewed some of the most important existing eco-toxicological studies, performed both *in vitro* and *in vivo*. What follows, is a brief summary on these and some additional relevant studies and subsequent results and conclusions.

In Vitro Studies

Several UV filters have been reported to display estrogenic activity *in vitro* [7, 44-48]. The *in vitro* models applied or used on these and other studies, often revolve around the highly efficient, sensitive, fast and inexpensive recombinant yeast assay [44, 47, 48], MCF-7 breast cancer cells [45, 48], the human embryonic kidney 293 reporter gene assay (HEK293) [7], the human endometrial Ishikawa cell line [46], or rat and human primary hepatocytes [46].

Regarding the UV filters commonly approached in *in vitro* studies, benzophenones seem to be quite popular in that regard, with Schultz [44] investigating their estrogenic activity in specific, although the compounds have been addressed in many other studies, in particular BZ3 [7, 45, 47].

MBC has also been the subject of some particular studies, regarding its interaction towards estrogenic receptors [46, 48], amongst other more generic *in vitro* eco-toxicological studies [7, 45, 47]. Amidst the most popular UV filters, one must also underline the UV filters EMC, BDM and EDP, also investigated as to their estrogenic activity [7, 45, 47].

As for the relevant eco-toxicological conclusions arisen from these studies, all have emphasized the issues subsequent to this context of investigation. These problems include noncommittal results or the clear inability of the general *in vitro* models to account for the toxico-kinetics and toxico-dynamics of complex whole organisms, which highlights their prominent limitations as to relevant predictive value for a mammalian *in vivo* context. Overall, nearly all filters have demonstrated dose-dependent estrogenic activity, with benzophenones being amongst the most active, as was the case of BZ3 [7, 45], with EMC [7] and BDM [45] being the least active and inactive, respectively, in the same type of studies. The estrogenic activity seems to be directly linked to the presence of benzene rings substituted with polar functional groups, particularly in *para-* position, as well as with the presence of symmetry in the molecule [44]. MBC, one of the filters studied in specific, has demonstrated either estrogenic activity analogous to that of other know weak estrogens [46] or ambiguous results occurring at extremely high levels [48].

Possible effects on thyroid hormonal regulation have also been mentioned [43, 48], but the data on the subject are rather scarce [49]. This study used a new human recombinant thyroid peroxidase stably transfected into a human follicular thyroid carcinoma cell line (FTC-238), in order to assess the possible effects of the filter BZ2.

Very significant disturbance of thyroid hormone homeostasis by inhibition of thyroid peroxidase was reported, making BZ2 the most potent thyroid peroxidase inhibitor found to date [49]. A similar study using human FTC-133 thyroid carcinoma cells [50] showed the opposite results for EMC and MBC.

Evaluation of mere estrogenic activity of UV filters has always been the main focus of hormonal activity studies of these compounds, but multiple combined hormonal effects (estrogenic, anti-estrogenic, androgenic and anti-androgenic effects) have seldom been investigated. Several UV filters have been recently shown to display multiple endocrine-disrupting behaviour like MBC, which displayed estrogenic and anti-estrogenic activities, or BZ3 and HS, which demonstrated estrogenic, anti-estrogenic and anti-androgenic activities [7, 51-53].

In another study [54], out of 19 UV filters and two benzophenone metabolites, all displayed some kind of hormonal effect, merely two (P25 and PAB) did not demonstrate multiple hormonal effects, while the vast majority demonstrated multiple effects. However, as Díaz-Cruz and Barceló argue [43], these effects might be subjective, since individual activities are directly and significantly dependent on the type of tests conducted.

Regarding the *in vitro* studies on UV filters' transformation or degradation by-products, seldom has it been the subject of any studies. The exceptions are a study by Butt and Christensen [12], which dealt with the toxicity of photo-degradation by-products of EMC and BDM in a mouse lymphoma cell line (L5178Y-R), and a more recent study from Nakajima [38], which focused on the mutagenic activity of EMC and EDP using a mutagenic assay on a *Salmonella typhimurium* strain (TA100).

Butt and Christensen [12] demonstrated that exposure to irradiated solutions of UV filter resulted in increased cell mortality, independently of the irradiation time. Regarding Nakajima's study [38], both EMC and EDP were not mutagenic in the referred assay, with the opposite being exhibited after chlorination. EMC's mutagenic by-products of chlorination however, proved to be unstable after 6 hours of completion of the chlorination reactions, since the mutagenicity of the solutions decreased subsequently.

In Vivo Studies

Díaz-Cruz and Barceló [43] mention that benzophenones are the essential focus of study, regarding *in vivo* investigations, and these are mostly centered on evaluation of hormonal effects, effects on reproduction or fertility [54-64].

The usual *in vivo* models of investigation include mostly fish, particularly juvenile or mature fathead minnows (*Pimephales promelas*) [54-58], Japanese rice fish (*Oryzias latipes*) [58, 62] or rainbow trout (*Oncorhynchus mykiss*) [58], with some existing studies also in ovariectomized rats [59, 60, 61], tadpoles [57, 63] or even fetal rats [64]. Benzophenones are indeed a special focus of these studies, particularly BZ2 [56, 59, 60] and BZ3 [58, 60], given the fact that the molecular structure of this class of compounds is quite similar to other known estrogenic chemicals. But camphor derivatives have also been approached often, with particular emphasis on MBC [57, 62-64] and 3BC [55, 57, 63, 64]. There are two existing studies on the extremely popular EMC [61, 62].

Regarding the conclusions of these studies, all have emphasized concerning considerations, and in general, dose-dependent: significant bioaccumulation factors [55, 56], which has also been approached in previous chapters (see Table 1 and corresponding references [3, 6]); quite significant decrease in fecundity or complete cessation of reproductive ability [55-58]; demasculinization of secondary sexual characteristics [55, 57]; significant induction of Vitellogenin [54, 55, 57, 58]; prominent effects in the masculine and feminine gonad histology [55, 56, 57]; and development of both oocytes and spermatocytes, as well as egg production, inhibited [55, 56, 57, 58].

On the other hand, MBC and 3BC displayed no accountable effects on tadpole's hormonal and thyroidal systems during metamorphosis [57], which was described as a critical stage quite susceptible to endocrine disruptions. The filter Ethyl-*p*-aminobenzoate (yet another *p*-aminobenzoic acid derivative) also did not exhibit negative effects on fathead minnows' weight and length development, and mortality was not verified either, upon exposure to the compound [54].

As a counterweight to all the concerning findings, some authors argue that many of the toxicological effects are found and reported at extremely high levels, sometimes as high as 75 fold the levels previously reported for wastewater effluents [58]. At environmental levels, however, MBC and 3BC were both studied as to their effects on the hormonal, thyroidal and sexual systems of tadpoles, during metamorphosis, and after 35 days of exposure, no relevant negative effects were found [63]. Contrary to this fact, studies have also reported that significant toxicological effects may indeed be found at low levels, as was the case with 3BC, which induced prominent histological and reproductive effects in fish and at low concentrations [57].

FUTURE PERSPECTIVES

In light of what was approached in this review, it is important to emphasize that very little is still known about the aqueous degradation reactions of UV filters induced by disinfecting agents. Very few filters have been studied in this context (essentially EMC, BDM and EDP), and considering the findings of these studies, it is imperative to focus even more on this context and extend the investigation towards other filters amongst the most popular.

Special attention should also be given to the determination of their DBP's, which is a field of special concern given their potential hazardous toxicological effects.

Considering the eco-toxicological reviews, it seems clear that additional studies are also required, given the ambiguous results obtained so far. Both the *in vitro* and *in vivo* contexts of toxicological investigation are of paramount importance, and should therefore be used in succession in order to achieve a reliable assessment of the eco-toxicity of UV filters and by-products. However, there are still many issues to consider and solve, particularly regarding the *in vitro* models: the typical models used carry significant unclearness regarding procedures and protocols; many display limited predictive value towards the *in vivo* results; and none reflect or replicate the metabolic processes of complex whole organisms, which is clear from the usually conflicting *in vitro* and *in vivo* results.

Naturally, the *in vitro* models lack the capacity to account for the toxico-kinetics and dynamics of complete organisms, which represents a comprehensive disadvantage. This fact stresses the need to carry out studies *in vivo*, following the investigations made *in vitro*, for these often generate inconclusive results and that do not necessarily reflect what may indeed occur in whole organisms.

Acknowledgments

A. J. M. Santos wishes to acknowledge Fundação para a Ciência e Tecnologia (FCT) for the Ph.D. Program in Sustainable Chemistry grant PD/BD/52530/2014.

References

[1] Chisvert, A., Salvador, A. (2007), *Analysis of Cosmetic Products*, Chapter 3, Elsevier, Amsterdam, The Netherlands.

[2] Salvador, A., Chisvert, A. (2005), Sunscreen analysis – a critical survey on UV filter determination, *Anal. Chim. Acta* 537, 1-14.

[3] Díaz-Cruz, M. S., Llorca, M., Barceló, D. (2008), Organic UV filters and their photodegradates, metabolites and disinfection by-products in the aquatic environment, *Trends in Analytical Chemistry* 27 (10), 873-887.

[4] Shaath, N. A. (2010), Ultraviolet filters, Photochem. *Photobiol.* 9, 464-469.

[5] Shaath, N. A. (2005), The chemistry of UV filters, in: Sunscreens: Regulations and Commercial Development, 3rd Edition, *Taylor and Francis*, New York, USA, pp. 217-238.

[6] Giokas, D. L., Salvador, A., Chisvert, A. (2007), UV filters: from sunscreens to the human body and the environment, *Trends in Analytical Chemistry* 26 (5), 360-374.

[7] Schreurs, R., Lanser, P., Seinen, W., Van der Burg, B. (2002), Estrogenic activity of UV filters determined by an in vitro reporter gene assay and an in vivo transgenic zebrafish assay, *Arch. Toxicol.* 76 (5-6), 257-261.

[8] La Farré, M., Pérez, S., Kantiani, L., Barceló, D. (2008), Fate and toxicity of emerging pollutants, their metabolites and transformation products in the aquatic environment, *Trends in Analytical Chemistry* 27 (11), 991-1007.

[9] Lam, M. W., Tantuco, K., Mabury, S. A. (2003), PhotoFate: a new approach in accounting for the contribution of indirect photolysis of pesticides and pharmaceuticals in surface waters, *Environ. Sci. Technol.* 37 (5), 899-907.

[10] Serpone, N., Salinaro, A., Emeline, A. V., Horikoshi, S., Hidaka, H., Zhao, J. (2002), An in vitro systematic spectroscopic examination of the photostabilities of a random set of commercial sunscreen lotions and their chemical UVB/UVA active agents, *Photochem. Photobiol. Sci.* 1 (12), 970-981.

[11] Serpone, N., Dondi, D., Albini, A. (2007), Inorganic and organic UV filters: their role and efficacy in sunscreens and suncare products, *Inorganica Chim. Acta* 360 (3), 794-802.

[12] Butt, S. T., Christensen, T. (2000), Toxicity and phototoxicity of chemical sun filters, *Radiat. Prot. Dosim.* 91 (1-3), 283-286.

[13] Sayre, R. M., Dowdy, J.C., Gerwig, A.J., Shields, W.J., Lloyd, R.V. (2005), Unexpected photolysis of the sunscreen octinoxate in the presence of the sunscreen avobenzone, *Photochem. Photobiol.* 81 (2), 452-456.

[14] Rohatgi-Mukherjee, K.K. (1978), *Fundamentals of Photochemistry* (Revised Edition), New Age International Limited Publishers.

[15] Sakkas, V.A., Giokas, D.L., Lambropoulou, D.A., Albanis, T.A. (2003), Aqueous photolysis of the sunscreen agent octyl-dimethyl-p-aminobenzoic acid. Formation of disinfection by-products in chlorinated swimming pool water, *J. Chromatogr.* A 1016, 211-222.

[16] Broadbent, J.K., Martincigh, B.S., Raynor, M.W., Salter, L.F., Moulder, R., Sjoberg, P. and Markides, K.E. (1996), Capillary supercritical fluid chromatography combined with atmospheric pressure chemical ionisation mass spectrometry for the investigation of photoproduct formation in the sunscreen absorber 2-ethylhexyl-p-methoxycinnamate, *J. Chromatogr.* A 732 (1), 101-110.

[17] Deflandre, A. and Lang, G. (1988), Photostability assessment of sunscreens. Benzylidene camphor and dibenzoylmethane derivatives, *Int. J. Cosmet. Sci.* 10 (2), 53-62.

[18] Plaguellat, C., Kupper, T., Furrer, R., Alencastro, L., Grandjean, D. and Tarradellas, J. (2006), Concentrations and specific loads of UV filters in sewage sludge originating from a monitoring network in Switzerland, *Chemosphere* 62 (6), 915-925.

[19] Poiger, T., Buser, H.R., Balmer, M.E., Bergqvist, P.A. and Müller, M.D. (2004), Occurrence of UV filter compounds from sunscreens in surface waters: regional mass balance in two Swiss lakes, *Chemosphere* 55 (7), 951-963.

[20] Ariens, E. J. (1989), Stereoselectivity of bioactive agents, general aspects, in: *Stereochemistry and Biological Activity of Drugs*, Ariens, E.J., Soudijn, W., Timmermann, P.B.M.W.M. (Editors), Blackwell, Oxford, UK.

[21] Buser, H.-R., Müller, M.D., Balmer, M.E., Poiger, T., Buerge, I.J. (2005), Stereoisomer Composition of the chiral UV filter 4-Methylbenzylidene camphor in environmental samples, *Environ. Sci. Technol.* 39 (9), 3013-3019.

[22] Pattanaargson, S.T., Munhapol, T., Hirunsupachot, P. and Luangthongaram, P. (2004), Photoisomerization of octyl methoxycinnamate, *J. Photochem. Photobiol.* A 161 (2-3), 269-274.

[23] Pattanaargson, S.T., Limphong, P. (2001), Stability of octyl methoxycinnamate and identification of its photo-degradation product, *Int. J. Cosmet. Sci.* 23 (3), 153-160.

[24] Huong, S.P., Andrieu, V., Reynier, J.-P., Rocher, E., Fourneron, J.-D. (2007), The photoisomerization of the sunscreen ethylhexyl p-methoxy cinnamate and its influence on the sun protection factor, *J. Photochem. Photobiol.* A 186 (1), 65-70.

[25] Rodil, R., Moeder, M., Altenburger, R., Schmitt-Jansen, M. (2009), Photostability and phytotoxicity of selected sunscreen agents and their degradation mixtures in water, *Anal. Bioanal. Chem.* 395 (5), 1513-1524.

[26] Maier, H., Schauberger, G., Brunnhofer, K. and Honigsmann, H. (2001), Change of ultraviolet absorbance of sunscreens by exposure to solar-simulated radiation, *J. Invest. Dermatol.* 117 (2), 256-262.

[27] Gaspar, L.R., Maia Campos, P.M.B.G. (2006), Evaluation of the photostability of different UV filter combinations in a sunscreen, *Int. J. Pharm.* 307 (2), 123-128.

[28] Huong, S.P., Rocher, E., Fourneron, J.-D., Charles, L., Monnier, V., Bun, H., Andrieu, V. (2008), Photoreactivity of the sunscreen butylmethoxydibenzoylmethane (DBM) under various experimental conditions, *J. Photochem. Photobiol. A* 196 (1), 106-112.

[29] Mturi, G.J. and Martincigh, B.S. (2008), Photostability of the sunscreening agent 4-tert-butyl-4′-methoxydibenzoylmethane (avobenzone) in solvents of different polarity and proticity, *J. Photochem. Photobiol. A* 200 (2-3), 410-420.

[30] Hojerová, J., Medovcíková, A., Mikula, M. (2011), Photoprotective efficacy and photostability of fifteen sunscreen products having the same label SPF subjected to natural sunlight, *Int. J. Pharm.* 408 (1-2), 27-39.

[31] Perugini, P., Simeoni, S., Scalia, S., Genta, I., Modena, T., Conti, B., Pavanetto, F. (2002), Effect of nanoparticle encapsulation on the photostability of the sunscreen agent, 2-ethylhexyl-p-methoxycinnamate, *Int. J. Pharm.* 246 (1-2), 37-45.

[32] Scalia, S., Mezzena, M. (2010), Photostabilization effect of quercetin on the UV filter combination, Butyl methoxydibenzoylmethane-Octyl Methoxycinnamate, *Photochem. Photobiol.* 86 (2), 273-278.

[33] Gopal, K., Tripathy, S.S., Bersillon, J.L., Dubey, S.P. (2007), Chlorination by-products, their toxico-dynamics and removal from drinking water, *J. Hazard. Mater.* 140 (1-2), 1-6.

[34] Scholz, M. (2006), *Wetland Systems To Control Urban Runoff*, Chapter 22, Elsevier, Amsterdam, The Netherlands, pp. 155-162.

[35] Richardson, S.D. (2005), New disinfection by-product issues: emerging DBPs and alternative routes of exposure, *Global NEST J.* 7 (1), 43-60.

[36] Ates, N., Kaplan, S.S., Sahinkaya, E., Kitis, M., Dilek, F.B., Yetis, U. (2007), Occurrence of disinfection by-products in low DOC surface waters in Turkey, *J. Hazard. Mater.* 142 (1-2), 526-534.

[37] Negreira, N., Canosa, P., Rodríguez, I., Ramil, M., Rubí, E., Cela, R. (2008), Study of some UV filters stability in chlorinated water and identification of halogenated by-products by gas chromatography–mass spectrometry, *J. Chromatogr. A* 1178 (1-2), 206-214.

[38] Nakajima, M., Kawakami, T., Niino, T., Takahashi, Y., Onodera, S. (2009), Aquatic fate of sunscreen agents Octyl-4-methoxycinnamate and Octyl-4-dimethylaminobenzoate in model swimming pools and the mutagenic assays of their chlorination by-products, *J. Health Sci.* 55 (3), 363-372.

[39] Santos, A.J.M., Crista, D.M.A., Miranda, M.S., Almeida, I.F., Sousa e Silva, J.P., Costa, P.C., Amaral, M.H., Lobão, P.A.L., Sousa Lobo, J.M., Esteves da Silva, J.C.G.

(2013), Degradation of UV filters 2-Ethylhexyl-2-methoxycinnamate and 4-tert-Butyl-4'-methoxydibenzoylmethane in chlorinated water, *Environ. Chem.* 10 (2), 127-134.

[40] Santos, A.J.M., Miranda, M.S., Esteves da Silva, J.C.G. (2012), The degradation products of UV filters in aqueous and chlorinated aqueous solutions, *Water Res.* 46 (10), 3167-3176.

[41] Balmer, M.E., Buser, H.R., Müller, M.D., Poiger, T. (2004), Occurrence of organic UV filter compounds BP-3, 4-MBC, EHMC and OC, in wastewater, surface waters and in fish from Swiss lakes, Agroscope, Swiss Federal Research Station for Horticulture, *Plant Protection Chemistry*, CH-8820 Wädenswill, Switzerland.

[42] Giokas, D.L., Sakkas, V.A., Albanis, T.A. (2004), Determination of residues of UV filters in natural waters by solid-phase extraction coupled to liquid chromatography–photodiode array detection and gas chromatography–mass spectrometry, *J. Chromatogr. A* 1026 (1-2), 289-293.

[43] Díaz-Cruz, M.S., Barceló, D. (2009), Chemical analysis and ecotoxicological effects of organic UV-absorbing compounds in aquatic ecosystems, *Trends in Analytical Chemistry* 28 (6), 708-717.

[44] Schultz, T.W., Seward, J.R., Links, G.D. (2000), Estrogenicity of benzophenones evaluated with a recombinant yeast assay: Comparison of experimental and rules-based predicted activity, *Environ. Toxicol. Chem.* 19 (2), 301-304.

[45] Schlumpf, M., Cotton, B., Consciente, M., Haller, V., Steinmann, B., Linchtesteiger, W. (2001), In vitro and in vivo estrogenicity of UV screens, *Environ. Health Perspect.* 109 (3), 239-244.

[46] Müller, S.O., Kling, M., Firzani, P.A., Mecky, A., Durante, E., Shields-Botella, J., Delansorne, R., Broschard, T., Kramer, P.J. (2003), Activation of estrogen receptor α and β by 4-methylbenzylidene-camphor in human and rat cells: comparison with phyto- and xenoestrogens, *Toxicol. Lett.* 142 (1-2), 89-101.

[47] Kunz, P.Y., Galicia, H.F., Fent, K. (2006), Comparison of In Vitro and In Vivo Estrogenic Activity of UV Filters in Fish, *Toxicol. Sci.* 90 (2), 349-361.

[48] Tinwell, H., Lefevre, P.A., Moffat, G.J., Burns, A., Odum, J., Spurway, T.D., Orphanides, G., Sabih, J. (2002), Confirmation of uterotrophic activity of 3-(4-methylbenzylidine)camphor in the immature rat, Environ. *Health Perspect.* 110 (5), 533-536.

[49] Schmutzler, C., Bacinski, A., Gotthardt, I., Huhne, K., Ambrugger, P., Klammer, H., Schlecht, C., Hoang-Vu, C., Grüters, A., Wuttke, W., Jarry, H., Köhrle, J. (2007), The ultraviolet filter benzophenone-2 interferes with the thyroid hormone axis in rats and is a potent in vitro inhibitor of human recombinant thyroid peroxidase, *Endocrinology* 148 (6), 2835-2844.

[50] Schmutzler, C., Hamann, I., Hofmann, P.J., Kovacs, G., Stemmler, L., Memtrup, B., Schomburg, L., Ambrugger, P., Grüters, A., Seidlova-Wuttke, D., Jarry, H., Wuttke, W., Köhrle, J. (2004), Endocrine active compounds affect thyrotropin and thyroid hormone levels in serum as well as endpoints of thyroid hormone action in liver, heart and kidney, *Toxicology* 205 (1-2), 95-102.

[51] Schreurs, R., Sonneveld, E., Hansen, J.H.J., Seeinen, W., Van der Burg, B. (2005), Interaction of Polycyclic Musks and UV Filters with the Estrogen Receptor (ER), Androgen receptor (AR), and progesterone receptor (PR) in reporter gene bioassays, *Toxicol. Sci.* 83 (2), 264-272.

[52] Ma, R., Cotton, B., Lichtensteiger, W., Schlumpf, M. (2003), UV Filters with antagonistic action at androgen receptors in the MDA-kb2 cell transcriptional-activation assay, *Toxicol. Sci.* 74 (1), 43-50.

[53] Schlumpf, M., Schmid, P., Durres, S., Consciente, M., Maerkel, K., Henseler, E., Gruetter, M., Herzog, I., Reolon, S., Ceccatelli, R., Faass, O., Stutz, O., Jarry, H., Wuttke, W., Lichtensteiger, W. (2004), Endocrine activity and developmental toxicity of cosmetic UV filters—an update, *Toxicol.* 205 (1-2), 113-122.

[54] Kunz, P.Y., Fent, K. (2006), Multiple hormonal activities of UV filters and comparison of in vivo and in vitro estrogenic activity of ethyl-4-aminobenzoate in fish, *Aquatic* Toxicol. *79 (4), 305-324.*

[55] *Kunz, P.Y., Gries, T., Fent, K. (2006), The ultraviolet filter 3-Benzylidene Camphor* adversely affects reproduction in fathead minnow (Pimephales promelas), Toxicol. Sci. 93 (2), 311-321.

[56] Weisbrod, C.J., Kunz, P.Y., Zenker, A.K., Fent, K. (2007), Effects of the UV filter benzophenone-2 on reproduction in fish, *Toxicol. Appl. Pharmacol.* 225, 255-266.

[57] Fent, K., Kunz, P.Y., Gomez, E. (2008), UV filters in the aquatic environment induce hormonal effects and affect fertility and reproduction in fish, *Chimia* 62, 368-375.

[58] Coronado, M., De Haro, H., Deng, X., Rempel, M.A., Lavado, R., Schlenk, D. (2008), UV filters in the aquatic environment induce hormonal effects and affect fertility and reproduction in fish, *Aquatic Toxicol.* 90, 182-187.

[59] Jarry, H., Christofell, J., Rimoldi, G., Koch, L., Wuttke, W. (2004), Multi-organic endocrine disrupting activity of the UV screen benzophenone 2 (BP2) in ovariectomized adult rats after 5 days treatment, *Toxicol.* 205, 87-93.

[60] Schlecht, C., Klammer, H., Jarry, H., Wuttke, W. (2004), Effects of estradiol, benzophenone-2 and benzophenone-3 on the expression pattern of the estrogen receptors (ER) alpha and beta, the estrogen receptor-related receptor 1 (ERR1) and the aryl hydrocarbon receptor (AhR) in adult ovariectomized rats, *Toxicol.* 205, 123-130.

[61] Klammer, H., Schlecht, C., Wuttke, W., Schmutzler, C., Gotthardt, I., Köhrle, J., Jarry, H. (2007), Effects of a 5-day treatment with the UV-filter octyl-methoxycinnamate (OMC) on the function of the hypothalamo-pituitary–thyroid function in rats, *Toxicol.* 238, 192-199.

[62] Inui, M., Adachi, T., Takenaka, S., Inui, H., Nakazawa, M., Ueda, M., Watanabe, H., Mori, C., Iguchi, T., Miyatake, K. (2003), Effect of UV screens and preservatives on vitellogenin and choriogenin production in male medaka (Oryzias latipes), *Toxicol.* 194, 43-50.

[63] Kunz, P.Y., Galicia, H.F., Fent, K. (2004), Assessment of hormonal activity of UV filters in tadpoles of frog Xenopus laevis at environmental concentrations, *Mar. Environ. Res.* 58, 431-435.

[64] Hofkamp, L., Bradley, S., Tresguerres, J., Lichtensteiger, W., Schlumpf, M., Timms, B. (2008), Region-specific growth effects in the developing rat prostate following fetal exposure to estrogenic ultraviolet filters, *Environ. Health. Perspect.* 116 (7), 867-872.

In: Encyclopedia of Dermatology (6 Volume Set)
Editor: Meghan Pratt
ISBN: 978-1-63483-326-4

Chapter 69

Assessment of Sunscreen Safety by Skin Permeation Studies: An Update

Lucia Montenegro*
Department of Drug Sciences, University of Catania, Catania, Italy

Abstract

One of the major concern about the use of sunscreens is their safety. Many investigations performed with different techniques have addressed this issue providing conflicting results. To be safe and effective, sunscreens should remain on the skin surface without penetrating into the underlying living tissue. As these products are normally applied on large skin areas, even small amounts of UV-filters permeating the skin could lead to their systemic absorption, making controversial their safety after topical application. To overcome real or perceived human health concerns arising from the use of sunscreen products, their margin of safety (MoS) can be easily estimated by assessing UV-filters skin permeation using *in vitro* techniques. At present, several *in vitro* and *in vivo* test systems that provide reliable and reproducible results are used by cosmetic and pharmaceutical industries.

In this chapter, physical and chemical parameters affecting UV-filters ability to permeate the skin will be discussed, and *in vitro* and *in vivo* skin permeation studies performed on the most commonly used UV-filters will be reviewed. Estimations of UV-filter MoS from skin permeation studies will highlight the safety of currently used sunscreen formulations.

Introduction

The increasing incidence of skin cancer has led the international health authorities to recommend protection measures to prevent the harmful effects of skin exposure to UV-radiation. Such measures include avoidance of sun exposure, especially at times when

* Phone: + 39 095 738 4010, Fax: + 39 095 738 4211, E-mail: lmontene@unict.it

disease-inducing wavelengths are more intense, wearing protective clothing and use of topical sunscreens (González et al., 2008; Lautenschlager et al., 2007).

As sunscreen products have gained the public favor, in the last decades there has been a notable increase of their consumption and of the number and content of UV-filters present in cosmetics and toiletries, thus enhancing the potential human exposure to sun-protecting active ingredients.

To be effective, ideally sunscreens should remain on the skin surface, without penetrating into the deep skin layers. As these products are often applied to large skin areas, even small amounts of UV-filters permeating the skin could lead to their systemic absorption and to adverse reactions.

Reports on the ability of some UV-filters to permeate the skin (Hayden et al., 1997; Janjua et al., 2004) and on their estrogenic effects (Klann et al., 2005; Koda et al., 2005; Kunz and Fent, 2006; Schlumpf and Cotton, 2001; Schlumpf et al., 2004) have given rise to a great concern about the safety of sunscreen products. Therefore, the need to guarantee the safety of sunscreen products has boosted toxicity studies on UV-filters. A recent review (Gilbert et al., 2013), illustrating the available toxicity data on the most commonly used UV-filters, evidenced that their potential estrogenic effects as well as their entrapment into vital organs are still very controversial.

To perform a risk assessment of sunscreen products, reliable information on the toxicological profile of individual sunscreen actives are required as well as data from percutaneous absorption studies designed to mimic actual product use. Therefore, understanding the basic concept of skin penetration/permeation is an essential requisite to conduct a rigorous evaluation of the actual safety of sunscreen agents.

The Process of Percutaneous Absorption

In recent years, a growing attention has been focused on the evaluation of permeation through human skin of exogenous compounds. This evaluation is of significance both in the pharmaceutical and cosmetic fields to assess the efficacy and the safety of products intended for application onto the skin. Predicting skin delivery of active ingredients is still a challenge as many factors are involved in the process of percutaneous absorption. This process relates to the entering of a molecule from the external environment within the skin (penetration) and it can be described as permeation if the molecule reaches the systemic circulation. An exhaustive knowledge of the skin's barrier function is fundamental both in evaluating the (trans)dermal delivery of drugs and in making a risk assessment following dermal exposure to chemicals.

It is well known that the outermost layer of the epidermis, the stratum corneum (SC), limits skin permeation of xenobiotics, acting as the rate-controlling barrier to skin delivery of most drugs (Förster et al., 2009). This thin ($15 - 30\mu m$) and highly hydrophobic layer consists of dead keratin cells embedded in a lipid domain and arranged in the so-called bricks and mortar model (Bouwstra et al., 2000; Wertz, 2000). Lipid content and organization within the SC and skin thickness are among the factors affecting drug skin permeation and vary for different anatomical regions in the same individual (intra-subject variability), the same region of different individuals (inter-subject variability) and among species (Akomeah et al., 2007).

The underneath viable epidermis is mostly hydrophilic as its water content is > 50% while in the dermis the water content reaches 70%, thus favoring the uptake of hydrophilic molecules in these skin layers. Variables such as SC water content, skin extensibility, recovery and elasticity in individuals of different sex and race could play a significant role, as well (Berardesca et al., 1991).

Key factors affecting the process of percutaneous absorption involve physicochemical properties of the applied molecule and type and composition of the vehicle.

As reported in the literature (Guy and Hadgraft 1988; Schaefer and Riedelmayer, 1996), the physicochemical properties that determine the skin permeation of an active ingredient include hydrophilic-lipophilic balance, molar mass, molecular size, dipole moment, vapor pressure and extent of ionization. Molecules showing partition coefficient (log P octanol/water) values in the range 1-3 have been reported to permeate the skin better than very lipophilic compounds as they have a sufficient solubility in the lipid domains of the SC while still having a sufficient hydrophilicity to allow their partitioning into the viable tissue of the epidermis (Beetge et al., 2000; Bunge and Cleek, 1995). Therefore, depending on its lipophilic or hydrophilic properties, an active ingredient will accumulate in the SC (very lipophilic molecules), or remain on the surface (very hydrophilic molecules) or penetrate into the skin (amphiphilic molecules).

The molar mass and the molecular size of a molecule affect mainly its ability to diffuse within the SC. Experiments on drugs with different molecular weights evidenced that the optimal permeability is achieved with molar mass lower than 500 Da (Bos and Meinardi, 2000) while the upper limit for drug ability to penetrate the skin is regarded to be 5000 Da (Schaefer and Riedelmayer, 1996).

In Table 1, calculated partition coefficients (Log P) (www.chemspider.com) and molecular weights of some of the most commonly used UV-filters are reported. All these sunscreen agents show molecular weights lower that 500 Da, suggesting that they would be able to penetrate the skin. However, penetration of the most lipophilic and the most hydrophilic UV-filters is likely to be minor as they should accumulate into the SC or remain on the skin surface, respectively.

The importance of partition coefficients and molecular weights in the structure-skin permeability relationships has been widely reported (Hadgraft and Lane, 2005; Patel et al., 2002). In 1992, Potts and Guy made the first attempt at predicting skin permeability from Log P and molecular weights, calculating the best linear fit for a data set of 93 compounds. The regression coefficient (0.67) obtained from this data set points at a non-linear relationship, with the involvement of other physicochemical features of the permeating molecule.

In the same year, Watkinson et al. (1992) developed a mathematical model to predict the extent of percutaneous absorption of sunscreen agents based on their physicochemical properties. In this model, some of the most common UV-filters such as benzophenone-3 (BP-3), octyl methoxycinnamate (OMC), butyl methoxydibenzoylmethane (BMBM), octyl salicylate (OS), octocrylene (OC), octyl dimethylPABA (OPABA), were analyzed. A rate constant was assigned to each process involved in skin absorption (partitioning of UV-filter from the vehicle to the SC; diffusion across the SC; partitioning from the SC to the viable epidermis; uptake into local circulation and elimination; back partitioning from the viable epidermis to the SC and from the SC to the vehicle). Rate constants were calculated considering molecular weight, melting point, and calculated partition coefficients of the UV-filters. Based on this model, sunscreen absorption ranging from 0.0033 to 83 mg/1.4m^2 after a

12-hour application was predicted, indicating a potential significant uptake in the systemic circulation after application to a large surface area for prolonged periods. However, this model did not account for variables such as effect of the vehicle, repeated application, skin metabolism of UV-filters or binding to skin sites, evidencing the need for well-designed *in vivo* and *in vitro* studies to perform an accurate evaluation of UV-filter skin absorption, and of the influence of physiological and formulation factors.

Table 1. Physicochemical properties, molecular weight (MW), partition coefficient (Log P), water solubility (S_w), UV absorption, maximum concentration allowed (Max conc.), of commonly used UV-filters

UV-filter	Key	CAS	Max conc.	Physical form	Absorption[a]	MW	Log P[b]	S_w (mg/L)
Octyl methoxycinnamate	OMC	5466-77-3	10	Oily liquid	UVB	290.41	5.66	0.15
Buthyl methoxydi-benzoylmethane	BMBM	70356-09-1	5	Crystalline solid	UVA	310.39	4.81	1.52
Octyl saliclylate	OS	118-60-5	5	Oily liquid	UVB	250.34	5.95	<0.1
Benzophenone-3	BP-3	131-57-7	6	Crystalline solid	UVB-UVAII	228.25	3.64	68.56
Benzophenone-4	BP-4	4065-45-6	5	Crystalline solid	UVB-UVAII	308.31	0.89	$25x10^4$
4-Methylbenzilydene camphor	BC	36861-47-9	4	Crystalline solid	UVB	254.37	4.95	0.57
Octyl dimethyl PABA	OPABA	58817-05-3	8	Oily liquid	UVB	277.41	6.15	0.20
Octocrylene	OC	6197-30-4	10	Oily liquid	UVB	361.48	7.53	<0.1

[a] UVB (290– 320 nm); UVAII (320– 340 nm); UVA (320– 400 nm).
[b] Calculated from www.chemspider.com.

As the main barrier to skin penetration is the non-viable SC, a drug applied in a vehicle on the skin surface penetrates into the skin by a passive mechanism depending on its physicochemical properties and according to Fick's First Law (equation 1).

$$J = -D \frac{\delta C}{\delta x}$$

Equation 1

Equation 1 shows that the flux (rate of transfer per unit area of a chemical at a given time and position) is proportional to the differential concentration change δC over the differential distance δx. Therefore, the driving force of the percutaneous absorption process is the concentration gradient of the active compound between the vehicle and the SC. In Equation 1, D represents the diffusion coefficient and the negative sign indicates that the flow is in the direction of decreasing concentration.

When the flux is constant (steady state), it can be calculated from equation 2:

$$J_{ss} = \frac{D(C_1 - C_2)}{L} \qquad \text{Equation 2}$$

J_{ss} represents flux at steady state; C_1 and C_2 represent the concentration of the permeating molecule in the vehicle and in the SC, respectively; L is the length of the diffusion pathway in the SC.

C_1 depends on the partition coefficient of the active ingredient between the SC and vehicle (considered equal to Log P for topical formulations) (Roberts et al., 1996) and on the concentration of the ingredient in the formulation.

Therefore, the extent of skin penetration and/or permeation depends not only on the physicochemical properties of the active ingredient but also on the vehicle in which it is formulated and on the interactions between the vehicle and the skin. After topical application of a pharmaceutical or cosmetic product onto the skin, the first critical step that determines the skin absorption level of an active ingredient is its release from the formulation and partitioning between the vehicle and the SC. The vehicle could alter the partitioning of the compound into the SC lipids and the solubility of the active ingredient in the vehicle will determine the thermodynamic driving force governing release of the chemical from the formulation to the skin. In addition, the vehicle itself could modify skin permeability, thus affecting skin penetration of the active compound.

Additional factors that may affect percutaneous absorption include the way of application of the formulation onto the skin, the presence of penetration modifiers in the vehicle (Trommer and Neubert, 2006), which could alter the barrier properties of the SC, the processes occurring in viable tissues such as metabolism, and biological factors.

SKIN PERMEATION OF UV-FILTERS

Skin permeation can be determined using different methodologies performing a) *in vivo* studies in animals or human volunteers, b) *in vitro* experiments employing excised skin from human or animal sources, or synthetic model membranes (Godin and Touitou, 2007; Rai et al., 2010; Varvaresou, 2006).

Because percutaneous absorption depends on the passive diffusion of the permeating molecule and not on an active transport, the viability of the skin is not a prerequisite for penetration testing, making the results of *in vitro* studies predictive of *in vivo* permeation (Bronaugh et al., 1982a; Franz, 1975).

Although *in vitro* tests are preferable for ethical reasons and feasibility and are well accepted in the European Union, regulatory authorities in the United States and Japan suggest *in vivo* penetration studies in a rodent model (EPA 1992).

Skin from a great variety of animals (e.g., pigs and guinea pigs, rats, rabbits, snakes) has been investigated as a model for human skin (Bartek et al., 1972; Bronaugh et al., 1982b; Chow et al., 1978; Harada et al., 1993; Itoh et al., 1990; Lin et al., 1992). Pigs and rats show the most similar skin barrier to that of human skin and therefore are most commonly used for skin penetration/permeation studies. However, due to the complex nature of the human SC, animal skin provides only an indication of the diffusion characteristics of chemicals, requiring a careful extrapolation to humans. In the following sections, *in vitro* and *in vivo* evaluations of percutaneous absorption through human or animal skin of the most commonly used UV-filters will be illustrated.

Human Studies

The most widely used sunscreen active ingredients such as octylmethoxycinnamate (OMC), benzophenone-3 (BP-3), benzophenone-4 (BP-4), octylsalicylate (OS), octyl dimethylPABA (OPABA), butyl methoxydibenzoylmethane (BMBM), octocrylene (OC), 3-(4-methylbenzylidene) camphor (BC), have been extensively investigated *in vitro* and *in vivo* in humans to assess their retention into the different skin layers and their permeation through the skin into the systemic circulation, applying representative vehicles of cosmetic formulations.

In vivo skin permeation of OMC, BP-3, and BC was evaluated on 32 healthy volunteers (15 men and 17 postmenopausal women) following daily whole-body topical application of a cream (2 mg/cm^2) without (week 1) or with (week 2) the three sunscreens, each at 10% w/w (Janjua et al., 2004). At the end of the study, all the sunscreens were detected in urine. Maximum plasma concentrations were similar for OMC (10 ng/mL in females and 20 ng/mL in males) and BC (20 ng/mL both in females and males) while they were significantly higher for BP-3 (200 ng/mL in females and 300 ng/mL in males). The authors observed minor differences in serum estradiol and inhibin B levels in men only but they concluded that these differences in hormone levels were not related to sunscreen exposure.

An interesting study on the relationship between *in vitro* skin penetration and cytotoxicity of sunscreens was performed to ensure that *in vitro* cytotoxicity studies examined relevant doses of these agents to which viable epidermal cells were realistically exposed. With this aim, *in vitro* percutaneous absorption through human skin of five commonly used sunscreen agents (BMBM, OMC, OC, BP-3 and OPABA) was assessed from mineral oil. After 24 hours, 95-98% of the sunscreen agents was recovered on the surface of the epidermis and detectable amounts of all UV-filters were found in the SC and viable epidermis. BP-3 showed the most evident epidermal penetration. After determining sunscreen concentration-human keratinocyte culture response curves, the authors concluded that the concentrations of each sunscreen found in human viable epidermis after topical application were at least 5-fold lower than those appearing to cause toxicity in cultured human keratinocytes (Hayden et al., 2005).

Due to its high photo-stability, BP-3 is widely used in commercial sunscreen products. However, several studies evidenced a higher skin permeation ability of this UV-filter compared to other commonly used sunscreens. BP-3 percutaneous absorption was evaluated in nine healthy volunteers after topical application (12.4 mg/cm^2) onto the entire surface of their forearms of a commercial available sunscreen lotion containing BP-3 6% (w/v), OMC 7.5% (w/v), OS 5% (w/v) and OC 7% (w/v) (Hayden et al., 1997). BP-3 was recovered in urine for 48 h as unchanged BP-3 and as metabolites and the authors concluded that the actual amount absorbed through the skin over a 10-h period was 1-2% of the applied amount contained in the product. However, in this study, the amount of formulation applied on the skin was about six-fold higher than that recommended to evaluate the sun protection factor of sunscreen products under realistic condition of use (2 mg/cm^2).

An *in vitro* study through excised human skin was performed to assess skin penetration/permeation from six commercial milk/lotion sunscreen products for adults and children of BP-3, along with other UVB-filters (OMC, OS, OC) (Jiang et al., 1999). All these sunscreens were recovered into the skin (14% of the applied dose) but only BP-3 was able to permeate through the skin (10% of the applied dose), thus confirming the results obtained from previous *in vivo* studies.

A further *in vivo* investigation on BP-3 skin permeation was carried out on eleven healthy volunteers who were instructed to apply a commercially available sun-protecting lotion containing 4% BP-3 over the whole body (2 mg/cm^2). Under these experimental conditions, the average total amount excreted in urine was approximately 0.4% of the applied amount of BP-3 (Gustavsson Gonzalez et al., 2002).

In vitro studies through human skin proved that BP-3 skin permeation was enhanced by the concomitant application of the insect repellent N,N-diethyl-m-toluamide (DEET) (Wang and Gu, 2007). DEET permeation was greater than that of BP-3 and a synergistic percutaneous enhancement of both compounds was observed when used simultaneously. The authors reported that the extent of the enhancement effect was dependent on the type of vehicle (lotion or spay) containing the active ingredients.

Synergy effects on *in vitro* absorption through human skin between UV filters and other compounds such as herbicides (Pont et al., 2004) have also been reported.

Vehicle effects on skin permeation of UV-filters have been investigated in many papers. Chatelain et al. (2003) evaluated the skin penetration of five UV- filters (BP-3, OMC, BMBM, OS, homosalate) from an O/W emulsion gel and a petrolatum jelly both *in vitro* and *in vivo*. The results of *in vitro* experiments showed that after applying the formulations under investigation for 30 min and 6 h, only BP-3 and to a lesser extent OMC were detectable in the dermis while no skin permeation of these UV filters was observed after 6 h application. In addition, the authors reported a greater BP-3 penetration from petrolatum. *In vivo i*nvestigations, performed by tape stripping of the SC, evidenced a clear vehicle effect on penetration of the UV-filters into the SC, being the amount of each UV-filter penetrated greater from the emulsion gel formulation compared to the petrolatum jelly. Treffel and Gabard (1996) reported similar results studying *in vitro* and *in vivo* skin penetration of BP-3 (5%), OMC (7.5%), and OS (3%) from two vehicles (an O/W emulsion-gel and petroleum jelly) applied (2 mg/cm^2) for 2 min to 6 h. The emulsion-gel provided higher epidermal concentrations of all UV-filters than the petroleum jelly both *in vivo* and *in vitro*. However, the authors noticed only for BP-3 a greater skin permeation from the petroleum jelly than from the emulsion gel.

The effects of emulsion composition on *in vitro* skin permeation of different UV-filters (OMC, BMBM) was evaluated evidencing differences in UV filter penetration/permeation among various emulsion-type formulations (Marginean-Lazar et al., 1996; Montenegro et al., 2004).

In vitro percutaneous absorption through human skin of OS was assessed from two representative sunscreen vehicles (an oil-in-water emulsion and a hydro-alcoholic formulation) using both the technique of finite and infinite dosing (Walters et al., 1997). The results of this study evidenced a low skin permeation of OS that was dependent on the amount of formulation applied (finite or infinite dosing) when a hydro-alcoholic vehicle was used.

Animal Studies

Several studies have validated pig skin as a suitable model for human skin to investigate percutaneous absorption of UV-filters.

Benech-Kieffer et al. (2000) performed *in vitro* experiments to compare skin permeation of two UV-filters (OMC and BP-4) through human abdominal skin and pig flank skin. The authors found a good agreement between data obtained from human and pig skin, as after 16 hours the percentage of the applied dose of OMC and BP-4 recovered in the skin was similar for both species. However, due to its lipophilicity, OMC showed a higher affinity for the SC than the hydrophilic BP-4.

Pigskin was used as model to evaluate BP-3 and OMC *in vitro* percutaneous absorption from two vehicles, a hydroacloholic and a diisopropyl adipate formulation (Gupta et al., 1999). BP-3 permeation was greater than that of OMC while OMC was retained to a greater extent in the SC. It is interesting to note that the authors found that permeation and SC retention were formulation dependent and the ratio of retained to permeated amount of sunscreen from a hydroalcoholic formulation after 10 hours was greater when these UV-filters were present together rather than alone.

Fernandez et al. (2000) evaluated the skin penetration of BP-3 *in vitro* and *in vivo* from six different vehicles, three solvents and three different types of emulsions. *In vitro* experiments were performed using pig skin while *in vivo* data were collected determining BP-3 concentration in the SC by the stripping method after 30-min application on the forearm of volunteers. Pig and human skin provided similar results, highlighting a good correlation between *in vitro* and *in vivo* data and between species. In both experiments, significant differences among the vehicles tested were observed as the highest concentration of BP-3 in the skin was obtained from the hydrophilic solvent (propylene glycol) and O/W submicron emulsion while the two oily solvents, W/O emulsion and O/W coarse emulsion provided lower concentrations of this UV-filter in the skin.

Another *in vitro* study on OMC percutaneous absorption through pig skin evidenced that microencapsulating this UV-filter reduced its absorption in comparison with an emulsion containing free OMC (Jimenez et al., 2004).

The effect two vehicles, an oil-in-water (O/W) emulsion and an alcoholic gel, on *in vitro* permeation of BC was assessed through pig ear skin. The results of this study showed that BC skin penetration was dependent on the vehicle, being more remarkable for alcoholic gel (Sasson et al., 2009).

In the last decade, several studies aimed at entrapping UV-filters in carriers such as cyclodextrins (Shokri et al., 2013), lipid microparticles (Scalia et al., 2007) lipospheres (Mew et al., 2007), lipid microspheres (Mestres et al., 2010; Yener et al., 2003), polymeric nanocapsules (Siqueira et al., 2011; Weiss-Angeli et al., 2010), microemulsions (Montenegro et al., 2011), solid lipid nanoparticles (Gulbake et al., 2010; Wissing and Muller, 2002), polymeric nanoparticles (Vettor et al., 2010) to avoid or at least to reduce skin permeation of sunscreens. Some of these investigations were performed *in vitro* or *in vivo* on rat skin, pointing out a good correlation between this animal model and human skin. In all these studies, incorporating UV-filters in different carriers resulted in a decrease of sunscreen release and penetration into the skin compared to conventional cosmetic formulations.

NOAEL AND RISK ASSESSMENT OF UV-FILTERS

The risk assessment of sunscreen products requires hazard identification and characterization, exposure assessment, and risk characterization, the last being a basic step that brings together hazard characterization and exposure assessment. For sunscreen products, such evaluations have to be performed taking into account the topical nature of human exposure.

While hazard identification and characterization lead to a qualitative assessment based on the available data of a specific chemical, safety evaluation provides a quantitative estimate of the intake that would not give rise to a significant risk of adverse effects in humans. Therefore, the margin of safety (MoS) is determined comparing the so-called no adverse effect level (NOAEL) to the potential human exposure, expressed as systemic exposure dose (SED).

NOAEL values are obtained from subchronic (90-180 days) or chronic (> 180 days) toxicity studies that are generally performed in animals, using different oral dosing. NOAEL is usually defined as the daily dose that does not elicit any toxic effect and is expressed in mg/kg body weight. However, the definition of NOAEL has been largely debated (Dorato and Engelhardt, 2005). According to the SCCS's notes of guidance for the testing of cosmetic substances and their safety evaluation (2012), the no observed (adverse) effect level is defined as the highest dose or exposure level where no (adverse) treatment-related findings are observed.

After establishing the NOAEL of UV-filters, their percutaneous absorption has to be quantified to determine SED, expressed in mg/kg body weight per single application. As sunscreen products are often applied to large skin areas, SED evaluations are performed considering the worst scenario, i.e., a total body application.

If the steady state flux through the skin (J_{ss}) is used to estimate SED, the weight and the skin surface area of a standard human are needed. According to SCCS's notes of guidance for the testing of cosmetic substances and their safety evaluation (2012), a weight of 60 kg and a skin area of 18.000 cm^2 (Timbrell, 2005) are used to calculate SED.

Therefore, the SED can be determined as follows:

$$SED = J_{ss} \times area_{exp} \times 24\ h\ /body\ weight \qquad \text{Equation 3}$$

where $area_{exp}$ is the exposed area of the skin. In addition, the SED can be estimated from the percentage of a topically applied dose that permeates the skin, according to equation 4:

$$SED = C_{product} \times A_{applied} \times n_{applications} \times area_{exp} \times Perm(\%)/body\ weight \qquad \text{Equation 4}$$

where $C_{product}$ is the concentration of UV-filter in the product (%w/w), $A_{applied}$ is the amount of product applied on the skin (mg/cm^2), $n_{applications}$ is the number of application per day and Perm(%) is the permeation percentage of UV-filter.

As many toxicological studies are carried out on animals, uncertainty factors (UF) have to be applied to convert animal data into an exposure level considered of no toxicological concern for humans; additional UF have to be considered to account for toxico-kinetic variability among healthy adults and in children (SCCS, 2012).

When NOAEL and SED are known, MoS can be calculated as follows:

$$MoS = NOAEL/SED \quad \text{Equation 5}$$

A MoS < 1 indicates a potential risk associated with a given scenario as the dose considered safe is lower than the SED. In the safety evaluation of cosmetic products in EU, to declare a product safe for use, MoS values greater than 100 are required (SCCS, 2012).

Several authors (Gonzalez 2010; Montenegro et al., 2013; Nohynek and Schaefer, 2001; Walters et al., 1997) have calculated MoS of UV-filters using SED values obtained from percutaneous absorption studies.

As BP-3 shows a greater skin permeation compared to other UV-filters, an extensive assessment of its safety has been carried out (El Dareer et al., 1986; Okereke et al., 1994). Okereke et al., (1995) performed a safety evaluation of BP-3 after topical application in rats and found it nontoxic when applied at a dose of 100 mg / kg body weight for 4 weeks. After evaluating *in vitro* and *in vivo* data on BP-3 skin permeation in animals and humans and the available toxicokinetic data, the Scientific Committee on Consumer Products (SCCP, 2008) concluded that the use of BP-3 up to 6% in cosmetic sunscreen products does not pose a risk to the health of the consumer, apart from its contact allergenic and photoallergenic potential. This conclusion was drawn considering that the mean percentage of the applied dose of BP- 3 permeated was 3.1% plus 2 standard deviations (3.4%). As shown in Table 2, in this condition a MoS value of 112 was obtained.

OMC and BMBM are the most commonly used UV-filters, being contained not only in sunscreen products but also in a great variety of cosmetics and toiletries. Although OMC demonstrated weak estrogenic effects *in vivo* and *in vitro* (Gomez et al., 2005; Klammer et al., 2005), it had no adverse effect on estrus cycle, sperm number, morphology and motility, differential follicle counts, mating, fertility, gestation and parturition (Schneider et al., 2005). The NOAEL for fertility and reproductive performance in rats and for systemic parental and developmental toxicity was determined to be 450 mg/kg/day. The same NOAEL has been reported for BMBM (Montenegro et al., 2013)

In vitro experiments showed that the percentage of the applied dose of OMC that permeated through the skin was 0.2–4.5%, using both human and porcine skin (Benech-Kieffer et al., 2000; Gupta et al., 1999). From *in vivo* studies, lower OMC skin permeation was observed (Chatelain et al., 2003; Janjua et al., 2004; Janjua et al., 2008).

As regards BMBM, *in vitro* studies evidenced that less than 1% of this UV-filter penetrated into the SC and epidermis while no skin permeation occurred (Montenegro et al., 2008; Simeoni et al., 2004; Weigmann et al., 2001).

Recently, Nohynek et al. (2010) have pointed out that *in vitro* experiments tend to overestimate human systemic exposure. According to the authors, this overestimation was supported by the results of a study performed in humans, both *in vivo* and *in vitro*, on the UV-filter Mexoryl SX®. In volunteers, 0.014% of the applied filter was systemically available, while parallel *in vitro* experiments, performed under identical exposure conditions, provided a skin penetration rate of 0.37%, suggesting that *in vitro* results produced a 25-fold overestimation of the human systemic exposure and of the potential human health risk (Benech-Kieffer et al., 2003).

Table 2. Systemic exposure dose (SED) and margin of safety (MoS) of UV-filters in adults

Parameter	UV-filter BP-3[a]	OMC[b]	BC-3[c]	BC-4[d]	OS[e]	BMBM[b]	Mexoryl XL (®)[f]
Typical adult body weight (Kg)	60	60	60	60	60	60	60
Body surface area (cm^2)	18000	18000	18000	18000	18000	18000	18000
Average amount (g) of sunscreen applied per day	18	36	18	36	16	36	18
Maximum allowable concentration in sunscreen products (%)	6	10	2	4	5	5	15
Maximum amount applied ultraviolet filter (g)	1.1	3.6	0.36	1.4	0.8	1.8	1.8
Maximum (*in vitro*) percutaneous absorption of UV filter (%)	9.9	4.5	3.29	2.45	0.65	1	0.8
Systemic Exposure Dose (SED) (mg/kg/day)	1.78	0.27	0.21	0.588	0.087	0.03	0.24
NOAEL of toxicity studies (mg/kg/day)	200	450	7.5	25	250	450	1000
Margin of Safety (MoS=NOAEL/SED)	112	1666	36	42.5	2900	15000	4170

[a] data obtained from Gonzalez (2010).
[b] data calculated from *in vitro* and *in vivo* experiments reported in the literature (see text for details).
[c] data obtained from SCCS/1513/13 (2013).
[d] data obtained from SCCP (2008).
[e] data obtained from Walters et al. (1997).
[f] data obtained from Nohynek and Schaefer (2001).

However, as according to SCCS (2012) the worst scenario has to be considered, calculating MoS of OMC and BMBM, the maximum percentage of the applied dose permeated (4.5% and 1%, respectively) was used (see Table 2). Based on a total body application of a formulation containing the maximum percentage of UV-filter allowed, the resulting MoS for OMC and BMBM were 1666 and 15000. A recent investigation on the effects of commercial O/W emulsions on *in vitro* skin permeation of OMC and BMBM evidenced that OMC permeation depended on both its concentration in the formulation and vehicle composition, while BMBM release from the vehicle was the key parameter that determined the permeation rate of this UV-filter (Montenegro et al., 2013). All the commercial products investigated proved safe under normal in use conditions as their MoS values were greater than 100.

Being one of the oldest UV-filters, the human safety of OS has been extensively reviewed, highlighting that this UV-filter is well tolerated (Nash, 2006). Investigating OS skin permeation, Walters et al., (1997) reported that less than 1% of the applied dose of OS penetrates through the human skin. Using these data, the authors demonstrated the safety of this sunscreen agent in cosmetic formulations.

Nohynek and Schaefer (2001) reported a thorough risk assessment of a new broad UVA filter, drometrizole trisiloxane (Mexoryl XL®), listing all the data needed to calculate its MoS, according to SCCS guidelines.

As illustrated In Table 2, apart from 3-benzilydene camphor (BC-3) and 4-methylbenzilydene camphor (BC-4), all the UV-filters mentioned above show MoS values greater than 100, evidencing their safety of use in sunscreen products at the maximum concentration allowed in EU.

As regards BC-3, Søeborg et al. (2006), studying *in vivo* skin permeation of BC-3 in rats, observed an accumulation of approximately 10% of the applied topical dose in various tissues after 65 days of treatment. Further studies (Søeborg et al., 2007) pointed out that skin permeation of BC-3 was higher than that of BC-4. As both UV-filters affected the endocrine activity, the risk associated with use of BC-3 and BC-4 in sunscreen products was found high. To evaluate the risk of human exposure to BC-3, the SCCP (2013) used a percentage of absorption of 3.29% and a NOAEL value of 7.5 mg/Kg/day obtained from maternal toxicity and embryo-toxicity studies in rats (15 mg/Kg/day), taking into account that BC-3 bioavailability was 50% of the administered dose. Based on the resulting MoS lower than 100, the SCCP declared that the use of BC-3 in cosmetic products in a concentration up 2.0% is not safe. Therefore, BC-3 has been withdrawn from the list of UV-filters approved in EU.

Using a percutaneous absorption rate of 1.9% along with a NOAEL of 25 mg/Kg/day (determined in rats) for human risk assessment of BC-4 (SCCP, 2008), a MoS below 100 was obtained, indicating that BC-4 cannot be considered safe as a UV filter in cosmetic sunscreen products at 4%. However, as detailed toxicokinetic studies in healthy volunteers demonstrated that the actual NOAEL in humans was 100 mg/Kg/day, a MoS value of 25 was considered safe for BC-4. Therefore, as the calculation of the MoS resulted in a value of 42.5, which was higher than the requested threshold of 25, the use of this UV-filter was regarded safe (SCCP, 2008).

CONCLUSION

In recent years, an increasing attention has been paid to the evaluation of UV-filter percutaneous absorption to assess the potential risk of human exposure to these sunscreen agents.

In vitro permeation experiments and animal models, with all their limitations, provide important tools for screening sunscreen products, making possible to estimate the rate and extent of percutaneous absorption of their active ingredients.

The safety evaluation of sunscreen products is based on the two factors that contribute to risk characterization, hazard characterization and potential human exposure and only UV-filters whose MoS are at least 100 times the NOAEL are accepted as safe.

As evidenced in this chapter, when comparing the toxicological properties of the most commonly used UV-A and UV-B filters to the potential human exposure, the human risk caused by exposure to sunscreen products is negligible. Furthermore, modern UV filters are formulated to be retained on or within the upper layers of the horny layer to achieve high protection factors, thus reducing their potential of skin permeation into the underlying living tissue.

Therefore, the benefits of sunscreen products to public health largely outweigh the risk of human topical exposure to such formulations, supporting the recommendation of a proper use of sunscreen products to prevent the deleterious effects of UV-radiation.

REFERENCES

Akomeah FK; Martin GP; Brown MB. Variability in human skin permeability in vitro: comparing penetrants with different physicochemical properties. *J. Pharm. Sci.*, 2007, 96, 824-834.

Bartek M J; LaBudde J A; Maibach HI. Skin permeability in vivo. Comparison in rat, rabbit, pig and man. *J. Invest. Dermatol.*, 1972, 58, 114-123.

Beetge E; Du Plessis J; Muller DG; Goosen C; Van Rensburg FJ. The influence of the physicochemical characteristics and pharmacokinetic properties of selected NSAID's on their transdermal absorption. *Int. J. Pharm.*, 2000, 193, 261-264.

Benech-Kieffer F; Wegrich P; Schwarzenbach R; Klecak G; Weber T; Leclaire J; Schaefer H. Percutaneous absorption of sunscreens in vitro: Interspecies comparison, skin models and reproducibility aspects. *Skin Pharmacol. Appl. Skin Physiol.*, 2000, 13, 324-335.

Benech-Kieffer F; Meuling WJA; Leclerc C; Roza L; Leclaire J; Nohynek G. Percutaneous absorption of Mexoryl SX® in human volunteers: comparison with in vitro data. *Skin Pharmacol. Appl. Skin Physiol.* 2003, 16, 343–355.

Berardesca E; De Rigal J; Leveque JL; Maibach HI. In vivo biophysical characterization of skin physiological differences in races. *Dermatologica*, 1991, 182, 89-93.

Bos JD; Meinardi MMHM. The 500 Dalton rule for the skin penetration of chemical compounds and drugs. *Exp. Dermato*, 2000, 9, 165-9.

Bouwstra JA; Dubbelaar FE; Gooris GS; Ponec M. The lipid organisation in the skin barrier. *Acta Derm Venereol Suppl* 2000, 208, 23–30.

Bronaugh RL; Stewart R F; Congdon ER; Giles AL. Methods for in vitro percutaneous absorption studies. I. Comparison with in vivo results. *Toxicol. Appl. Pharmacol.*, 1982a, 62, 474-480.

Bronaugh RL; Stewart R F; Congdon ER. Methods for in vitro percutaneous absorption studies. II. Animal models for human skin. *Toxicol. Appl. Pharmacol.*, 1982b, 62, 481-488.

Bunge AL; Cleek RL. A new method for estimating dermal absorption from chemical exposure: 2. Effect of molecular weight and octanol-water partitioning. *Pharm Res*, 1995, 12, 88-95.

Chatelain E; Gabarda B; Surber C. Skin penetration and sun protection factor of five UV filters: effect of the vehicle. *Skin Pharmacol. Appl. Skin Physiol.*, 2003, 16, 28–35.

Chow C; Chow AYK; Downie RH; Buttar HS. Percutaneous absorption of hexachlorophene in rats, guinea pigs and pigs. *Toxicology* 1978, 9, 147-154.

Dorato MA; Engelhardt JA. The no-observed-adverse-effect-level in drug safety evaluations: Use, issues, and definition(s). *Regul. Toxicol. Pharmacol.*, 2005, 42, 265–274.

El Dareer SM; Kalin JR; Tillery KF; Hill DL. Disposition of 2-hydroxy-4-methoxybenzophenone in rats dosed orally, intravenously, or topically. *J. Toxicol. Environ. Health* 1986, 19, 491–502.

EPA 1992 Dermal Exposure Assesment: Principles and applications, Interim Report EPA/600/8-91/011B. Exposure Assesment Group, Office of Health and Enviromental Assesment Group, U.S. Enviromental Protection Agency, Washington DC.

Fernández C; Marti-Mestres G; Ramos J; Maillols H. LC analysis of benzophenone-3: II application to determination of 'in vitro' and 'in vivo' skin penetration from solvents, coarse and submicron emulsions. *J. Pharm. Biomed. Anal.*, 2000, 24, 155–165.

Förster M; Bolzinger MA; Fessi H; Briançonet S. Topical delivery of cosmetics and drugs. Molecular aspects of percutaneous absorption and delivery. *Eur. J. Dermatol.*, 2009, 19, 309-23.

Franz TJ. Percutaneous absorption on the relevance of in vitro data. *J. Invest. Dermatol.*, 1975, 64, 190-195.

Gilbert E; Pirot F; Bertholle V; Roussel L; Falson F; Padois K. Commonly used UV filter toxicity on biological functions: review of last decade studies. *Int. J. Cosm. Sci.*, 2013, 35, 208–219.

Godin B; Touitou E. Transdermal skin delivery: Predictions for humans from in vivo, ex vivo and animal models. *Adv Drug Del Rev*, 2007, 59, 1152-61.

Gomez E; Pillon A; Fenet H; Rosain D; Duchesne MJ; Nicolas JC; Balauger P; Casellas C. Estrogenic activity of cosmetic components in reporter cell lines: parabens, UV screens, and musks. *J Toxicol Environ Health*, 2005, 68, 239-251.

Gonzalez H. Percutaneous absorption with emphasis on sunscreens. *Photochem. Photobiol. Sci.*, 2010, 9, 482–488.

González S; Fernández-Lorente M; Gilaberte-Calzada Y. The latest on skin photoprotection. *Clin. Dermatol.*, 2008, 26, 614–626.

Gulbake A; Jain A; Khare P; Jain SK. Solid lipid nanoparticles bearing oxybenzone: in-vitro and in-vivo evaluation. *J. Microencapsul.*, 2010, 27, 226–233.

Gupta VK; Zatz JL; Rerek M. Percutaneous absorption of sunscreens through micro-Yucatan pig skin in vitro. *Pharm. Res.*, 1999, 16, 1602-1607.

Gustavsson Gonzalez H; Farbrot A; Larko O. Percutaneous absorption of benzophenone-3, a common component of topical sunscreens. *Clin. Exp. Dermatol.*, 2002, 27, 691-694.

Guy RH; Hadgraft J. Physicochemical aspects of percutaneous penetration and its enhancement. *Pharm Res*, 1988, 5, 753-8.

Hadgraft J; Lane ME. Skin permeation: The years of enlightenment. *Int. J. Pharm.*, 2005, 305, 2–12.

Harada K; Murakami T; Kawasaki E; Higashi Y; Yamamoto S; Yata N. In-vitro permeability to salicylic acid of human, rodent, and shed snake skin. *J. Pharm Pharmacol.*, 1993, 45, 414-418.

Hayden CG; Roberts MS; Benson HA. Systemic absorption of sunscreen after topical application. *Lancet* 1997, 350, 863-4.

Hayden CGJ; Cross SE; Anderson C; Saunders NA; Roberts MS. Sunscreen penetration of human skin and related keratinocyte toxicity after topical application. *Skin Pharmacol. Physiol.*, 2005, 18, 170-174.

Iannucelli V; Coppi G; Sergi S; Mezzena M; Scalia S. In vivo and in vitro skin permeation of butyl methoxydibenzoylmethane from lipospheres. *Skin Pharmacol. Physiol.*, 2007, 21, 30–38.

Itoh T; Xia J; Magavi R; Nishihata T; Rytting JH. Use of shed snake skin as a model membrane for in vitro percutaneous penetration studies: Comparison with human skin. *Pharm. Res.*, 1990, 7, 1042-1047.

Janjua NR; Mogensen B; Andersson AM; Petersen JH; Henriksen M; Skakkebaek NE; Wulf HC. Systemic absorption of the sunscreens benzophenone-3, octyl-methoxycinnamate, and 3-(4-methyl-benzylidene) camphor after whole-body topical application and reproductive hormone levels in humans. *J. Invest Dermatol.* 2004, 123, 57– 61.

Janjua NR; Kongshoj B; Andersson AM; Wulf, HC. Sunscreens in human plasma and urine after repeated whole-body topical application. *J. Eur. Acad. Dermatol. Venereol*, 2008, 22, 456–61.

Jiang R; Roberts MS; Collins DM; Benson HA. Absorption of sunscreens across human skin: an evaluation of commercial products for children and adults. *Br. J. Clin. Pharmacol.*, 1999, 48, 635–7.

Jimenez MM; Pelletier J; Bobin MF; Martini MC. Influence of encapsulation on the in vitro percutaneous absorptionof octyl methoxycinnamate. *Int. J. Pharm.*, 2004, 272, 45-55.

Klammer H; Schlecht C; Wuttke W; Jarry H. Multi-organic risk assessment of estrogenic properties of octyl-methoxycinnamate in vivo. A 5-day sub-acute pharmacodynamic study with ovariectomized rats. *Toxicology*, 2005, 215, 90-96.

Klann A; Levy G; Lutz I; Müller C; Kloas W; Hildebrandt JP. Estrogen-like effects of ultraviolet screen 3-(4-methylbenzylidene)-camphor (Eusolex 6300) on cell proliferation and gene induction in mammalian and amphibian cells. *Environ Res.* 2005, 97, 274– 81.

Koda T; Umezu T; Kamata R; Morohoshi K; Ohta T; Morita M. Uterotrophic effects of benzophenone derivatives and a p-hydroxybenzoate used in ultraviolet screens. *Environ Res*, 2005, 98, 40 –5.

Kunz PY; Fent K. Estrogenic activity of UV filter mixtures, *Toxicol. Appl. Pharmacol.*, 2006, 217, 86–99.

Lautenschlager S; Wulf HC; Pittelkow MR; Photoprotection. *Lancet* 2007, 370, 528–37.

Lin S Y; Hou S J; Hsu TH; Yeh FL. Comparisons of different animal skins with human skin in drug percutaneous penetration studies. *Methods Find Exp. Clin. Pharmacol.*, 1992, 14, 645-654.

Marginean-Lazar G; Baillet A; Fructus AE; Arnaud-Battandier J; Ferrier D; Marty JP. Evaluation of in vitro percutaneous absorption of UV filters used in sunscreen formulations. *Drug Cosm. Ind*, 1996, 158, 50–62.

Mestres JP; Duracher L; Baux C; Vian L; Marti-Mestres G. Benzophenone-3 entrapped in solid lipid microspheres: formulation and in vitro skin evaluation. *Int. J. Pharm.*, 2010, 400, 1-7.

Montenegro L; Paolino D; Puglisi G. (2004). Effects of silicone emulsifiers on in vitro skin permeation of sunscreens from cosmetic emulsions. *J. Cosmet Sci*, 2004, 55, 509–518.

Montenegro L.; Carbone C.; Paolino D.; Drago R.; Stancampiano A.H.; Puglisi G. *In vitro* skin permeation of sunscreen agents from O/W emulsions. Int. J. Cosmet. Sci., 2008, 30, 57-65.

Montenegro L; Carbone C; Puglisi G. Vehicle effects on in vitro release and skin permeation of octylmethoxycinnamate from microemulsions. *Int. J. Pharm.*, 2011, 405, 162-8.

Montenegro L; Puglisi G. Evaluation of sunscreen safety by in vitro skin permeation studies: effects of vehicle composition. *Pharmazie*, 2013, 68, 34-40.

Nash JF. Human safety and efficacy of ultraviolet filters and sunscreen products. *Dermatol. Clin.*, 2006, 24, 35 – 51.

Nohynek GJ; Schaefer H. Benefit and Risk of Organic Ultraviolet Filters. *Regul. Toxicol. Pharmacol.*, 2001, 33, 285–299.

Nohynek GJ; Antignac E; Re T; Toutain H. Safety assessment of personal care products/cosmetics and their ingredients. *Toxicol. Appl. Pharmacol.*, 2010, 243, 239–259.

Okereke CS, Abdel-Rhaman MS, Friedman MA. Disposition of benzophenone-3 after dermal administration in male rats. *Toxicol. Lett.* 1994, 73, 113– 22.

Okereke CS; Barat SA; Abdel-Rahman MS. Safety evaluation of benzophenone-3 after dermal administration in rats. *Toxicol. Lett.* 1995, 80, 61–7.

Patel H; Berge W; Cronin MTD. Quantitative structure-activity relationships (QSARs) for the prediction of skin permeation of exogenous chemicals. *Chemosphere,* 2002, 48, 603-613.

Pont AR; Charron AR; Brand RM. Active ingredients in sunscreens act as topical penetration enhancers for the herbicide 2,4-dichlorophenoxyacetic acid. *Toxicology Appl. Pharmacol.,* 2004, 195, 348–354.

Potts RO; Guy RH. Predicting skin permeability. *Pharm. Res.*, 1992, 9, 663- 669.

Rai V;, Ghosh I; Bose S; Silva SMC; Chandra P; Michniak-Kohn B. A transdermal review on permeation of drug formulations, modifier compounds and delivery methods. *J. Drug Del. Sci. Tech.*, 2010, 20, 75-87.

Roberts MS; Pugh WJ; Hadgraft J. Epidermal permeability: Penetrant structure relationships. 2. The effect of h-bonding groups in penetrants on their diffusion through the stratum corneum. *Int. J. Pharm.*, 1996, 132, 23-32.

Sasson CS; Sato ME; da Silva Beletti K; Cunha Mota F; Dakiw Piaceski A. Influence of cosmetics vehicles on 4-methylbenzylidene-camphor's skin penetration, in vitro. *Braz. Arch. Biol. Technol.*, 2009, 52, 299-303.

Scalia S; Mezzena M; Iannuccelli V. Influence of solid lipid microparticle carriers on skin penetration of the sunscreen agent, 4-methylbenzylidene camphor. *J. Pharm. Pharmacol.,* 2007, 59, 1621–1627.

SCCP Opinion on 4-Methylbenzylidene camphor (4-MBC) COLIPA n° S60, 24 June 2008.

SCCS's notes of guidance for the testing of cosmetic substances and their safety evaluation SCCS/1501/12, 8th Revision, 11 December 2012.

SCCS/1513/13 Opinion ion 3-Benzylidene camphor COLIPA n° S61, 18 June 2013.

Schaefer H; Riedelmayer TE. Skin Barrier: Principles of Percutaneous Absorption. Karger, Basel, 1996, pp. 118–28.

Schlumpf M, Schmid P, Durrer S, Conscience M; Maerkel K; Henseler M; Gruetter M; Herzog I; Reolon S; Ceccatelli R; Faass O; Stutz E; Jarry H; Wuttke W; Lichtensteiger W. Endocrine activity and developmental toxicity of cosmetic UV filters—an update. *Toxicology,* 2004, 205,113–22.

Schlumpf M; Cotton B; Conscience M; Haller V; Steinmann B; Lichtensteiger W. In vitro and in vivo estrogenicity of UV screens. *Environ Health Perspect*, 2001, 109, 239– 44.

Schneider S; Deckardt K; Hellwig J; Kuttler K; Mellert W; Schulte S; van Ravenzwaay B. Octyl methoxycinnamate: Two-generation reproduction toxicity in Wistar rats by dietary administration. *Food Chem. Toxicol.*, 2005, 43, 1083-1092.

Shokri J; Hasanzadeh D; Ghanbarzadeh S; Dizadji-Ilkhchi M; Adibkia K. The effect of Beta-cyclodextrin on percutaneous absorption of commonly used Eusolex® sunscreens. *Drug Res*, 2013, 63, 591-6.

Siqueira NM; Contri RV; Paese K; Beck RCR; Pohlmann AR; Guterres SS. Innovative sunscreen formulation based on benzophenone-3-loaded chitosan-coated polymeric nanocapsules. *Skin Pharmacol. Physiol.*, 2011, 24, 166–174.

Simeoni S; Scalia S; Benson HA. Influence of cyclodextrins on in vitro human skin absorption of the sunscreen, butylmethoxydibenzoylmethane. *Int. J. Pharm.*, 2004, 280, 163–71.

Søeborg T; Ganderup NC; Kristensen JH; Bjerregaard P; Pedersen KL; Bollen P; Hansen SH; Halling-Sørensen B. Distribution of the UV filter 3-benzylidene camphor in rat following topical application. *J. Chromatogr B,* 2006, 834, 117–121.

Søeborg T; Hollesen Basse L; Halling-Sørensen B. Risk assessment of topically applied products. *Toxicology,* 2007, 236, 140–148.

Timbrell, J. Principles of Biochemical Toxicology, 3rd ed. Taylor & Francis, New York, 2005.

Treffel P; Gabard B. Skin penetration and sun protection factor of ultra- violet filters from two vehicles. *Pharm. Res.,* 1996, 13, 770–774.

Trommer H; Neubert RHH. Overcoming the stratum corneum: the modulation of skin penetration. *Skin Pharmacol. Physiol.* 2006, 19, 106–121.

Varvaresou A. Percutaneous absorption of organic sunscreens. *Journal of Cosmetic Dermatology,* 2006, 5, 53–57.

Vettor M; Bourgeois S; Fessi H; Pelletier J; Perugini P; Pavanetto F; Bolzinger MA. Skin absorption studies of octyl-methoxycinnamate loaded poly(D,L-lactide) nanoparticles: estimation of the UV filter distribution and release behaviour in skin layers. *J. Microencapsul,* 2010, 27, 253–262.

Walters KA; Brain KR; Howes D; James VJ; Kraus AL; Teetsel NM; Toulon M; Watkinson AC; Gettings SD. Percutaneous penetration of octyl salicylate from representative sunscreen formulations through human skin in vitro. *Food Chem. Toxicol.*, 1997, 35, 1219-25.

Wang T; Gu X. In vitro percutaneous permeation of the repellent DEET and the sunscreen oxybenzone across human skin. *J. Pharm. Pharm. Sci.*, 2007, 10, 17-25.

Watkinson AC; Brain KR; Walters KA; Hadgraft J. Prediction of the percutaneous penetration of ultraviolet filters used in sunscreen formulations. *Int. J. Cosmet Sci.* 1992, 14, 265–75.

Weigmann HJ; Lademann J; Schanzer S; Lindemann U; von Pelchrzim R; Schaefer H; Sterry W; Shah V. Correlation of the local distribution of topically applied substances inside the stratum corneum determined by tape-stripping to differences in bioavailability. *Skin Pharmacol. Appl. Skin Physiol.*, 2001, 14 (Suppl 1), 98–102.

Weiss-Angeli V; Bourgeois S; Pelletier J; Guterres SS; Fessi H; Bolzinger MA. Development of an original method to study drug release from polymeric nanocapsules in the skin. *J. Pharm. Pharmacol.*, 2010, 62, 35–45.

Wertz PW. Lipids and barrier function of the skin. *Acta Derm Venereol Suppl* (Stockh) 2000, 208, 7-11.

Wissing S A; Muller RH. Solid lipid nanoparticles as carrier for sunscreens: in vitro release and in vivo skin penetration. *J. Control Rel.*, 2002, 81, 225–233.

Yener G; Incegül T; Yener N. Importance of using solid lipid microspheres as carriers for UV filters on the example octyl methoxy cinnamate. *Int. J. Pharm.*, 2003, 258, 203–207.

In: Encyclopedia of Dermatology (6 Volume Set)
Editor: Meghan Pratt
ISBN: 978-1-63483-326-4

Chapter 70

UV PROTECTION BY WOOLEN FABRIC DYED WITH NATURAL DYESTUFF

Ana Sutlović, Anita Tarbuk*, Ana Marija Grancarić and Đurđica Parac-Osterman
University of Zagreb, Faculty of Textile Technology,
Department of Textile Chemistry and Ecology, Zagreb, Croatia

ABSTRACT

The UV protection by textiles highly depends on large number of factors such are type of fiber, fabric surface, construction, porosity, density, moisture content, type and concentration of dyestuff, fluorescent whitening agents (FWA), UV-B protective agents (UV absorbers), as well as nanoparticles, if applied. The dyes are selective absorbers. They all absorb visible light, but some absorb light in the near ultraviolet region, as well. Even though synthetic dyes are cheaper, their usage led to such consequences as carcinogenicity and some of them are toxic to the environment. Due to increased awareness of the environmental and health hazards associated with the synthesis, processing and use of synthetic dyes, most of the commercial dyers have started to re-looking to the maximum possibilities of using natural dyes for dyeing and printing of different textiles for targeting niche market. Natural dyes are usually derived from the plants, animal and mineral sources. The shades produced by natural dyes are usually soft, lustrous and soothing to the human eye, can be produced a wide range of colors by mix and match system and are usually renewable and biodegradable. However, it needs longer dyeing time and excess cost for mordants and mordanting. Applied on textiles, provide some UV blocking which depends on the structure of dye molecules, type of dye or pigment, present absorptive groups, depth of dyeing and the uniformity. According to colour physic principles, darker colors (e.g., black, navy blue and dark red) absorb UV-R much more strongly than light pastel colors. For that reason, in this chapter the UV protection by woolen fabric dyed with natural dyestuff extracted from European Ash bark (*Fraxinus excelsior)* and European black elderberry berries (*Sambucus nigra)* was researched. Since these natural dyes, as most of the natural dyes, are non-substantive and must be applied on textiles in the combination with mordants i.e., metallic salts, 4

* Corresponding address: Prilaz baruna Filipovića 28a, HR-10000 Zagreb, Croatia; E-mail: anita.tarbuk@ttf.hr.

different mordants were applied. The color parameters were measured on remission spectrophotometer. The fabric UV protection was determined according to AS/NZS 4399:1996 *Sun Protective Clothing: evaluation and classification*, by UV-A and UV-B transmission measurement on transmission spectrophotometer and calculation of Ultraviolet protection factor (UPF).

Keywords: Wool, UV protection, natural dyestuff, *Sambucus nigra, Fraxinus excelsior*

INTRODUCTION

The application of a number of synthetic dyes is associated with allergies, toxic and carcinogenic effect as well as impact on the environment. Due to increased awareness of the environmental and health hazards associated with the synthesis, processing and use of synthetic dyes, most of the commercial dyers have started to re-looking to the maximum possibilities of using natural dyes for dyeing and printing of different textiles for targeting niche market [1-6]. Natural dyes are usually derived from the plants, animal/insects and mineral sources, and can be classified according to dyeing properties, chemical structure, origin, hue or application area [1-6]. In regards to dyeing properties, most natural dyes can be sorted into group of mordant dyes; some can be classified as vat, while a small number of natural dyes belong to groups of direct and basic dyes [6-13].

Table 1. Review of main groups of natural dyes according hues [6, 12, 13, 26, 27]

Name	Colour Index	Source	Mordant	Main colouring matters
Red colour hues				
Alkanet root *(Anchusa tinctoria L.)*	Natural Red 20	roots	Al	alkannin
Henna *(Lawsonia inrmis L.)*	Natural Orange 6	leaves	Al	lawsone
Kermes *(Coccus ilicis L.)*	Natrual Red 3	insect	Al, Sn, Cu, Fe	kermesic and flavokermesic acid
Cochineal *(Coccus cacti L.)*	Natural Red 4	insect	Al, Sn, Cu, Fe	carminic acid
Madder *(Rubia tinctorum L.)*	Natural Red 8	root	Al, Fe, Sn	alizarin, pseudopurpurin, purpurin, xanthopurpurin
Brazilwood *(Caesalpinia sappan L.)*	Natural Red 24	wood	Al, Fe, Sn	brazilin, brazilein
Yellow colour hues				
Tree of Sorrow *(Nyctanthes arbor-tristis L.)*	Natural Yellow 19	flower	Al	crocetin
Chamomile *(Chamaemelum recutica L.)*	Natural Yellow 1	flowers and leaves	Sn, Al	luteolin, palulitrin, rutin
Jasmine *(Gardenia jasminoides L.)*	Natural Yellow 6	fruit	Sn, Al	crocetin

Name	Colour Index	Source	Mordant	Main colouring matters
Saffron *(Crocus sativus)*	Natural Yellow 6	stigmas	Al	crocetin
Pomegranate *(Punica granatum)*	Natural Yellow 3	fruit	Al	gallotannins, anthocyanins, betalains
Curcuma *(Curcuma longa)*	Natural Yellow 3	root	Al, Cu	curcumin
Marygold (Calendula officinalis L.)	Natural Yellow 27	flower	Al	rubixanthin
Ashtree *(Fraxinus excelsior)*	Natural Yellow 10	bark	Sn, Al	quercitrin, isoquercitrin
Spanish broom *(Spartium junceum L.)*	Natural Yellow 2	flower	Al, Cu	isoflavon, genistin
Blue colour hues				
Logwood *(Haematoxylum campenhianum L.)*	Natural Black 1	heartwoo d	Al, Sn, Cu, Fe	haematoxylin, haematein
Indigo *(Indigofera tinctoria L.)*	Natural Blue 1	leaves	-	indigotin, indirubin
Purple colour hues				
Tyrian purple *(Murex brandraris L. and Murex trunculus L.)*	Natural Violet 1	shellfish	-	6,6′-dibromoindigotin, 6,6′-dibromoindirubin, 6-bromoindigotin
Brown colour hues				
Walnut-tree *(Junglans regia)*	Natural Brown 7	green scale or leaves	Fe	juglone
Sicilian Sumac *(Ruhus coriaria L.)*	Natural Brown 6	leaves	Fe	chebulinic acid - eutannin

Complexing with metal salts, mordant dyes give different colorations. Aluminum, copper, iron and tin salts are most usually used mordants. Mordants are usually applied in protein fiber dyeing as mordant pre-treatment of fibres (prior to dyeing); during the process of dyeing, or mordant after-treatment. The most common source of these dyestuffs are madder (*Rubia tinctorum*), cochenil bug (*Dactylopius coccus*), as well as herbs from which most widely used mordant dyes are obtained – flavonoid dyes [14-19]. Second important group of natural textile dyes are in water insoluble vat dyes, which have to be transformed into soluble form with the addition of reduction agent and alkali. Most commonly known representatives of this group are indigo and purple 6,6'-dibromindigo dye obtained from murex sea snail (*Murex brandaris and Murex trunculus*) [7, 20-23]. Among most important natural direct dyes are turmeric or yellow root (*Curcuma longa*) and powderd bark or roots of common barberry (*Berberis vulgaris*) [7, 24, 25]. Review of main groups of natural dyes [6,12,13,26,27] is shown in Table 1. Some other plants commonly used as natural dyes are: Dyer's woad (*Isatis tinctoria L.),* Lipsticktree (*Bixa orellana L.*), Brasilwood (*Caesalpina brasiliensis L.*), Weld (*Reseda luteola L.*), Juniper (*Juniperus Communis*); Elder (*Sambucus Nigra*), Oak (Quercus Aegilops), Bramble (*Rubus fruticosus*), Nettle (*Urtica dioica*), St. John

Wart (*Hypericum perforatum*), Hibiscus (*Hibiscus L.*), Oak (*Quercus Aegilops*), Bottlebrush (*Callistemon citrinus*), Eucalyptus (*E. Camaldulensis),* etc. [1-37].

When classifying natural dyes according to color hue, the type and process of mordant should be regarded. Only a few natural dyes are substantive (direct and vat dyes), whilst all other require inorganic oxides or salts – metal salts (mordant dyes). Division of natural dyes according to chemical constitution is in accordance to botanical nomenclature. Most important chemical groups of natural dyes are: carationoide, diaril-methane, benzoquinone, anthraquinone, indigoide, flavonoide, anthociane, betalaine, neoflavonoide, basic, alcaloide, benzofenon, galotannine, tannins, chlorophyll, natural pigments, etc. [7,8]. Flavonoids and flavonoid derivatives are most represented compounds in watery herbal extracts [38-42]. In regards to dyeing properties flavonoids belong to a group of mordant dyes. Most commonly used dyeing method uses a pretreatment process in which wool is mordanted in watery solution of metal salts, followed by a process of dyeing in the solution of watery extracted natural dyes [7, 10-13, 38-41]. The combination dye-metal salt has a strong infuence on the color hue and color fastness properties [10]. Depending on the structure of flavonoid derivative metal complexes 1:1 or 1:2 may be formed [38] (Figure 1).

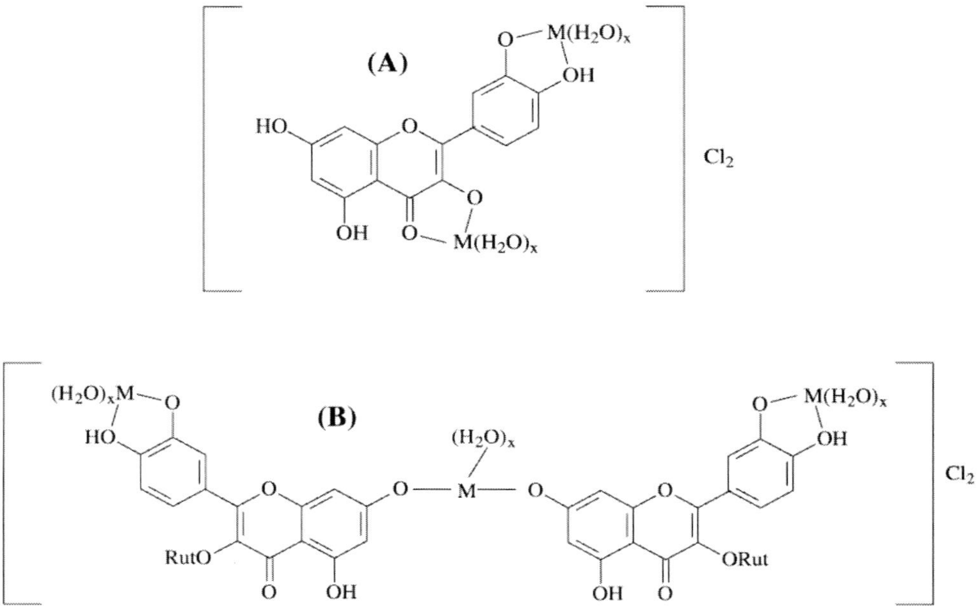

Figure 1. Tentative structures of the complexes: (A) quercetin complexes (1:1); (B) rutin complexes (1:1 and 1:2). x =2 for M = Cu (II); x = 4 for M = Fe(II) [42].

Natural dyes represent renewable and sustainable bioresource products with minimum environmental impact and as such are a potential 'Green chemistry' option as an alternative/co-partner to some extent to synthetic dyes [43-45]. The shades produced by natural dyes are usually soft, lustrous and soothing to the human eye, can be produced a wide range of colors by mix and match system and are usually renewable and biodegradable. However, it needs longer dyeing time and excess cost for mordants and mordanting. There are some issues yet to be solved regard optimization of the amount and contents of natural extracts, increase of dye exhaustion to material, increase in colour fastness, selection and optimization of mordants used. Although, water is the most usual solvent used to prepare natural extract it is being substituted with another solvent (ethanol, methanol) in the aim of increasing the overall amount of the extract, isolation of certain extract components or simply to remove unwanted impurities such as waxes and lipids from watery extracts [46-49].

During the last few decades, increasing attention has been paid by researchers to various aspects of natural dye applications. A large number of plant and animal/insect sources have been identified for extraction of color [2,3] and their diversified use in textile dyeing [9, 29] and functional finishing [30, 31, 50-56], food coloration, cosmetics, and other application disciplines [5]. Natural dyes in functional finishing of textiles has become as a result of a careful balance between compatibility of different finishing products and treatments and the application processes used to provide eco-friendly textiles with desirable properties, such as antimicrobial [30, 31, 43, 49-56], insect repellent, deodorizing and UV-protective [54-64] properties. Several new techniques of modern innovative finishing have been added to dyeing technologies: CO_2, chitosan treatment [65], enzymatic treatment [66, 67], plasma treatment [68, 69], cationization [70-72], microencapsulation and cross-linking [73], etc. for enhancement of protective properties of naturally dyed textile materials, e.g., antimicrobial and UV protection.

The primary cause of skin cancer is believed to be a long exposure to solar ultraviolet (UV) radiation crossed with the amount of skin pigmentation in the population [74-76]. Intermittent sun exposure in childhood and adolescence is considered to be a stronger risk factor for melanoma than continuous exposure. In addition to some beneficial effects of UV radiation it may cause skin and eye damage, especially during the summer time. The proper and early photoprotection may reduce the risk of subsequent occurrence of skin cancer [76]. Therefore, photoprotection is based on protection from UV-B (from 280 nm to 320 nm) and UV-A (from 320 nm to 400 nm) radiation, which are reaching the Earth due to diminishing of the ozone layer.

Textile and clothing show some UV protection, but in the most cases it does not provide full sun screening properties. A good fabric UV protection depends on a large number of factors, such as, the type of fiber, fabric surface and construction, porosity, density, moisture content, type and concentration of dyestuff, fluorescent whitening agent (FWA), UV-B protective agents, as well as nanoparticles, if applied [57, 77-91].

The dyestuffs are selective absorbers. They all absorb visible light, but some absorb light in the near ultraviolet region, as well. Applied on textiles, provide some UV blocking which depends on the structure of dye molecules, type of dye or pigment, present absorptive groups, depth of dyeing and the uniformity. According to colour physic principles, darker colors (e.g., black, navy blue and dark red) absorb UV-R much more strongly than light pastel colors. Therefore, dyed fabrics protect more than undyed ones and their protection levels rise with the increase in dye concentration [57-60, 64, 77]. However, most of these results concern synthetic dyes.

There are only few studies that focused on the UV protection properties of natural dyes. Sarkar [57] characterized UV protection of plain, twill or sateen weave cotton fabrics dyed with colorants of plant (madder and indigo) and insect (cochineal) origins. Feng et al. [58] in an experiment conducted to evaluate UV protection properties of two natural dyes (Rheum and Lithospermum erythrorhizon) applied on cotton and silk found that these natural dyes exhibit a comparable UV-absorption performance to benzophenone. Results demonstrated that UV-protective effect was strongly dependent on absorption characteristics of natural dyes for UVR. Grifoni et al. [59, 60] studied the effect of color on UVR transmission of cotton, flax, hemp and ramie fabrics with different construction parameters dyed with some common natural dyes: dyer's woad, madder, logwood, lipsticktree, brasilwood, weld and cochineal by in vitro and outdoor assessments. Metallic salt mordants have been reported to enhance UV-protective properties of naturally dyed cotton [55], wool and silk [61-63] fabrics to a substantial account depending on nature of fibre, mordant and natural dye used. Recently, Hou et al. [75] used natural dyes extracted from orange peel, an abundant, cheap and readily available agricultural byproduct, for producing highly durable UV protective wool fabrics. The authors could not found any research considering UV protection of fabric dyed with European Ash bark *(Fraxinus excelsior)*. On the other hand, there has been ne report regarding European black elderberry berries *(Sambucus nigra)* in photoprotective UVA and UVB; photostability in cosmetic emulsions [92].

For that reason, in this chapter the UV protection by woolen fabric dyed with natural dyestuff extracted from European Ash bark *(Fraxinus excelsior)* and European black elderberry berries *(Sambucus nigra)* was researched. Since these natural dyes are non-substantive and must be applied on textiles in the combination with mordants i.e., metallic salts, 4 different mordants were applied. Additionally, color parameters were measured.

EXPERIMENTAL

Materials

Fabric

Twill woven fabric of 100% wool fibers, having mass per unit area of 162 g/m^2 was used for this research. Warp in the fabric was 30 tex, of density 33 yarns/cm; and weft 25 tex, of density 28 yarns/cm.

Plant Selection

Natural dyestuff was extracted from European Ash bark *(Fraxinus excelsior)* and European black elderberry berries *(Sambucus nigra)* from Croatia.

Mordants

The chemicals (from Kemika, Zagreb) used as mordants in this research were: $KAl(SO_4)_2 \cdot 12H_2O$, $CuSO_4 \cdot 5H_2O$, $FeSO_4 \cdot 7H_2O$ and $SnCl_2 \cdot 2H_2O$.

Procedure

The dyeing of the wool fabric was done in 3 stages: extraction of dyes from the plant, mordanting in pre-treatment or after-treatment, and dyeing.

Extraction of Dyestuff

Air-dryed and powered plants were dried 6 hours at 105°C and cooled. Water extract of European Ash bark (*Fraxinus excelsior)* and European black elderberry berries (*Sambucus nigra*) was performed in deionized water for 1 hour at the 100°C, in bath ratio (BR) 1:20. The solution was cooled down and filtered.

Mordanting

The woolen fabrics were treated with metal salts – mordants:

$KAl(SO_4)_2 \cdot 12H_2O$, $CuSO_4 \cdot 5H_2O$, $FeSO_4 \cdot 7H_2O$ and $SnCl_2 \cdot 2H_2O$ as pre-treatment or after-treatment for wool fabric dyed with water extract of European Ash bark (Fraxinus excelsior); and as pre-treatment for wool fabric dyes with water extract of European black elderberry berries (*Sambucus nigra*) due to it is more effective. In pre-treatment, woolen fabrics were treated with metal salts, followed by dyeing in a water extract of natural dyes. In after-treatment mordants were applied after the dyeing process.

Procedure of mordating

Mordant was dissolved in deionized water to make the liquor. pH 4.5 was set by adding 2% oxalic acid and 2 % tartaric acid. Wool fabrics were mordanted for 60 min at 100°C using laboratory dyeing machine (Polycolor, Mathis) at a material to BR 1:20. Mordanting was carried out with 4 different mordants: Pottasium alum dodecahydrate ($KAl(SO_4)_3 \cdot 12\ H_2O$), Copper (II) sulfate pentahydrate ($CuSO_4 \cdot 5H_2O$), Iron (II) sulfate heptahydrate ($FeSO_4 \cdot 7\ H_2O$) and Tin(II) chloride dihydrate ($SnCl_2 \cdot 2H_2O$)in wide concentration range (0.1% - 5% owf – over weigth of fabric). The mordant material was than rinsed and dried.

Dyeing

Untereated and woolen fabric treated with mordants were dyed with plant extract solution of pH value 6.5. Dyeing process was done in laboratory dyeing machine (Polycolor, Mathis) at a material to liquor ratio of 1:20. The dye bath temperature was raised at a rate of 3°C/min to 100°C, maintained at this temperature for 60 min and cooled down to room temperature. Dyed fabrics were rinsed in cold and hot water and allowed to air-dry.

Measurements

The electrokinetic (zeta) potential is part of the total potential drop occurring in the intermediate surface layer at the boundary of the solid/liquid phases as a consequence of the ions distribution from the solid surface to the liquid mass. It was measured by streaming potential/current method using Brookhaven-Paar Electrokinetic Analyzer with a stamp cell and calculated according to Helmholtz-Smoluchowsky equation [93]. Isoelectric Point (IEP) is a numeric value of pH where electrokinetic surface potential equals zero and indicate the nature of solid surface. Therefore, the zeta potential (ZP) was investigated versus pH, and the Isoelectric Point (IEP) of woolen fabric was determined.

HPLC of plant water extract using Shimadzu HPLC system of LC-10 series was performed to determine composition of primary dyeing agent in natural dyestuffs. Based on the best selectivity of flavonoides that should contain these plant extracts, measurement was performed at 300 nm, bandwidths of 10 nm, in time of 15 min. Column C18 Shodex RSpak DS-613 were used. Analysis was performed by binary system where the mobiles phase included water (pH 2 adjusted with phosphoric acid) and acetonitrile in a ratio of 77,5:22,5; at a flow rate 1 ml/min.

Color parameters of woolen fabrics after dyeing were measured using remission spectrophotometer SF 600 PLUS CT (Datacolor) under illuminant D65, 8° standard observer with the specular component excluded and the UV component included. The coordinates used to determine color values are "L*" for lightness, "a*" for redness (positive value) and greenness (negative value), "b*" for yellowness (positive value) and blueness (negative value), "C*" for chroma and "h°" for hue angle in the range of 0° to 360°.

Colour strength (K/S) was calculated by the Kubelka-Munk equation:

$$K/S = (1-R)^2/2R \tag{1}$$

where R is the remission value (reflectance of the dyed fabric) at λ_{max}, K is the absorption coefficient.

The fabric UV protection was determined according to AS/NZS 4399:1996 *Sun Protective Clothing: evaluation and classification.* UVA and UVB transmission through fabric were measured on Varian Cary 50 Spectrophotometer. The *ultraviolet protection factor* (*UPF*) was calculated automatically. Fabrics UV protection was rated accordingly (Table 2).

Table 2. UV protection rating according to AS/NZS 4399:1996

UPF range	UPF rating	UV-R protection category	UV-R blocking [%]
< 14	0, 5, 10	non-rateable	<93,3
15-24	15, 20	good	93,3-95,8
25-39	25, 30, 35	very good	95,9-97,4
> 40	40, 45, 50, 50+	excellent	> 97,5

RESULTS AND DISCUSSION

In this chapter the UV protection by woolen fabric dyed with natural dyestuff extracted from European Ash bark (*Fraxinus excelsior)* and European black elderberry berries (*Sambucus nigra)* was researched. Prior to dyeing with these natural dyes, the zeta potential and Isoelectric Point (IEP), a numeric value of pH where electrokinetic surface potential equals zero, were determined by streaming potential/current method using Brookhaven-Paar Electrokinetic Analyzer with a stamp cell. The results are shown in Figure 2.

The wool fibre has an anionic character at pH 10 due to the presence of numerous carboxylate groups. The is also a large number of other chargeable groups, including nitrogen containing groups, that will protonate and give rise to positive charge at lower pH values. All these groups result in a high ZP of wool fabric (-48 mV) and IEP = 4.3. The net charge is due to the balance of these different groups and is the reason for positive zeta potential of wool at low pH. Isoelectric point, IEP, depends on molecular and supramolecular structure of fibres in textile fabric. It is important parameter for fabric dyeability and finishing process. Therefore, mordating was performed near the isoelectric point, at pH 4.5, what resulted in yellow shade; whilst in alkali medium it would be brown.

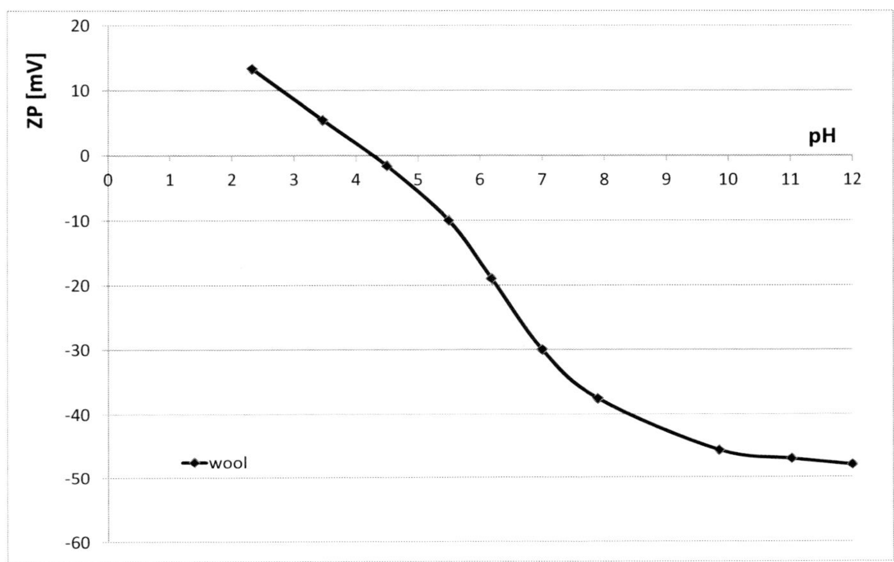

Figure 2. Zeta potential (ZP, ζ) of the wool fabrics vs. pH of 0.001 M KCl (IEP=4.3).

Based on the retention times of occurrence of peaks of standard solutions of flavonoids proved to be in alcocholic extract of European Ash bark obtained the strongest signal in the retention time of 2.61 min, which corresponds to the rutine and less intensity at retention times 3.44 and 4.40 min corresponding isoquercitrin and quercetin. In the alcoholic extract of European black elderberry berries resulted in two spades and at retention time 2.61 min (characteristic of rutin) and 1.85 min which corresponds to anthocyanines. Based on literature data and HPLC measurement in European Ash bark (*Fraxinus excelsior)* extract primary dyeing agents are rutin, quercetin and isoquercitrin [6, 30, 94], and in European black elderberry berries (*Sambucus nigra)* rutine and anthocyanin, especially Cyanidin 3-glucoside and Cyanidin 3-sambubioside [6, 94-96]. The chemical structures of primary dyeing agents are listed in the Table 3. These compounds were taken account when applied to textiles in the combination with 4 different mordants.

Natural dyes derived from plants are usually acid mordant dyes which create metal-flavonoid complexes with metal ions. Depending on the chosen metal the different tones of the coloration can be obtained. Since all these flavonoid pigments belong to the group of mordant dyes, 4 different mordants were used in pre-treatment or after-treatment. The woolen fabrics were pre-treated with metal salts, followed by dyeing in an aqueous extract of natural dyes. In after-treatment mordants (metal salts) were applied after the dyeing process. In both cases, it was essential that the flavonoid component from the extract creates colored metal complex where, depending on the structure of flavonoid derivatives, metal complexes 1:1 or 1:2 may arise.

Table 3. The primary dyeing agents in European Ash bark (*Fraxinus excelsior)* and European black elderberry berries (*Sambucus nigra)*

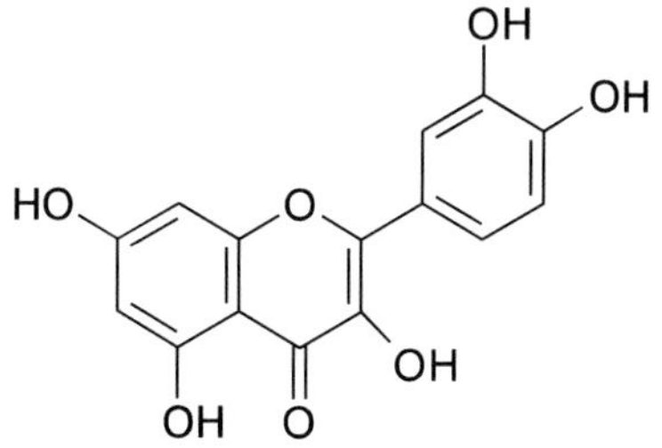 quercetin dihydrate *3,3',4',5,7-pentahydroxyflavon*	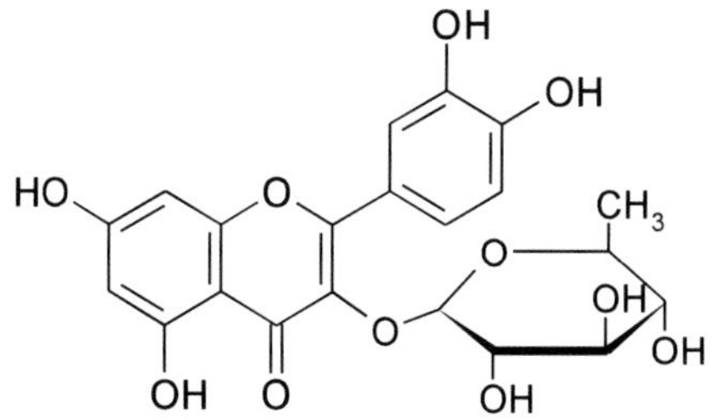 isoquercitrin *quercetin 3-glucoside*
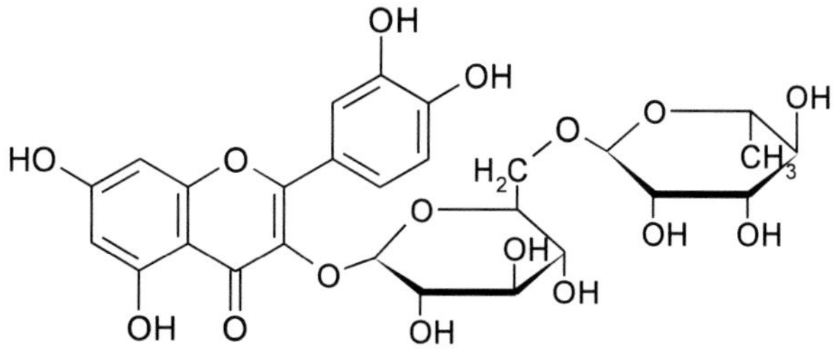 rutin trihydrate *quercetin -3-rutinoside*	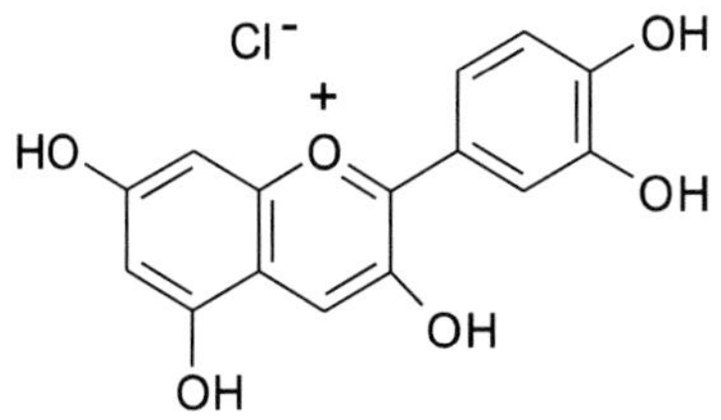 Anthocyanin *Cyanidin*

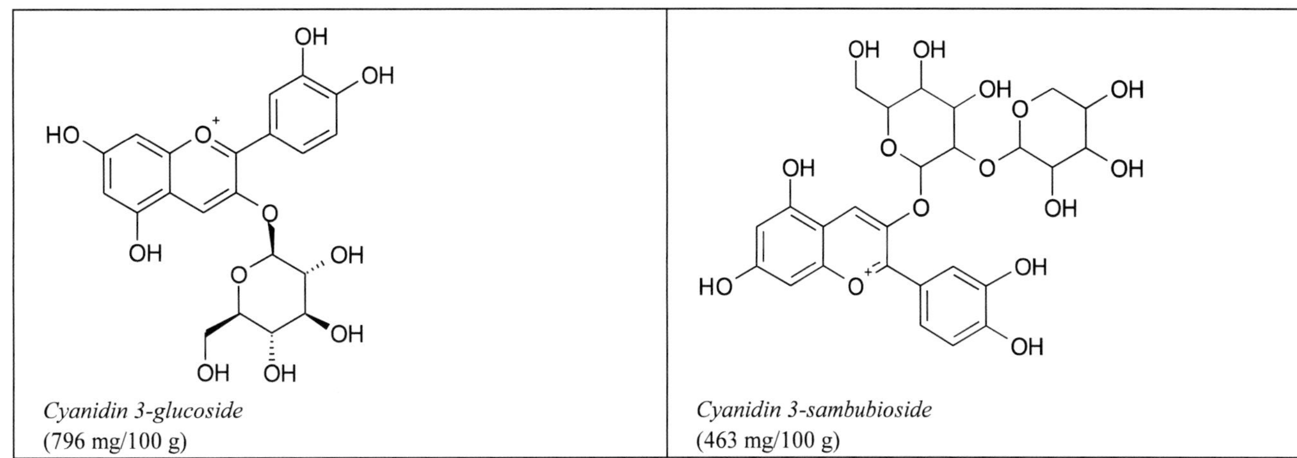

Cyanidin 3-glucoside
(796 mg/100 g)

Cyanidin 3-sambubioside
(463 mg/100 g)

Possible copper complexes with quercetin and rutin are shown in Figures 3 and 4. In neutral aglycone quercetin dihydrate reactivity is [94]: $Sn^{2+} > Al^{3+} > Fe^{2+} > Cu^{2+}$. On the other hand, glycoside rutin trihydrate and isoquercetin showed oposite reactivity: $Cu^{2+} > Fe^{2+} > Al^{3+} > Sn^{2+}$. The resulting inverse selectivity of aglycone and glycosides in favor of "natural series" H. Irving and R.J.P. Williams who proved that the stability of metal complexes is growing in a number of divalent central ions: $Mn^{2+}<Fe^{2+}<Co^{2+}<Ni^{2+}<Cu^{2+}$.

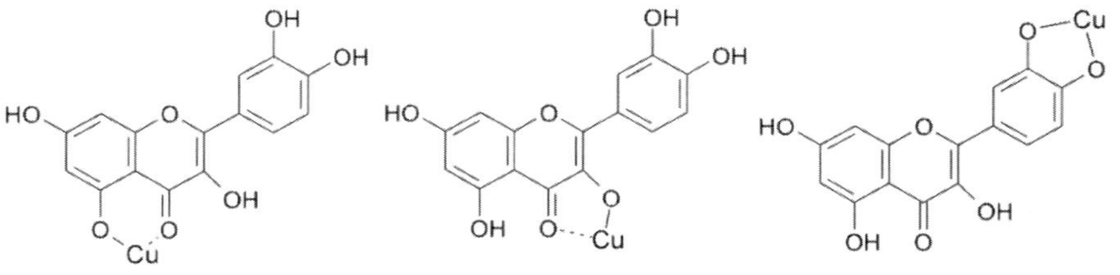

Figure 3. Possible quercetin:copper complex (1:1).

In order to confirm the formation of the colored complex on the dyed woolen fabric, samples were analyzed with a remission spectrophotometer SF 600 PLUS CT (Datacolor). The coloristic parameters are given in Tables 4-6. Color depth (K/S) of all dyed woolen fabrics is presented in Figures 5-9.

From the Tables 4 and 5 can be seen that woolen fabrics dyed in water extract of European Ash bark (*Fraxinus excelsior)* resulted with tones in yellow-orange region, a range of values tons h* = 77 – 87 regardless of mordant or procedure of its application. The effect of mordant concentration and its application procedure to saturation (C*) can be observed. The maximum differences are observed for the metal salts of iron and copper which is in correlation with their ionic potential.

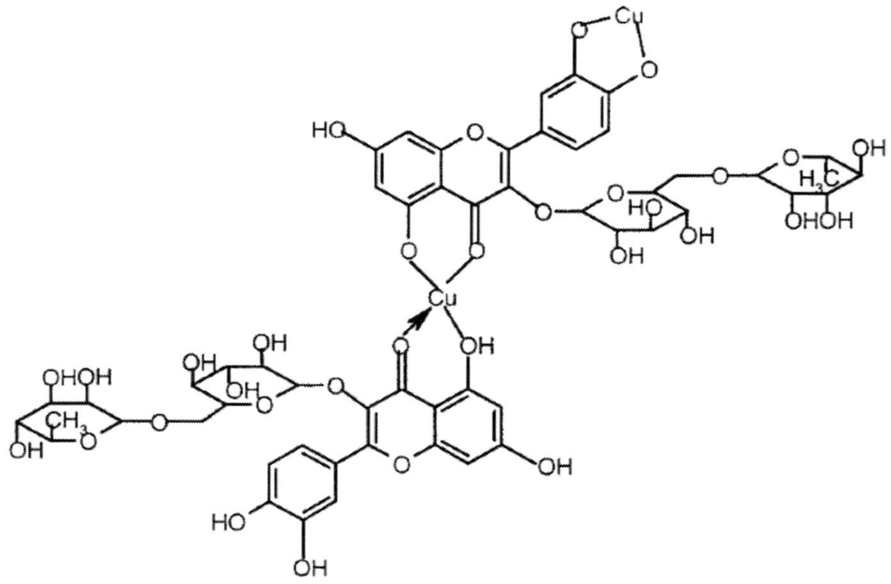

Figure 4. Possible rutin:copper complex (1:1 and 1:2) [97].

Table 4. Color parameters of woolen fabrics dyed in water extract of European Ash bark (*Fraxinus excelsior*) with $KAl(SO_4)_2{\cdot}12H_2O$ and $CuSO_4{\cdot}5H_2O$ as mordants

Mordant	a*	b*	L*	C*	h*	X	Y	Z	x	y
No mordant	4.42	24.38	61.29	24.78	79.72	30.44	29.58	13.42	0.41	0.40
Pre-treatment $KAl(SO_4)_2{\cdot}12H_2O$										
0.1%	5.61	25.77	53.41	26.37	77.71	22.40	21.42	8.61	0.43	0.41
0.5%	5.87	26.36	52.61	27.01	77.44	21.71	20.69	8.08	0.43	0.41
1.0%	5.77	26.41	53.48	27.04	77.68	22.51	21.49	8.47	0.43	0.41
1.5%	5.49	26.23	53.27	26.80	78.17	22.25	21.29	8.42	0.43	0.41
2.0%	5.62	26.28	53.20	26.88	77.94	22.21	21.23	8.38	0.43	0.41
3.0%	5.75	26.25	52.42	26.87	77.65	21.51	20.52	8.02	0.43	0.41
4.0%	5.63	25.99	51.86	26.59	77.79	20.96	20.02	7.84	0.43	0.41
5.0%	5.90	26.27	50.89	26.92	77.35	20.16	19.18	7.35	0.43	0.41
After-treatment $KAl(SO_4)_2{\cdot}12H_2O$										
0.1%	4.66	24.07	67.84	24.52	79.05	38.81	37.76	18.19	0.41	0.40
0.5%	4.88	23.74	67.92	24.24	78.39	38.99	37.86	18.40	0.41	0.40
1.0%	5.05	24.02	67.24	24.55	78.13	38.11	36.95	17.75	0.41	0.40
1.5%	4.77	25.03	63.98	25.48	79.21	33.79	32.78	14.96	0.41	0.40
2.0%	5.13	25.03	63.55	25.55	78.41	33.35	32.25	14.66	0.42	0.40
3.0%	4.61	25.43	61.51	25.84	79.72	30.75	29.83	13.18	0.42	0.40
4.0%	4.84	25.68	62.03	26.13	79.32	31.42	30.43	13.42	0.42	0.40
5.0%	4.85	24.31	63.45	24.79	78.73	33.15	32.12	14.87	0.41	0.40
Pre-treatment $CuSO_4{\cdot}5H_2O$										
0.1%	4.27	23.99	54.54	24.37	79.90	23.20	22.49	9.68	0.42	0.41
0.5%	4.60	24.38	54.30	24.81	79.31	23.04	22.26	9.45	0.42	0.41
1.0%	3.85	24.10	54.45	24.40	80.92	23.01	22.40	9.60	0.42	0.41
1.5%	4.10	24.85	53.30	25.18	80.62	21.97	21.32	8.82	0.42	0.41
2.0%	3.84	24.61	53.97	24.91	81.13	22.55	21.95	9.21	0.42	0.41
3.0%	4.23	24.62	54.48	24.99	80.25	23.13	22.43	9.46	0.42	0.41
4.0%	4.58	24.95	55.20	25.37	79.61	23.91	23.12	9.73	0.42	0.41
5.0%	4.54	25.93	54.45	26.32	80.07	23.17	22.40	9.07	0.42	0.41
After-treatment $CuSO_4{\cdot}5H_2O$										
0.1%	3.77	24.20	62.06	24.49	81.16	31.17	30.48	13.99	0.41	0.40
0.5%	3.16	22.63	65.05	22.85	82.06	34.66	34.10	16.70	0.41	0.40
1.0%	2.08	23.00	61.45	23.09	84.82	30.00	29.77	14.05	0.41	0.40
1.5%	1.20	21.37	61.35	21.40	86.79	29.64	29.64	14.61	0.40	0.40
2.0%	1.78	22.56	58.60	22.63	85.50	26.75	26.60	12.41	0.41	0.40
3.0%	2.47	23.24	59.30	23.38	83.94	27.68	27.35	12.59	0.41	0.40
4.0%	1.56	22.48	63.53	22.53	86.04	32.31	32.22	15.67	0.40	0.40
5.0%	2.37	23.36	61.64	23.48	84.22	30.29	29.98	14.03	0.41	0.40

Table 5. Color parametres of woolen fabrics dyed in water extract of European Ash bark (*Fraxinus excelsior*) with $FeSO_4{\cdot}7H_2O$ and $SnCl_2{\cdot}2H_2O$ as mordants

MORDANT	a*	b*	L*	C*	h*	X	Y	Z	x	y
Pre-treatment $FeSO_4{\cdot}7H_2O$										
0.1%	2.33	15.71	45.23	15.89	81.58	14.93	14.70	7.54	0.40	0.40
0.5%	1.04	12.75	41.77	12.80	85.32	12.37	12.35	6.81	0.39	0.39
1.0%	0.58	10.66	37.55	10.67	86.91	9.80	9.84	5.67	0.39	0.39
1.5%	0.59	9.99	36.98	10.00	86.63	9.50	9.53	5.60	0.39	0.39
2.0%	0.42	10.31	37.54	10.31	87.65	9.78	9.83	5.74	0.39	0.39
3.0%	0.80	10.97	37.04	11.00	85.81	9.55	9.56	5.42	0.39	0.39
4.0%	0.89	12.03	38.52	12.07	85.78	10.39	10.38	5.73	0.39	0.39
5.0%	0.99	12.53	38.20	12.56	85.46	10.22	10.20	5.51	0.39	0.39

Table 5. (Continued)

MORDANT	a*	b*	L*	C*	h*	X	Y	Z	x	y
After-treatment $FeSO_4 \cdot 7H_2O$										
0.1%	2.02	16.47	54.91	16.59	83.01	23.05	22.84	12.31	0.40	0.39
0.5%	1.29	13.90	53.72	13.96	84.70	21.76	21.71	12.50	0.39	0.39
1.0%	1.39	14.92	51.12	14.98	84.66	19.44	19.38	10.66	0.39	0.39
1.5%	1.22	16.43	46.74	16.47	85.76	15.86	15.82	8.03	0.40	0.40
2.0%	1.07	16.21	49.21	16.25	86.23	17.77	17.76	9.26	0.40	0.40
3.0%	1.50	17.02	46.50	17.09	84.96	15.73	15.64	7.77	0.40	0.40
4.0%	1.47	18.29	47.34	18.35	85.39	16.37	16.28	7.82	0.40	0.40
5.0%	1.96	18.53	45.32	18.63	83.96	14.94	14.77	6.90	0.41	0.40
Pre-treatment $SnCl_2 \cdot 2H_2O$										
0.1%	6.13	30.06	59.18	30.67	78.48	28.49	27.23	10.27	0.43	0.41
0.5%	5.94	30.46	60.05	31.03	78.97	29.42	28.18	10.61	0.43	0.41
1.0%	5.99	30.86	61.56	31.44	79.01	31.18	29.89	11.32	0.43	0.41
1.5%	6.18	31.49	62.20	32.09	78.90	32.01	30.64	11.48	0.43	0.41
2.0%	6.44	32.62	62.29	33.25	78.83	32.18	30.74	11.15	0.43	0.42
3.0%	6.45	32.42	62.43	33.05	78.74	32.36	30.90	11.30	0.43	0.41
4.0%	6.53	31.59	60.98	32.25	78.33	30.65	29.22	10.76	0.43	0.41
5.0%	7.00	31.75	59.60	32.51	77.57	29.18	27.68	9.97	0.44	0.41
After-treatment $SnCl_2 \cdot 2H_2O$										
0.1%	5.10	24.81	66.92	25.33	78.38	37.70	36.53	17.16	0.41	0.40
0.5%	4.99	26.23	65.64	26.70	79.22	35.98	34.86	15.63	0.42	0.40
1.0%	4.88	26.41	66.08	26.86	79.54	36.52	35.43	15.87	0.42	0.40
1.5%	4.27	25.70	71.05	26.05	80.58	43.25	42.27	20.02	0.41	0.40
2.0%	5.53	26.84	66.99	27.41	78.36	37.93	36.62	16.34	0.42	0.40
3.0%	5.39	26.64	62.12	27.18	78.56	31.69	30.54	13.12	0.42	0.41
4.0%	4.93	26.12	62.40	26.58	79.32	31.89	30.87	13.49	0.42	0.40
5.0%	5.26	26.71	68.00	27.22	78.86	39.22	37.97	17.14	0.42	0.40

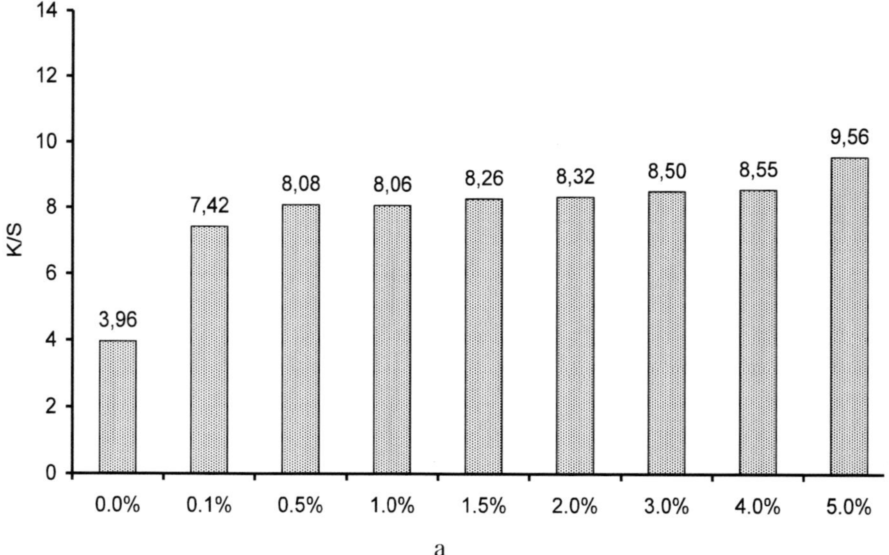

Figure 5. (Continued).

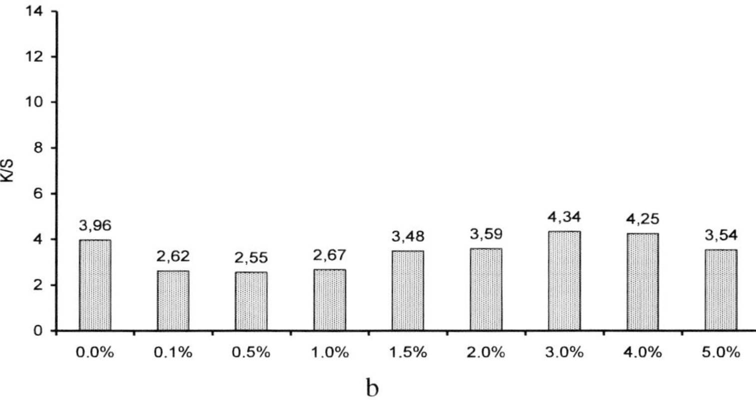

Figure 5. K/S values of woolen fabrics dyed in water extract of European Ash bark (*Fraxinus excelsior)* mordanted with $KAl(SO_4)_2{\cdot}12H_2O$ (0.1% - 5% owf) in a. pre-treatment and b. after-treatment.

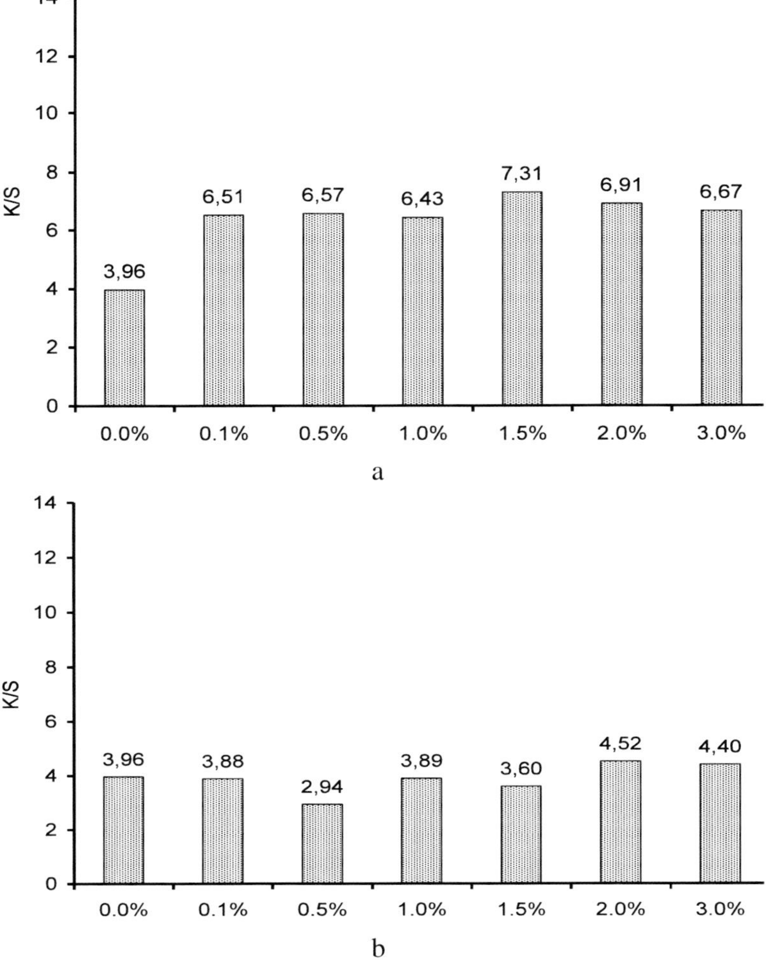

Figure 6. K/S values of woolen fabrics dyed in water extract of European Ash bark (*Fraxinus excelsior)* mordanted with $CuSO_4{\cdot}5H_2O$ (0.1% - 5% owf) in a. pre-treatment and b. after-treatment.

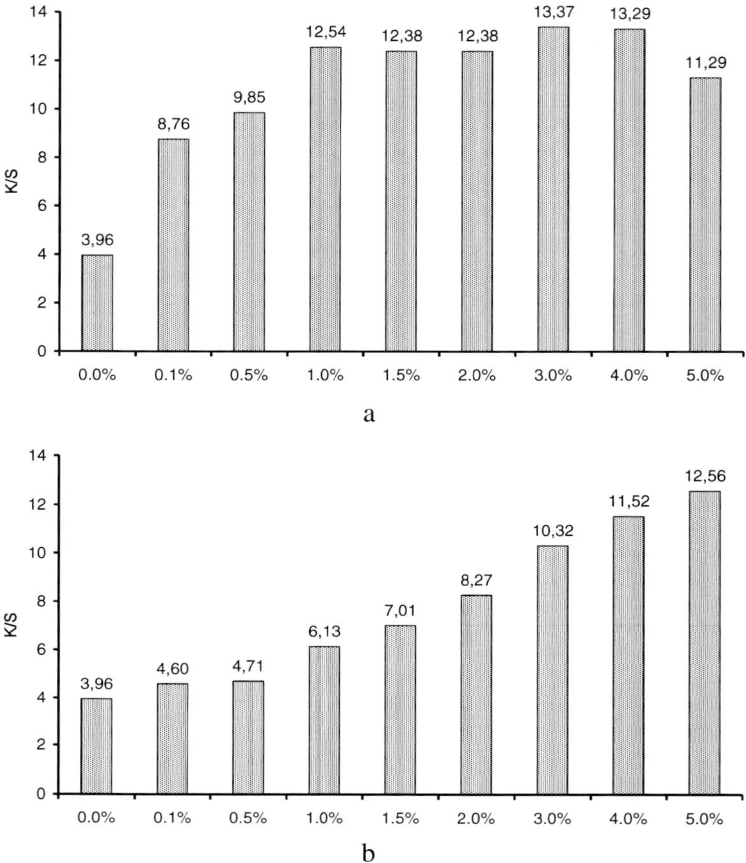

Figure 7. K/S values of woolen fabrics dyed in water extract of European Ash bark (*Fraxinus excelsior)* mordanted with $FeSO_4 \cdot 7H_2O$ (0.1% - 5% owf) in a. pre-treatment and b. after-treatment.

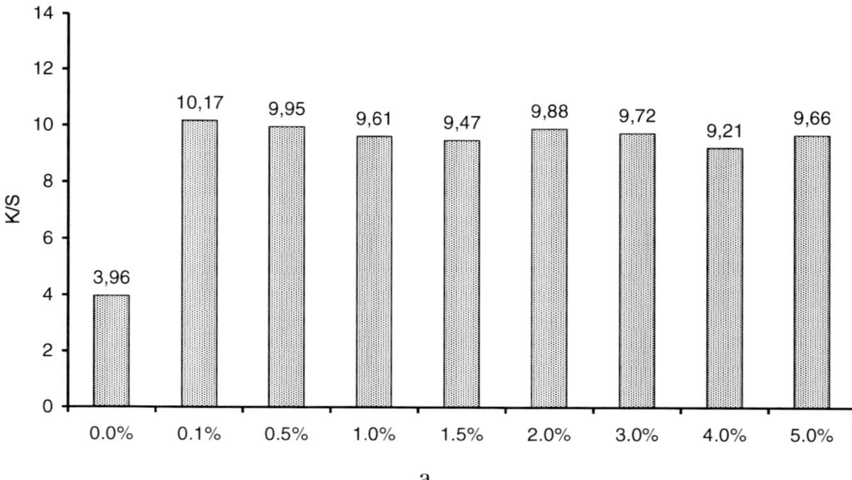

Figure 8. (Continued).

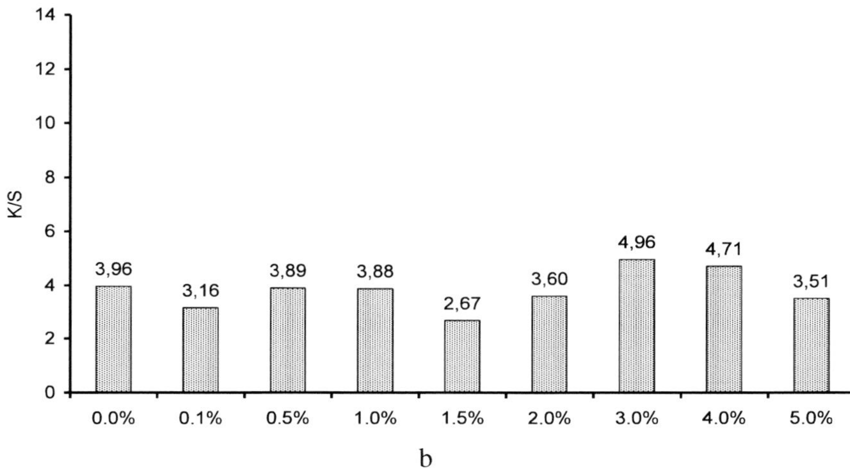

Figure 8. K/S values of woolen fabrics dyed in water extract of European Ash bark (*Fraxinus excelsior)* mordanted with $SnCl_2 \cdot 2H_2O$ (0.1% - 5% owf) in a. pre-treatment and b. after-treatment.

However, two-dimensional relationship between hue and saturation, can not make conclusive experience of color without the third dimension - the ligthness (L*). In general, on the basis of the coloristic parameters for all samples the $L^* > 60$, except for samples processed with salt $FeSO_4 \cdot 7H_2O$, $L^* < 40$. It is recognized, based on the x and y, these color samples are closer to achromatic point, resulting in olive shade. This pheomenon is more evident if the mordant was applied in pre-treatment. Comparing the procedures of applying mordants it is evident that pre-treatment results in better saturation than if applied in after-treatment. This can be considered from two aspects: 1st supstantivity of plant extract to the wool substrate and 2nd stability of resulting metal complexes. In the complexing was done in solution of quercetin dihydrate, and isoquercitrin, rutin trihydrate, the highest reactivity was obtained with the copper salt [94]. However, according to the color measurement, these results are not the best ones. This confirms that all components in plant extract, as well as the textile substrate, participate in creating of colored complex on the fiber/textile material. Mechanism of dyeing with flavonoid dyes is similar to the mechanism of antiradical behaviour of flavonoids in biological system and chelat bonding of metal ions. In biological systems the mechanism has not yet been completely explained on molecular level since there are great differences in chemical properties and significant structural heterogenity. However, the relationship between the structure and activity of the flavonoid and certain structural components and properties of bonding free radicals, formation of chelate complexes and anti oxidation activities have been proofed. Depending on chemical structure and chemico-morphological characteristics of the fibres being dyed by flavonoid dyes, following chemical bond are formed: hydrogen bonds are formed among poliphenol hydroxyl groups with free amino and amid groups of the protein fibre; ionic bonds are formed among free and available anionic groups in poliphenols and cationic groups of protein fibre [41, 97-100].

Table 6. Color parameters of woolen fabrics dyed in water extract of European black elderberry berries (*Sambucus nigra)*

MORDANT	a*	b*	L*	C*	h*	X	Y	Z	x	y
No mordant	7.29	21.07	52.10	22.30	70.91	20.65	20.23	11.99	0.39	0.38
Pre-treatment $KAl(SO_4)_2 \cdot 12H_2O$										
0.1%	6.67	18.57	45.65	19.74	70.24	12.60	12.28	7.08	0.39	0.38
0.5%	7.58	19.83	44.17	21.23	69.09	14.43	13.96	7.92	0.40	0.38
2.0%	6.45	18.97	42.91	20.04	71.23	13.39	13.10	7.56	0.39	0.38
Pre-treatment $CuSO_4 \cdot 5H_2O$										
0.1%	7.51	18.60	43.17	20.06	68.00	13.73	13.27	7.78	0.39	0.38
0.5%	7.25	18.45	42.73	19.83	68.56	13.39	12.98	7.62	0.39	0.38
2.0%	7.46	19.11	40.58	20.51	68.68	12.05	11.61	6.48	0.40	0.39
Pre-treatment $FeSO_4 \cdot 7H_2O$										
0.1%	6.67	18.57	41.65	19.74	70.24	12.60	12.28	7.08	0.39	0.38
0.5%	5.46	15.62	38.37	16.54	70.72	10.46	10.30	6.40	0.39	0.38
2.0%	4.00	12.88	33.96	13.48	72.75	8.01	7.99	5.28	0.38	0.38
Pre-treatment $SnCl_2 \cdot 2H_2O$										
0.1%	6.67	18.57	41.65	19.74	70.24	12.60	12.28	7.08	0.39	0.38
0.5%	5.61	17.64	42.20	18.51	72.36	12.80	12.63	7.59	0.39	0.38
2.0%	4.82	17.38	40.56	18.04	74.49	11.66	11.59	6.90	0.39	0.38

Considering the mordant concentration, it is evident that optimal color was obtained for samples pre-treated with 2% of metal salts. By increasing the concentration of mordant, no significant change in color depth (K/S) occured. If mordant applied in wide concentration range in after-treatment, the significant change in color parameters occurred if salt $FeSO_4 \cdot 7H_2O$ was applied. The obtained K/S values can be used as an indicator of water plant extract supstantivity. Approximately the same color depth (K/S) of woolen fabric achieved by pre-treated with 2%, and after-treated with 5% of $FeSO_4 \cdot 7H_2O$, can be attributed to the reactivity of the whole system. If pre-treated with 2% $FeSO_4 \cdot 7H_2O$ whole system is more reactive, because in the chelating participate both, the textile substrate and the plant extract. Considering these observations, mordating was performed only in pre-treatment prior to dyeing with European black elderberry berries (*Sambucus nigra)* water extract. Color parameters are collected in Table 6, and color depth (K/S) is shown in Figure 9.

Considering the color parameters of woolen fabrics dyed with European black elderberry berries (*Sambucus nigra)* it can be seen that fabrics have yellow-orange to yellow coloration ($h^* = 68 - 75$). Samples with the highest lightness values were obtained using aluminum salts as mordant ($L = 45$) and the darkest samples were obtained using copper and iron salts, e.g., $L = 34$, respectively.

Considering color depth (K/S) of woolen fabrics dyed in water extract of European black elderberry berries (*Sambucus nigra)* mordanted in pre-treatment with $KAl(SO_4)_2 \cdot 12H_2O$, $CuSO_4 \cdot 5H_2O$; $FeSO_4 \cdot 7H_2O$ and $SnCl_2 \cdot 2H_2O$ it can be seen that the highest K/S value has fabric mordaned with iron salt.

However, these samples showed lower chromaticity and the subjective visual assessment noted that the samples have more pronounced grey shade. It is to point out mordating with $SnCl_2 \cdot 2H_2O$ as well, which resulted in high K/S value of 13.33. Other properties and observations are similar to the ones dyes with water extract of European Ash bark (*Fraxinus excelsior).*

It is to notice lower reactivity of water extract of European black elderberry berries (*Sambucus nigra)* than European Ash bark (*Fraxinus excelsior).*

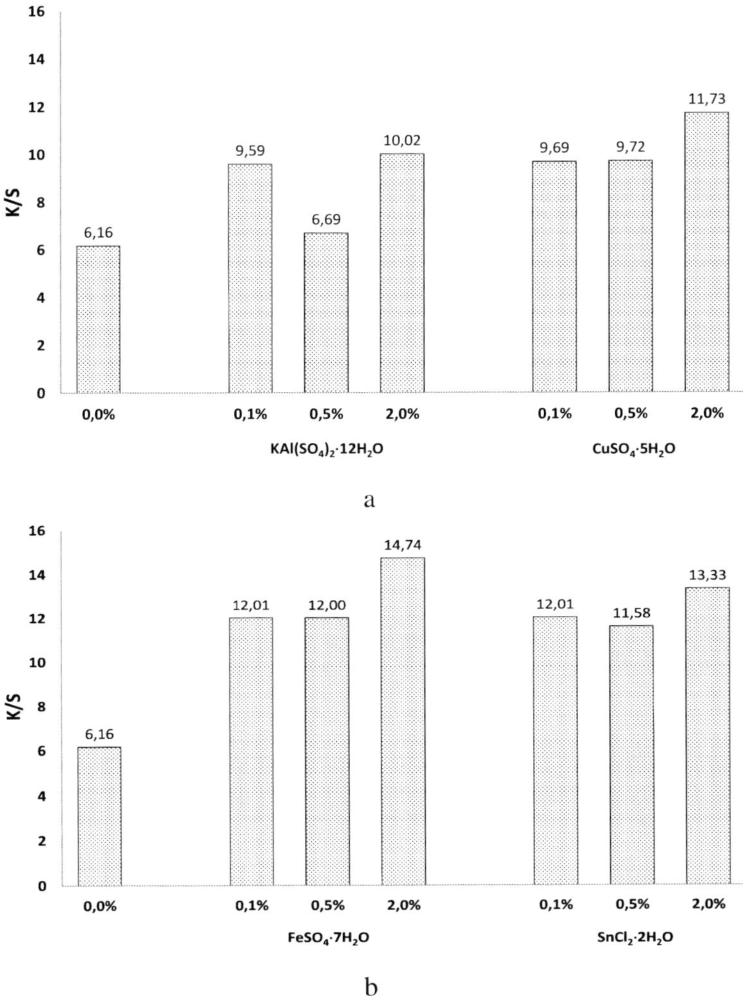

Figure 9. K/S values of woolen fabrics dyed in water extract of European black elderberry berries (*Sambucus nigra)* mordanted in pre-treatment with: a. $KAl(SO_4)_2{\cdot}12H_2O$ and $CuSO_4{\cdot}5H_2O$; b. $FeSO_4{\cdot}7H_2O$ and $SnCl_2{\cdot}2H_2O$ (0.1%, 0.5%, 2% owf).

On the basis of the literature, this lower reactivity of isoquercitrin and rutin trihydrate is a result of flavonoid glycosidation. Additionally, the berries in a greater proportion contain anthocyanosides and betalaines, which are considerably more reactive towards metal ions [6, 94-96].

The most of results of the UV protective fabrics concern application of synthetic dyes, whilst only few studies reports of natural dyes. Since it was found that European black elderberry berries (*Sambucus nigra)* helps in cosmetic emulsions giving of photoprotection to UV-A and UV-B irradiation, its application and European Ash (*Fraxinus excelsior)* bark were choosen for the application on light woollen fabric which could protect from harmful UV radiation.

The fabric UV protection was determined according to AS/NZS 4399:1996 *Sun Protective Clothing: evaluation and classification*, by UV-A and UV-B transmission measurement on transmission spectrophotometer and calculation of Ultraviolet protection factor (UPF). The results are presented in Tables 7-9.

Table 7. UV protection of woolen fabrics dyed in water extract of European Ash bark (*Fraxinus excelsior*) with $KAl(SO_4)_2 \cdot 12H_2O$ and $CuSO_4 \cdot 5H_2O$ as mordants

MORDANT	Mean UPF	τ UVA	τ UVB	Stand. Dev.	Stand. Err.	Calc. UPF	UV protection
Wool	32.070	7.634	2.194	1.069	1.326	30.744	30
No mordant	54.800	5.043	1.103	1.481	2.444	52.356	50
Pre-treatment $KAl(SO_4)_2 \cdot 12H_2O$							
0.1%	210.273	0.574	0.455	64.604	80.109	130.163	50+
0.5%	188.651	0.651	0.509	47.362	58.728	129.922	50+
1.0%	188.513	0.615	0.481	15.142	18.776	169.737	50+
1.5%	96.801	1.031	0.981	3.529	4.376	92.425	50+
2.0%	134.488	0.812	0.700	12.303	15.256	119.232	50+
3.0%	77.371	1.300	1.237	6.584	8.164	69.207	50+
4.0%	147.360	0.124	0.634	7.927	9.829	137.531	50+
5.0%	70.494	1.449	1.367	7.667	9.507	60.987	50+
After-treatment $KAl(SO_4)_2 \cdot 12H_2O$							
0.1%	344.562	0.630	0.206	1.160	54.465	290.097	50+
0.5%	427.916	0.527	0.193	43.923	189.108	238.808	50+
1.0%	265.127	0.771	0.336	152.506	130.034	135.093	50+
1.5%	197.291	0.910	0.418	104.866	64.764	132.528	50+
2.0%	197.056	0.855	0.391	52.229	15.342	181.714	50+
3.0%	364.845	0.567	0.209	12.373	124.600	240.245	50+
4.0%	308.848	0.698	0.299	144.756	179.498	129.350	50+
5.0%	158.789	1.027	0.496	12.907	16.005	142.785	50+
Pre-treatment $CuSO_4 \cdot 5H_2O$							
0.1%	204.600	0.600	0.440	34.831	43.191	161.409	50+
0.5%	147.816	0.759	0.616	10.199	12.647	135.168	50+
1.0%	105.849	1.008	0.890	13.102	16.246	89.648	50+
1.5%	119.909	0.924	0.787	19.677	24.400	95.509	50+
2.0%	150.996	0.752	0.601	12.028	14.915	136.081	50+
3.0%	147.508	0.787	0.642	31.394	38.928	108.579	50+
4.0%	103.013	1.057	0.909	7.773	9.639	93.374	50+
5.0%	140.480	0.786	0.656	10.790	13.379	127.101	50+
After-treatment $CuSO_4 \cdot 5H_2O$							
0.1%	456.846	0.446	0.239	250.687	310.852	145.993	50+
0.5%	408.100	0.529	0.206	152.717	189.369	218.731	50+
1.0%	335.774	0.600	0.303	166.050	205.902	129.872	50+
1.5%	546.108	0.416	0.138	111.925	138.787	407.321	50+
2.0%	488.220	0.398	0.154	58.708	72.798	415.422	50+
3.0%	772.257	0.230	0.116	184.463	228.734	543.523	50+
4.0%	347.056	0.573	0.229	93.859	116.385	230.671	50+
5.0%	939.780	0.163	0.100	15.416	19.115	920.665	50+

Table 8. UV protection of woolen fabrics dyed in water extract of European Ash bark (*Fraxinus excelsior*) with $FeSO_4 \cdot 7H_2O$ and $SnCl_2 \cdot 2H_2O$ as mordants

MORDANT	Mean UPF	τ UVA	τ UVB	Stand. Dev.	Stand. Err.	Calc. UPF	UV protection
Pre-treatment $FeSO_4 \cdot 7H_2O$							
0.1%	156.575	0.699	0.604	28.632	35.504	121.071	50+
0.5%	288.053	0.395	0.306	30.565	37.901	250.153	50+
1.0%	102.195	0.972	0.935	8.843	10.966	91.230	50+
1.5%	125.637	0.786	0.760	2.921	3.622	122.051	50+
2.0%	167.955	0.599	0.570	20.070	24.887	143.068	50+
3.0%	146.659	0.681	0.645	3.414	4.234	142.426	50+
4.0%	168.330	0.593	0.576	18.537	22.986	145.344	50+
5.0%	99.988	0.945	0.970	5.214	6.465	93.523	50+
After-treatment $FeSO_4 \cdot 7H_2O$							
0.1%	665.082	0.275	0.125	83.611	103.677	561.404	50+
0.5%	982.979	0.116	0.100	19.794	24.544	958.435	50+
1.0%	734.727	0.249	0.116	86.981	107.857	626.870	50+
1.5%	967.769	0.119	0.101	41.580	51.559	916.210	50+
2.0%	953.918	0.127	0.101	71.234	60.330	893.588	50+
3.0%	999.824	0.100	0.100	0.497	0.616	999.209	50+
4.0%	949.955	0.119	0.104	66.391	82.325	867.630	50+
5.0%	987.772	0.105	0.101	16.573	20.551	967.222	50+
Pre-treatment $SnCl_2 \cdot 2H_2O$							
0.1%	221.733	0.468	0.419	46.565	57.741	163.991	50+
0.5%	167.333	0.581	0.560	13.917	17.257	150.076	50+
1.0%	136.940	0.700	0.689	12.894	15.989	120.951	50+
1.5%	696.052	0.194	0.128	61.790	76.619	619.433	50+
2.0%	791.720	0.160	0.117	124.593	154.495	637.225	50+
3.0%	305.541	0.345	0.309	66.323	82.241	223.300	50+
4.0%	660.171	0.204	0.138	107.995	133.913	526.258	50+
5.0%	254.974	0.432	0.397	62.367	77.335	168.639	50+
After-treatment $SnCl_2 \cdot 2H_2O$							
0.1%	594.845	0.344	0.128	41.231	514.127	543.719	50+
0.5%	218.308	0.657	0.384	33.397	41.413	176.896	50+
1.0%	317.715	0.512	0.235	27.706	34.355	283.360	50+
1.5%	681.892	0.412	0.106	50.341	62.423	619.469	50+
2.0%	612.764	0.357	0.125	90.445	112.152	500.612	50+
3.0%	443.513	0.384	0.168	15.942	19.769	423.745	50+
4.0%	257.243	0.549	0.325	54.372	67.422	189.821	50+
5.0%	756.154	0.279	0.107	40.552	50.284	821.869	50+

Since no UV-C radiation reaches the earth's surface due to absorption by oxygen and ozone in the upper atmosphere, the transmittance of ultraviolet including UV-A and UV-B through the fabrics was measured on transmission spectrometer Cary 50 (Varian). The ultraviolet transmittance spectra of the woolen fabric without dyeing and after mordating and dyeing with European black elderberry berries (*Sambucus nigra)* and European Ash bark (*Fraxinus excelsior)* was compared. As can be seen from Tables 7-9, there was a significant difference between the dyed fabrics and un-dyed one. Even thoug woolen fabric is the only one that absorbs radiation throughout the entire UV spectrum even when completely untreated due to its chemocal composition, it transmit 7.6% of UV-A nad 2.2% UV-B radiation, resulting in very good UV protection (UPF=32.070).

Table 9. UV protection of woolen fabrics dyed in water extract of European black elderberry berries (*Sambucus nigra)*

MORDANT	Mean UPF	τ UVA	τ UVB	Stand. Dev.	Stand. Err.	Calc. UPF	UV protection
Wool	32.070	7.634	2.194	1.069	1.326	30.744	30
No mordant	59.489	4.949	0.826	2.371	1.460	58.029	50+
Pre-treatment $KAl(SO_4)_2 \cdot 12H_2O$							
0.1%	856.997	0.167	0.107	76.302	94.689	762.307	50+
0.5%	743.963	0.193	0.124	185.664	230.223	513.739	50+
2.0%	482.273	0.275	0.189	96.842	120.084	362.181	50+
Pre-treatment $CuSO_4 \cdot 5H_2O$							
0.1%	399.652	0.366	0.314	245.563	304.498	95.154	50+
0.5%	164.585	0.616	0.567	10.381	12.872	151.677	50+
2.0%	439.309	0.349	0.309	289.529	359.016	80.293	50+
Pre-treatment $FeSO_4 \cdot 7H_2O$							
0.1%	847.995	0.143	0.112	161.190	199.876	648.119	50+
0.5%	279.710	0.394	0.347	60.479	74.994	204.717	50+
2.0%	952.089	0.119	0.102	49.075	60.853	891.236	50+
Pre-treatment $SnCl_2 \cdot 2H_2O$							
0.1%	740.017	0.179	0.139	247.636	307.068	432.949	50+
0.5%	735.046	0.181	0.140	245.511	304.433	430.613	50+
2.0%	996.544	0.102	0.100	3.978	4.933	991.612	50+

Dyeing with water extract of European Ash bark (*Fraxinus excelsior)* without mordant, results already in excellent UV protection (UPF=54.8). It is to point out that UV-B transmission is lower 50%, whilst UV-A transmission only 30%. As proved in cosmetics, dyeing with European black elderberry berries (*Sambucus nigra),* improve UV-B absorption for 63%, and UV-A for 35%, resulting in excellent UV protection (Highest class 50+).

From the Tables 7-9 it can be clearly seen that the values of spectral transmittance decrease with all mordants applied, resulting in excellent UV protection. However, it is possible to evaluate the influence of mordants to UV protection considering the mean UPF values. Considering mordant concentration, similar behaviour was noticed as for the color parameters. The concentration of 2% of mordant was selected as optimal one. Therefore, these results are presented in Figure 10.

The best UV protection has been achieved applying $FeSO_4 \cdot 7H_2O$ as mordant resulting in UPF almost 1000. The reason for that is the lowest ligthness, suggesting darkest shade with the highest absorption of UV radiation what results in the lowest UV transmittion. The results of color parameters confirm that.

For the difference of color depth which was achieved if mordant was applied in pre-treatment; the significantly better UV protection was achieved if mordant was applied in after-treatment. Ibrahim et al. [101] research of UV-protective finishing of cotton knits by addition of the metal-oxide into the finishing bath. It resulted in better UV protection probably because of ligth scattering [89, 90, 102]. Considering the metal-oxides applied, UV protection was the next: Cu > Zr > Zn ≫ Al ≈ none. For that reason, if the metal salts were applied as mordants in after-treatment, it is to assume that ligth scattering form the fabric surface was higher, what led to better UV protection. In the case of mordating in after treatment dyed fabrics with water extract of Fraxinus excelsior, UV protection was next: Fe > Sn > Cu > Al, and significantly higher than if applied as pre-treatment. Again, the difference in chelating played an important role. It is to point out mordating with $SnCl_2{\cdot}2H_2O$ as well, which resulted in higher K/S values, and the highest UV protection as well.

Comparing the influence of European Ash bark (*Fraxinus excelsior)* and European black elderberry berries (*Sambucus nigra),* it can be seen that *Sambuctus nigra* gave off better UV protection.

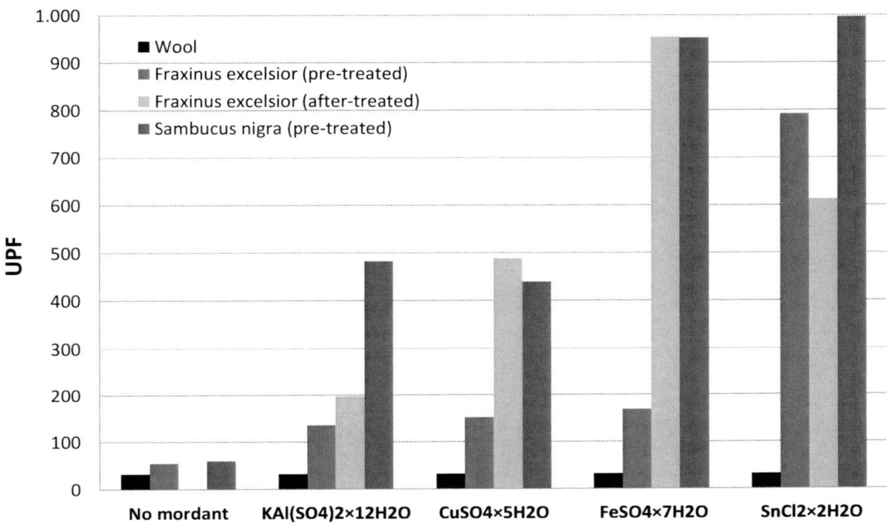

Figure 10. Mean UPF of woollen fabrics dyed with 2% water extracts of *Fraxinus excelsior* and *Sambuctus nigra* pre-treated or after-treated with 4 different mordants.

CONCLUSION

In this chapter the UV protection by woolen fabric dyed with natural dyestuff extracted from European Ash bark (*Fraxinus excelsior)* and European black elderberry berries (*Sambucus nigra)* was researched. As most of natural dyes water extracts were applied on textiles in the combination with mordants - $KAl(SO_4)_2{\cdot}12H_2O$, $FeSO_4{\cdot}7H_2O$, $CuSO_4{\cdot}5H_2O$ and $SnCl_2{\cdot}2H_2O$. The woolen fabric was characetrized by its zeta potential and isoelectric point; therefore mordants were applied at pH 4.5. The active components, which are the most responsible for achieved colour hue, respectively for the forming of coloured chelates, were determined for the *Fraxinus excelsior* and *Sambucus nigra* by HPLC. Analyzed extracts contained flavonoids substances: quercetin dihydrate, isoquercitrin and rutin trihydrate. It was confirmed that the water based herbal extracts has got certain substantivity towards woolen substrates. The influence of a sort of the metal on a hue of a coloured complexes was confirmed by the color parameters on remission spectrophotometer determination. For $KAl(SO_4)_2{\cdot}12H_2O$ and $SnCl_2{\cdot}2H_2O$ as mordants, the yellow – orange hues were obtained, for $CuSO_4{\cdot}5H_2O$ orange – brown, and for the $FeSO_4{\cdot}7H_2O$ achromatic – chromatic olive green hues. In dependence to reactivity and property of forming the coloured chelates, the largest colour depth (K/S) was achieved using Fe^{2+} ions.

Since flavonoids and anthocyanosides have an important role in protecting against harmful effects of UV radiation the fabric UV protection was determined according to AS/NZS 4399:1996 *Sun Protective Clothing: evaluation and classification*, by UV-A and UV-B transmission measurement on transmission spectrophotometer and calculation of Ultraviolet protection factor (UPF). It was confirmed that woolen fabrics dyed with natural dyes, extracted from *Fraxinus excelsior* and *Sambucus nigra, ensure* excellent UV protection (UPF > 50). It is to point out that it offers protection against UVB radiation as well, and therefore it may reduce the risk of subsequent occurrence of skin cancer. In the case of application, it is to suggest European black elderberry berries (*Sambucus nigra),* which gave maximum UV protection (UPF=1000).

REFERENCES

[1] Taylor G. W. 1986. Natural dyes in textile applications, *Rev. Prog. Coloration,* 16: 53-61.

[2] Kumar, J.K., Sinha, A.K., 2004. Resurgence of natural colourants: a holistic view. *Nat. Prod. Res.* 18: 59-84

[3] Samanta, A.K., Agarwal, P., 2009. Application of natural dyes on textiles. *Indian J. Fibre Text. Res.* 34: 384-399.

[4] Islam, S. U.; M. Shahid, F. Mohammad. 2013. Perspectives for natural product based agents derived from industrial plants in textile applications – a review. *Journal of Cleaner Production* 57: 2-18.

[5] Shahid, M.; S. U. Islam, F. Mohammad. 2013. Recent advancements in natural dye applications: a review. *Journal of Cleaner Production* 53: 310-331.

[6] Schweppe H. 1992. Handbuch der Naturfarbstoffe. Vorkommen, Verwendung, Nachweis, ecomed, *Landsberg/Lech.*

[7] Sekar, N. 1999. Application of natural colourants to textiles – principles and limitations. *Colourage* 46(7): 33-34.

[8] Teli, M. D.; Paul, R.; Pardeshi, P. D. 2000. Natural Dyes: Classification, chemistry and extraction methods, Part – I: Chemical classes, extraction methods and future prospects. *Colourage.* 47 (12): 43-48.

[9] Guinot, P., Roge, A., Gargadennec, A., Garcia, M., Dupont, D., Lecoeur, E., Candelier, L., Andary, C. 2006. Dyeing plants screening: an approach to combine past heritage and present development. Color. Technol. 122: 93-101.

[10] Tušek, L., Golob, V. 1998. Natural Dyes in textile in history and today (Naravna barvila v tekstilstvu včasih in danes). *Tekstilec* 41(3-4): 75-83.

[11] Fakin D., D. Tepeš, A. Majcen le Marechal, A. Ojstršek, M. Božič. 2010. Dyeing of Wool with Plant Dyes and Sample Evaluation with CIE Colour System, *Tekstilec* 53(7–9): 179–193.

[12] Parac-Osterman, Đ.; Karaman, B.; Horvat, A.; Pervan, M. 2001. Dyeing Wool with Natural Dyes in the Ligth of Ethnological Heritage of Lika (Bojadisanje vune prirodnim bojilima u svjetlu etnografske baštine Like). *Tekstil* 50: 339-344.

[13] Sutlović, A.; Đ. Parac-Osterman, V. Đurašević. 2011. Croatian Traditional Herbal Dyes for Textile Dyeing; TEDI 1:65-69. Available at: http://www.ttf.unizg.hr/tedi/pdf/TEDI-1-1-65.pdf; accesed: 2014-12-12.

[14] Bird, C. L., Boston W. S. 1975. The Theory of coloration of textiles. *Dyers Company Publications Trust,* Bradford.

[15] Zollinger, H. Color Chemistry. 1987. Syntheses, Properties and Applications of Organic Dyes and Pigments. VCH, New York.

[16] Goodwin, J. 1990. A Dyer's Manual. Pelham books, *Stephen Greene Press,* Middlesex

[17] Doran, A. 1993. Latest developments in the low-temperature dyeing of wool with 1:2 matal-complex and milling acid dyes. *JSDC* 109 (1): 15-20.

[18] Engeler, E. 1997. Wollfarbstoff – Gammen und ihr ökologisches Umfeld. *Texilveredlung* 32 (7-8): 156-161.

[19] Imming, P.; Zentgraf, M.; Imhof, I. 2000. Welche Farbe hatte der antike Purpur?. *Texilveredlung* 35 (9-10): 22-24.

[20] Grdenić, D. 2002. Purpur i grimiz. *Priroda,* 6-8.

[21] Pötsch, W. R. 2002. Naturfarbstoffherstellung aus Waidpflanzen: Gesank als Qualitätsmerkmal. *Melliand Textilberichte* 83 (3): 170-171.

[22] Lokhande, H. T.; Dorugade, V. A.; Sandeep R. N. 1998. Applicaton of Natural Dyes on Polyester. *American Dyestuff Reporter* 87 (9): 40-50.

[23] Samanta, A. K.; Singhee, D.; Sethia, M. 2003. Application of single and mixture of selected natural dyes on cotton fabric: A scientific approach. *Colourage* 50(10): 29-42.

[24] Ansari, A. A.; Thakur, B. D. 2000. Extraction, characterisation and application of a natural dye: The eco-friendly textile colorant. *Colourage* 47(7): 15-20.

[25] Grotewold, E. 2006. The Science of Flavonoids. *Springer.*

[26] Hofenk de Graaff, J.H. 2004. The Colourful Past: Origins, Chemistry, and identification of Natural Dyestuffs, Archetype Publications, Ltd., London, *Abegg-Stiftung,* Riggisberg.

[27] Nemeth E. Colouring (Dye) Plants. In Cultivated Plants, Primarly as Food Sources – Vol. II. EOLSS (Encyclopedia of Life Support Systems), available at: http://www.eolss.net/Sample-Chapters/C10/E5-02-05-08.pdf; accesed: 2014-11-12.

[28] Bechtold, T., Mussak, R. 2009. Handbook of Natural Colorants, *John Wiley and Sons,* Ltd. UK.

[29] Samanta, A. K., Konar, A. 2011. Dyeing of Textiles with Natural Dyes. In Natural Dyes, InTech, pp. 29-56. Available at: http://www.intechopen.com /books/natural-dyes/dyeing-of-textiles-with-natural-dyes, accessed: 2014-06-19.

[30] Bechtold T., A. Mahmud-Ali, R.A. M. Mussak. 2007. Reuse of ash-tree (Fraxinus excelsior L.) bark as natural dyes for textile dyeing: process conditions and process. *Coloration Technology* 123 (4): 271-279.

[31] Đorđević, D., Šmelcerović, M.; Tarbuk, A. 2009. Environmental-Friendly Cotton Fabric Finishing by Alcohol Extract of Hibiscus Flowers. *Proceedings of VIIIth Symposium, Tehnološki fakultet, Leskovac;* 226-232.

[32] Kovačević, Z; A. Sutlović, S. Bischof. 2014. Spartium Junceum L. as a Natural Dyestuff for Wool Dyeing. Book of *Proceedings 7th International Textile, Clothing & Design Conference – Magic World of Textiles, University of Zagreb, Faculty of Textile Technology, Zagreb;* 220-225.

[33] Kechi, A. R.B. Chavan, R. Moeckel. 2013. Dye Yield, Color Strength and Dyeing Properties of Natural Dyes Extracted from Ethiopian Dye Plants. *Textiles and Light Industrial Science and Technology* 2(3): 137-145.

[34] Baishya, D., J. Talukdar, S. Sandhya S. 2012. Cotton Dyeing with Natural Dye Extracted from Flower of Bottlebrush (Callistemon citrinus), Universal Journal of Environmental Research and Technology 2(5): 377-382.

[35] Deo H. T, Desai B. K. 1999. Dyeing cotton and jute with tea as a natural dye, *J. Soc. Dyers Color.* 115(7-8): 224-227.

[36] Bhattacharya N, Doshi B. A., Sahasrabudhe A. S. 1998. Dyeing jute with natural dyes, *Am. Dyst. Rep.,* 87(4): 26-29.

[37] Nishida K, Kobayashi K. 1992. Dyeing properties of natural dyes from vegetable sources, Part II, *Am. Days. Rep.* 81(9): 26-30.

[38] Kazaić, S. 2004. Antioxydative and antiradical activity of flavonoids. *Archives. of Industrial Hygiene and Toxicology* 55(4): 279-290.

[39] Malešev, D.; Kuntić, V. 2007. Investigation of metal-falvonoid chelates and the determination of flavonoids via matel-falvonoid complexing reactions *Serbian Soc. Chem. Ind. Jour.* 72(10): 921-939.

[40] Cornard, J. P.; Boudet, A. C.; Merlin, J. C. 2001. Complexes of Al(III) with 3′4′-dihydroxy-flavone: characterization, theoretical and spectroscopic study. *Spectrochemica Acta Part A* 57(3): 591-602.

[41] Raj Narayana, K.; Sripal Reddy, M.; Chaluvadi, M. R.; Krishna D. R. Bioflavonoids classification, pharmacological, biochemical effects and therapeutic potential. *Indian Journal of Pharmacology*, 2001, 33 (1), 2-16

[42] R.F. V. de Souza , E.M. Sussuchi, W. F. De Giovani. 2003. Synthesis, Electrochemical, Spectral, and Antioxidant Properties of Complexes of Flavonoids with Metal Ions. *Synthesis and Reactivity in Inorganic and Metal-Organic Chemistry* 33(7): 1125-1144.

[43] Kasiri, M.B., S. Safapour. 2014. Natural dyes and antimicrobials for green treatment of textiles, *Environ Chem Lett* 12: 1-13.

[44] Mirjalili, M., Nazarpoor, K., Karimi, L., 2011. Eco-friendly dyeing of wool using natural dye from weld as co-partner with synthetic dye. *J. Clean. Prod.* 19: 1045-1051.

[45] Yusuf, M., Shahid, M., Khan, M.I., Khan, S.A., Khan, M.A., Mohammad, F. 2011. Dyeing studies with henna and madder: a research on effect of tin (II) chloride mordant. *J. Saudi Chem. Soc.,* available at: http://dx.doi.org/10.1016/j.jscs.2011.12.020, accesed: 2014-12-12.

[46] Robinson, T.; Chandran, B.; Nigam, P. 2002. Removal of dyes from a synthetic textile dye effluent by biosorption on apple pomace and wheat straw. *Water Res.* 36(11): 2824-2830.

[47] Talreja, D.; Talreja, P.; Mathur, M. 2003. Eco-friendliness of natural dyes. *Colourage* 50(7): 35-44.

[48] Singh, R.; Jain, A.; Panwar, S.; Gupta, D.; Khare, S. K. 2005. Antimicrobial activity of some natural dyes. *Dyes and Pigments* 66(2): 99-102.

[49] Kosalec, I.; Pepeljnjak, S.; Bakmaz, M.; Vladimir-Knežević, S. 2005. Flavonoid analysis and antimicrobial activity of commercially available propolis products. *Acta Pharm.* 55(4): 423-430.

[50] Yusuf M., M. Shahid, S.A. Khan, M.I. Khan, S.U. Islam, F. Mohammad, M.A. Khan. 2013. Eco-Dyeing of Wool Using Aqueous Extract of the Roots of Indian Madder (Rubia cordifolia) as Natural Dye. *Journal of Natural Fibers* 10(1): 14-28.

[51] Yusuf, M., Ahmad, A., Shahid, M., Khan, M.I., Khan, S.A., Manzoor, N., Mohammad, F. 2012. Assessment of colorimetric, antibacterial and antifungal properties of woollen yarn dyed with the extract of the leaves of henna (Lawsonia inermis). *J. Clean. Prod.* 27: 42-50.

[52] Šmelcerović M., Mizdraković M., Đorđević D. 2007. Environmental-friendly wool fabric finishing by some water plant extracts. *Serbian Soc. Chem. Ind. Jour.* 61(5): 251-256.

[53] Šmelcerović M., D. Đorđević, A. M. Grancarić. 2009. Spectral properties of cotton fabric treated with marigold flowers water extract. *Zbornik radova Tehnološkog fakulteta u Leskovcu* 19: 315-321.

[54] Šmelcerović, M.; Đorđević, D.; Grancarić, A. M.; Tarbuk, A. 2009. Ecological Finishing of Woolen Fabric with Extracts of Marigold, St.-John's-Wart and Hibiscus Plants. *Book of Proceedings of 2nd Scientific-Professional Symposium Textile Science & Economy. University of Zagreb, Faculty of Textile Technology,* Zagreb, 163-166.

[55] Gupta, D., Jain, A., Panwar, S., 2005. Anti-UV and anti-microbial properties of some natural dyes on cotton. Indian J. Fibre Text. Res. 30: 190-195.

[56] Ibrahim N. A., S. Zhang, M. R. El-Zairy, H. A. Ghazal. 2013. Enhancing the UV-protection and Antibacterial Properties of Polyamide-6 Fabric by Natural Dyeing. *Textiles and Light Industrial Science and Technology* (TLIST) 2(1): 36-41.

[57] Sarkar, A.K., 2004. An evaluation of UV protection imparted by cotton fabrics dyed with natural colorant. *BMC Dermatol.* 4: 15.

[58] Feng, X.X., Zhang, L.L., Chen, J.Y., Zhang, J.C., 2007. New insights into solar UVprotective properties of natural dye. *J. Clean. Prod.* 15: 366-372.

[59] Grifoni, D., Bacci, L., Zipoli, G., Carreras, G., Baronti, S., Sabatini, F. 2009. Laboratory and outdoor assessment of UV protection offered by flax and hemp fabrics dyed with natural dyes. *Photochem. Photobiol.* 85: 313-320.

[60] Grifoni, D., Bacci, L., Zipoli, G., Albanese, L., Sabatini, F. 2011. The role of natural dyes in the UV protection of fabrics made of vegetable fibres. *Dyes Pigm.* 91: 279-285

[61] Mongkholrattanasit, R., Krystufek, J., Wiener, J. 2010. Dyeing and fastness properties of natural dyes extracted from eucalyptus leaves using padding techniques. *Fiber. Polym.* 11: 346-350.

[62] Mongkholrattanasit, R., Krystufek, J., Wiener, J., Vikova, M. 2011. Dyeing, fastness, and UV protection properties of silk and wool fabrics dyed with eucalyptus leaf extract by the exhaustion process. *Fibres Text. East. Eur.* 19(3): 94-99.

[63] Mongkholrattanasit, R., Krystufek, J., Wiener, J., Vikova, M. 2011. UV protection properties silk fabric dyed with eucalyptus leaf extract. *J. Text. Inst.* 102(3): 272-279.

[64] Hustvedt G., P. Cox Crews. 2005. The Ultraviolet Protection Factor of Naturally-pigmented Cotton. *The Journal of Cotton Science* 9: 47–55.

[65] Hou, X., Chen, X., Cheng, Y., Xu, H., Chen, L., Yang, Y. 2013. Dyeing and UV protection properties of water extracts from orange peel. *J. Clean. Prod.* 52: 410-419.

[66] Dev, V.R.G., Venugopal, J., Sudha, S., Deepika, G., Ramakrishna, S., 2009. Dyeing and antimicrobial characteristics of chitosan treated wool fabrics with henna dye. *Carbohydr. Polym.* 75, 646-650.

[67] Raja, A.S.M., Thilagavathi, G. 2011. Influence of enzyme and mordant treatments on the antimicrobial efficacy of natural dyes on wool materials. *Asian J. Text* 1: 138-144.

[68] Popescu A., L. Chirila; C. P. Ghituleasa; C. Hulea; M. Vamesu. 2014. Influence of enzyme pre-treatments on natural dyeing of proteinic substrates. *Annals of the University of Oradea, Fascicle of Textiles, Leatherwork* 15(1): 83-88.

[69] Ghoranneviss, M., Shahidi, S., Anvari, A., Motaghi, Z., Wiener, J., Slamborova, I., 2011. Influence of plasma sputtering treatment on natural dyeing and antibacterial activity of wool fabrics. *Prog. Org. Coat* 70: 388-393.

[70] Chen, C., Chang, W.Y., 2007. Antimicrobial activity of cotton fabric pretreated by microwave plasma and dyed with onion skin and onion pulp extractions. *Indian J. Fibre Text. Res.* 32: 122-125.

[71] Tarbuk, A., A. M. Grancarić, D. Đorđević, M. Šmelcerović. 2009. Adsorption of Plant Extracts on Cationized Cotton. *Zbornik radova Tehnološkog fakulteta u Leskovcu* 19: 257-264.

[72] Đorđević, D., Tarbuk, A., Grancarić, A. M., Šmelcerović, M. 2009. Ecological Finishing of Cationized Cotton Fabric with Extracts of Marigold, St.-John's- Wart and Hibiscus Plants, *Proceedings of 9th AUTEX Conference, Ege Univresity, Izmir,* 1441-1446.

[73] Hong, K.H., Bae, J.H., Jin, S.R., Yang, J.S., 2012. Preparation and properties of multifunctionalized cotton fabrics treated by extracts of gromwell and gallnut. *Cellulose* 19: 507-515.

[74] Sathiyanarayanan, M.P., Bhat, N.V., Kokate, S.S., Walnuj, V.E., 2010. Antibacterial finish for cotton fabric from herbal products. *Indian J. Fibre Text. Res.* 35: 50-58.

[75] Armstrong, B. K., Kricker, A. 1993. How much melanoma is caused by sun exposure? *Melanoma Res* 3(6): 395-401.

[76] Šitum M. 2012. Melanoma. Chapter 57 in Guidliness in common dermatoses and skin cancers diagnostics and treatments (in Croatian: Smjernice u dijagnostici i liječenju najčešćih dermatoza i tumora kože). *Naklada Slap, Jastrebarsko.*

[77] Tarbuk, A., Grancarić A. M., Šitum, M., Martinis M. 2010. UV Clothing and Skin Cancer. *Collegium Antropologicum.* 34(Suppl. 2): 179-183.

[78] Hoffmann, K., Laperre, J., Avermaete, A., Altmeyer, P., Gambichler, T. 2001. Defined UV protection by apparel textiles. *Arch Dermatol.* 137(8): 1089-1094.

[79] Reinert, G., Fuso, F., Hilfiker, R., Schmidt, E. 1997. UV-protecting properties of textile fabrics and their improvement. *Textile Chemist and Colorist* 29(12): 36-43.

[80] Gies, P. H., Roy, C. R., Toomey, S., Mclennan, A. 1998. Protection against solar ultraviolet radiation. *Mutation Research* 422: 15-22.

[81] Grancarić, A. M., Tarbuk, A., Dumitrescu, I., Bišćan J. 2006. UV Protection of Pretreated Cotton – Influence of FWA's Fluorescence. *AATCC Review* 6(4): 44-48.

[82] Tarbuk, A., Grancarić, A.M., Jančijev, I., Sharma, S. 2006. Protection against UV radiation using a modified polyester fabric. *Tekstil* 55(8): 383-394.

[83] Hilfiker, R., Kaufmann, W., Reinert, G., Schmidt, E. 1996. Improving sun protection factors of fabrics by applying UV- absorbers. *Text. Res. J.* 66(2): 61-70.

[84] Algaba, I., Riva, A., Cox Crews, P. 2004. Influence of Fiber Type and Fabric Porosity on the UPF of Summer Fabrics. *AATCC Review* 4(2):26-31.

[85] Grancarić, A.M., Penava, Ž., Tarbuk, A. 2005. UV Protection of Cotton – the Influence of Weaving Structure. *Serbian Soc. Chem. Ind. Jour.* 59(9-10): 230-234.

[86] Saravanan, D. 2007. UV protection textile materials. *AUTEX Research Journal* 7(1): 53-62.

[87] Zhou Y., Cox Crews P. 1998. Effect of OBAs and repeated launderings on UVR transmission through fabrics. *Textile Chemist and Colorist* 30(11): 19-24.

[88] Dekanić, T., Pušić, T., Soljačić I. 2014. Impact of artificial light on optical and protective effects of cotton after washing with detergent containing fluorescent compounds, *Tenside Surf. Det.* 51(5): 451-459.

[89] Farouk, A., Textor, T. Schollmeyer, E. Tarbuk, A. Grancarić, A. M. 2010. Sol-gel Derived Inorganic-organic Hybrid Polymers Filled with ZnO Nanoparticles as Ultraviolet Protection Finish for Textiles, *AUTEX research journal* 10(8): 58-63.

[90] Grancarić, A. M., Tarbuk, A., Kovaček, I. 2009. Nanoparticles of Activated Natural Zeolite on Textiles for Protection and Therapy, *Chem. Ind. & Chem. Engineering Quarterly.* 15(4): 203-210.

[91] Sundaresan, K., Sivakumar A., Vigneswaran, C., Ramachandran, T. 2012. Influence of nano titanium dioxide finish, prepared by sol-gel technique, on the ultraviolet protection, antimicrobial, and self-cleaning characteristics of cotton fabrics. *Journal of Industrial Textiles* 41(3): 259-277.

[92] Jarzycka A., Lewińska A., Gancarz R., Wilk K.A. 2013. Assessment of extracts of Helichrysum arenarium, Crataegus monogyna, Sambucus nigra in photoprotective UVA and UVB; photostability in cosmetic emulsions. *J Photochem Photobiol B.* 128: 50-7.

[93] Grancarić, A. M., Tarbuk, A., Pušić, T. 2005. Electrokinetic Potential of Some of the Most Important Textile Fabrics; *Coloration Technology* 121(4): 221-227.

[94] Sutlović, A. Study of Natural Dyestuff – Contribution to Human Ecology, Doctoral dissertation.University of Zagreb, Faculty of Textile Technology, Zagreb, July 2008.

[95] Häkkinen, S. Flavonols and Phenolic Acids in Berries and Berry Products. Doctoral dissertation, University of Kuopio, Kuopio, 2000

[96] Kananykhina, E. N.; Pilipenko I.V. 2000. Characteristics of the pigments from anthocyan-containing food plants, raw material for production of bioflavonoid dyes, *Chemistry of Natural Compounds* 36(2): 148-151.

[97] Bai Y, Song F, Chen M, Xing J, Liu Z, Liu S. 2004. Characterization of the rutin-metal complex by electrospray ionization tandem mass spectrometry. *Anal Sci.* 20(8): 1147-1151.

[98] Amić, D.; Davidović-Amić, D.; Bešlo, D.; Trinajstić, N. 2003. Structure-Radical Scavenging Activity Relationships of Flavonoids. *Croatica Chem. Acta* 76(1): 55-61.

[99] Dalby, G. 1993. Greener mordants for natural coloration. JSDC 109(1): 8-9.

[100] Glover, B.; Pierce, J. H. 1993. Are natural colorants good for your health? *JSDC* 109(1): 5-7.

[101] Ibrahim N. A., M. Gouda, Sh. M. Husseiny, A. R. El-Gamal, F. Mahrous. 2009. UV-protecting and antibacterial finishing of cotton knits. *Journal of Applied Polymer Science* 112(6): 3589-3596.

[102] Grancarić, A. M., A. Tarbuk, L. Botteri. 2014. Light Conversion and Scattering in UV Protective Textiles. *AUTEX research journal.* 14(4): 247-258.

In: Encyclopedia of Dermatology (6 Volume Set)
Editor: Meghan Pratt
ISBN: 978-1-63483-326-4

Chapter 71

LIGHT CONVERSION FOR UV PROTECTION BY TEXTILE FINISHING AND CARE

Tihana Dekanić, Anita Tarbuk**, Tanja Pušić, Ana Marija Grancarić and Ivo Soljačić
University of Zagreb, Faculty of Textile Technology,
Department of Textile Chemistry and Ecology, Zagreb, Croatia

ABSTRACT

The incidence of skin cancer is increasing by epidemic proportions. Its primary cause is a long exposure to solar ultraviolet (UV) radiation crossed with the amount of skin pigmentation in the population. It is believed that in childhood and adolescence 80% of UV-R gets absorbed, whilst in the remaining 20% gets absorbed later in the lifetime. This suggests that proper and early photoprotection may reduce the risk of subsequent occurrence of skin cancer. Textile and clothing can show UV protection, but in the most cases it does not provide full sun screening properties. UV protection highly depends on large number of factors such are type of fiber, fabric surface and construction, type and concentration of dyestuff, fluorescent whitening agent (FWA), UV-B protective agents, as well as nanoparticles, if applied. Based on electronically-excited state by energy of UV-R (usually 340-370 nm) the molecules of FWAs show the phenomenon of fluorescence giving to white textiles high whiteness of outstanding brightness by reemitting the energy at the blue region (typically 420-470 nm) of the spectrum, what leads to better UV protection. Molecules of UV absorbers are able to absorb the damaging UV-R range of 290 nm to 360 nm, and convert it into harmless heat energy. Latest research declares that FWA's and UV absorbers can be applied in textile care – washing process as well. Therefore, the UV protective properties of cotton and cotton/polyester blend fabrics achieved by light conversion in textile finishing and care was researched in this chapter. For that purpose, three stilbene derivative fluorescent compounds were selected – fluorescent whitening agent commonly used in textile finishing, the other one used in detergent formulations, and UV absorber. In textile finishing process fluorescent compounds were applied by exhaustion procedure in wide

* Corresponding address: Prilaz baruna Filipovića 28a, HR-10000 Zagreb, Croatia. E-mail: anita.tarbuk@ttf.hr, tpusic@ttf.hr

concentration range. In textile care fluorescent compounds were applied through 9 washing cycles at 60°C with standard ECE reference detergent and commercial detergent. UV protection was determined *in vitro* through Ultraviolet protection factor, UPF. Additionally the influence to fabric whiteness was researched. Since the fabric properties change in wet state, the discrepancy in whiteness and UV protection was research in distilled water as well as Adriatic Sea water.

Keywords: UV protection, cotton, polyester/cotton blend, FWA, UV absorber, wet state

INTRODUCTION

The incidence of skin cancer is increasing by epidemic proportions. Basal cell cancer remains the most common skin neoplasm, and simple excision is generally curative. On the other hand, aggressive local growth and metastasis are common features of malignant melanoma, which accounts for 75 percent of all deaths associated with skin cancer [1]. The reason for that is most likely that in the most cases melanoma was diagnosed in an advanced stage. The back sides in men and women, as well as the lower limbs in women, are the most common site for melanomas [2, 3]. The primary cause of skin cancer is believed to be a long exposure to solar ultraviolet (UV) radiation crossed with the amount of skin pigmentation in the population [1-6]. Melanoma incidence rates in white populations increase with proximity to the Equator, and vary across Europe, with the highest rates for both sexes in Switzerland, Denmark, Norway, Sweden and the Netherlands and the lowest rates in Central and Southeastern Europe [1].

UV as a whole does not exceed 5% of the total energy emitted by the sun, but their impact on the organic molecules is very important and it induces significant physiological responses in all areas of life. In addition to some beneficial effects of UV radiation (UV-R; wavelengths from 100 nm to 400 nm) on skin it may cause skin and eye damage, especially during the summer time (UV-C). The UV-C radiation (from 100 nm to 280 nm) is absorbed by atmosphere. However, diminishing of the Earth´s atmospheric ozone layer raised the UV exposure health risk, since both, UV-B (from 280 nm to 320 nm) and UV-A (from 320 nm to 400 nm) radiation, are reaching the Earth. Dangerous UV-B rays can cause acute and chronic reactions and damages such as erythema (sunburn), sun tanning, "photoaging," DNA and eye damage, photokeratitis and cataract, and photocarcinogenesis; increase risk factor for melanoma, or cause various skin cancers [3, 6-33]. Experts estimate about 90% of melanomas are associated with severe UV exposure and sunburns over a lifetime. Intermittent sun exposure, especially in childhood and adolescence is considered to be a stronger risk factor for melanoma than continuous exposure [1]. It is believed that in that period of life 80% of UV-R gets absorbed, whilst in the remaining 20% gets absorbed later in the lifetime. This suggests that proper and early photoprotection may reduce the risk of subsequent occurrence of skin cancer [2].

Textile and clothing are the most suitable interface between environment and human body. It can show UV protection, but in the most cases it does not provide full sun screening properties. Literature sources claim that only 1/3 of the spring and summer collections tested give off proper UV protection [11]. In contact with textile fabric, UV radiation can be reflected and/or scattered from fabric surface, or get absorbed or transmitted (Figure 1).

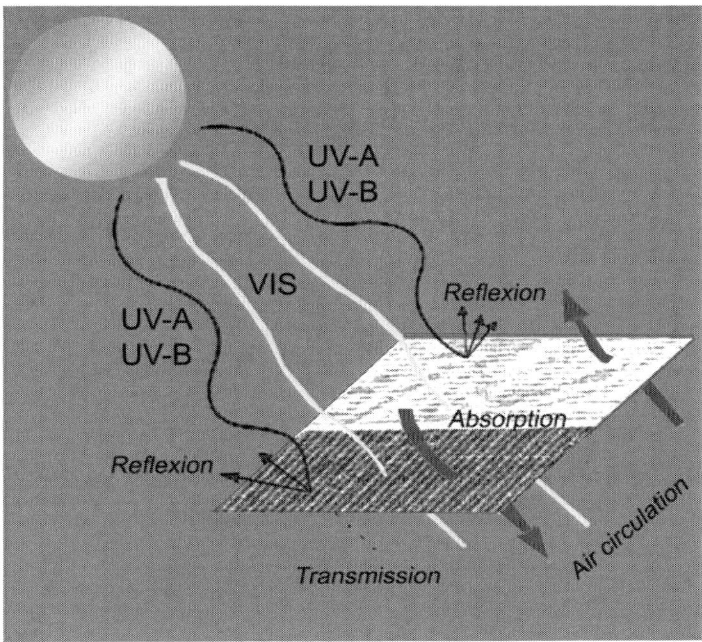

Figure 1. UV radiation in contact with textile fabric [28].

A good fabric UV protection depends on a large number of factors, such as, the type of fiber, fabric surface and construction, porosity, density, moisture content, type and concentration of dyestuff, fluorescent whitening agent (FWA), UV-B protective agents, as well as nanoparticles, if applied [13-37]. For example, polyester fabric gives off better UV protection than cellulose one, due to the polyester benzene rings [17, 30].

Fluorescent whitening agents (FWAs), commonly used for reaching higher whiteness degrees, are chemical compounds that absorb UV-R (usually 340-370 nm), show the phenomenon of fluorescence, and re-emit in the blue region (typically 420-470 nm) of the spectrum.

When P. Krais in 1929 discovered fluorescent compound *Aesculin* by water extraction from wild chestnut, he wrote "About the new white ...." It was the new white indeed, never seen before such high whiteness degree. However, he could never assume that this UV-A absorption of FWA's would result in better UV protection as well [6, 15-17, 26, 30, 32]. The phenomenon of fluorescence can be explained by modified diagram according Jablonski (Figure 2) [38].

The molecules of FWAs go to electronically-excited state by absorbing energy of UV-R. An electronically-excited molecule can lose its energy by emission of radiation which is known as "luminescence." In this case, the emission is fluorescence, which is, according to Figure 2, an emission process occurring from lowest excited state (S_1) to the ground state (S_0). The frequency of fluorescence radiation is lower than that of excitation light (which is known Stokes Law). For the same compound an ideal emission should be the mirror image of the absorption band system [39].

Textile finishing agents for UV protection can be incorporated into the fiber matrix, or it can be applied to the surface of the fabric [3]. Usually sun protection effect is achieved through the use of UV absorbers [6, 16-18].

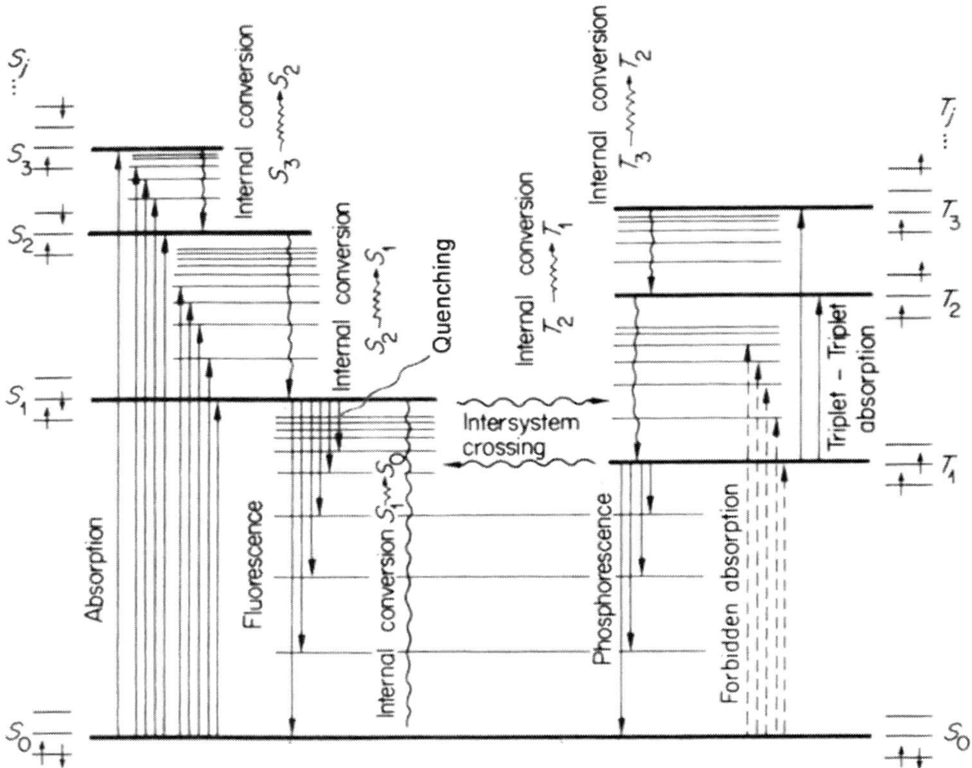

Figure 2. Modified Jablonski diagram [38].

UV absorbers are, as a matter of fact, a special type of fluorescent whitening agents and have the same or similar effect [6, 40]. Molecules of UV absorbers, such as benzotriazole and phenyl benzotriazole, are able to absorb the damaging UV-R range of 290 nm to 360 nm, and convert it into harmless heat energy. Therefore, they are even more effective than fluorescent whitening agents [3]. The impact of fluorescent whitening agents on the whiteness degree of cotton fabrics, as well as PES/cotton blends, in multiple washing cycles, has been comprehensively investigated together with the UV protection abilities [26, 29-33]. Recently, there has been an systematic investigation of the UV absorber resistance to light since the final effect of fluorescent whitening agents is affected by the exposal to sunlight and by drying after washing. Exposing the materials treated with fluorescent compounds to sunlight can cause various photochemical reactions as they are prone to absorb UV radiation [32, 41].

Since the latest research declare that FWAs and UV absorbers can be applied in washing process as well, the UV protective properties of cotton and cotton/polyester blend fabrics achieved by light conversion in textile finishing and care was researched in this chapter. UV protection was determined *in vitro* through Ultraviolet protection factor, UPF. Additionally the influence to fabric whiteness was researched. Since the fabric properties change in wet state, the discrepancy in whiteness and UV protection was research in distilled water as well as Adriatic Sea water.

EXPERIMENTAL

Materials

Two fabrics, cotton (C) and polyester/cotton (65/35) blend (P/C), such are frequently used during summer time, were used in the investigation. Both fabrics were pre-bleached, in plain weave, with the following properties: Cotton fabric surface mass of 175.6 g/m^2 and yarn density of (warp/weft 25/25 yarns/cm), and P/C blend fabric surface mass 155.1 g/m^2 and yarn density of (warp/weft 26/25 yarns/cm).

Three fluorescent compounds of stilbene type were used (Table 1): one fluorescent whitening agent (FWA) commonly used in textile finishing (F1), one FWA commonly used in textile care in detergent formulation (F2), and UV absorber (F3).

Table 1. Characteristics and structural formula of applied fluorescent compounds

Compound characteristic	Structural formula
F1 Fluorescent whitening agent (FWA) - stilbene type CI Fluorescent Brightener 336 Uvitex BAM (Ciba-Geigy AG) For textile finishing	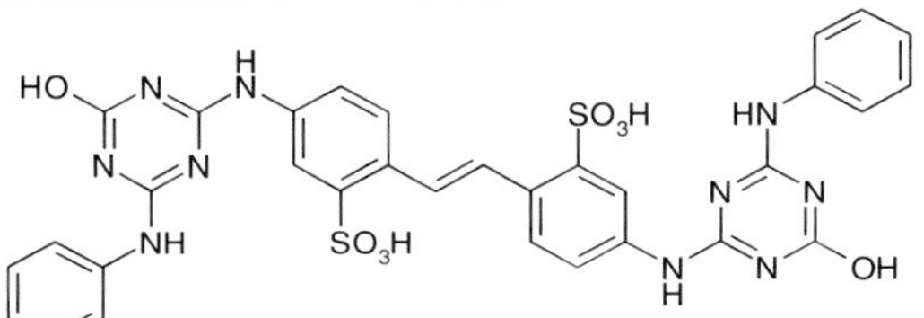 bis(4,4'-triazinylamino)-stilbene-2,2'-disulfonic acid derivative
F2 Fluorescent whitening agent (FWA) - stilbene type Optiblanc 2MG/LT Extra (Sigma 3V) In detergent formulation	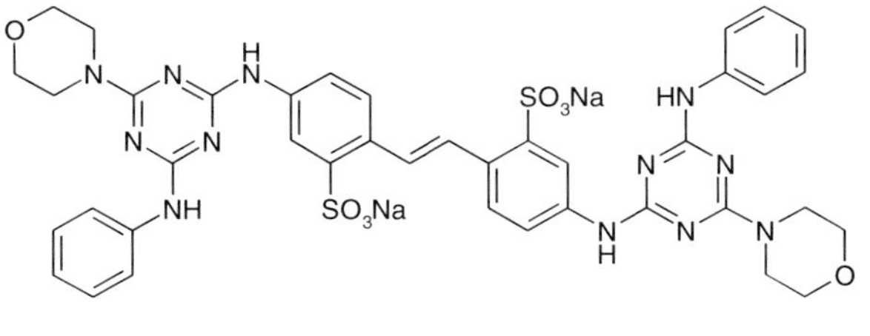 disodium 4.4'-bis[(4-anylino-6-morpholino-1.3.5-triazine-2-yl) amino]-stilbene-2.2'-disulphonate
F3 UV absorber - stilbene type Tinosorb FD (Ciba-Geigy AG)	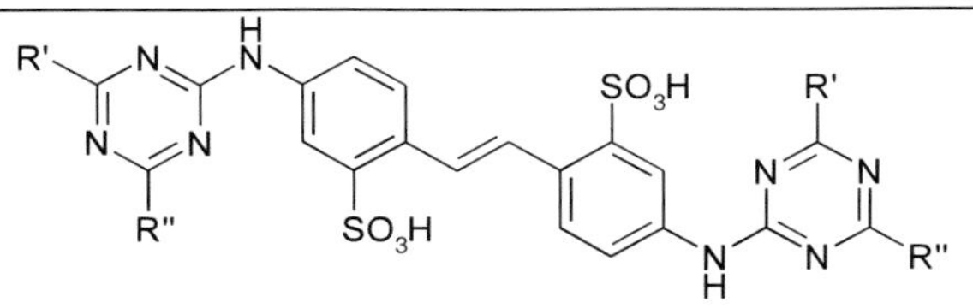 R', R'' - differently substituted amines stilbene disulphonic acid triazine derivative

Procedure

In this chapter, fluorescent compounds – two FWAs and UV absorber, all stilbene derivatives, were applied to cotton and cotton/polyester blend fabrics in textile finishing and care.

Textile Finishing

Fluorescent compounds were applied in wide concentration range ($c_1 = 0.004\%$ owf (over weight of fiber); $c_2 = 0.006\%$ owf; $c_3 = 0.0125\%$ owf; $c_4 = 0.1\%$ owf; $c_5 = 0.5\%$ owf; $c_6 = 1\%$ owf, $c_7 = 10\%$ owf, $c_8 = 50\%$ owf) by exhaustion procedure at 60°C for 30 minutes to achieve the best whiteness and UV protection. Afterwards, the discrepancy in whiteness and UV protection was research in distilled and Adriatic Sea water.

Textile Care - Laundering

In textile care fluorescent compounds were applied through 9 washing cycles with ECE reference detergent 77 for color fastness, without optical brightener, phosphate based, for application in ISO 105-C06:2010, ISO 6330:1984; and commercial detergent. Formulations of detergents are given in Table 2.

Table 2. Formulations of detergents

ECE reference detergent	Commercial detergent
- 8% Linear sodium alkyl benzene sulphonate (mean length of alkane chain $C_{11.5}$) - 2,9% Ethoxylated tallow alcohol (14 EO) - 3,5% Sodium soap, (chain length C_{12-16} 13% - 26% : C_{18-22} 74% - 87%) - 43,8% Sodium tripolyphosphate - 7,5% Sodium silicate (SiO_2:Na_2O = 3.3 : 1) - 1,9% Magnesium silicate - 1,2% Carboxy methyl cellulose (CMC) - 0,2% Etylene diamine tetra acetic acid, tetra sodium salt (TAED) - 21,2% Sodium sulphate - 9,8% Water *Added 1 g/l of sodium perborate	- 5% Anionic sufractant - 1% Nonionic sufractant - 2% Sodium soap - 20% Sodium tripolyphosphate - 5% Sodium silicate - 12% Sodium carbonate - 11% Sodium perborate - 1,2% Carboxy methyl cellulose (CMC) - 2% Etylene diamine tetra acetic acid, tetra sodium salt (TAED) - 0,6% Enzymes - up to 100%: Sodium sulphate and Water

The samples were laundered in the Linitest apparatus, Original Hanau, in the bath of a 5 g/l of detergent. The laundering bath was prepared in the ratio of 1:15, heated from the initial temperature of 25°C for 15 minutes to 60°C. The fabrics were laundered at 60°C for 15 minutes up to 9 laundering cycles. The samples were rinsed and dried in a Scholl drier for 45 minutes at 40°C. For the purpose of better visibility and review of the results, only the results after the 1st, 3rd, 6th and 9th laundering cycle are presented. Laundering was done with the addition of fluorescent whitening agent and UV absorber in different concentration over weight of detergent. FWA was applied in concentrations of 0.08%, 0.16% and 0.25%; UV absorber in concentration of 0.20%, and in combination 0.10% of each.

Methods

The fabric UV protection was determined according to AS/NZS 4399:1996 *Sun Protective Clothing: evaluation and classification.* UV-A and UV-B transmission through fabric were measured on Spectrophotometer Cary 50 (Varian). This instrument measures sunlight transmission in the range from 280 to 400 nm. The irradiation applied is a simulation of a part of sunlight spectrum, as measured at noon on January 17th 1990 in Melbourne, Australia, while the results obtained indicate the degree of protection offered by the fabric when worn directly to the skin.

The *ultraviolet protection factor* (*UPF*) was calculated automatically according to:

$$UPF = \frac{\sum_{\lambda=280}^{400} E(\lambda)\cdot\varepsilon(\lambda)\cdot\Delta\lambda}{\sum_{\lambda=280}^{400} E(\lambda)\cdot T(\lambda)\cdot\varepsilon(\lambda)\cdot\Delta\lambda} \tag{1}$$

where:

$E(\lambda)$ = Solar radiation [W m^{-2} nm^{-1}]
$\varepsilon(\lambda)$ = relative erythemal spectral effectiveness
$T(\lambda)$ = spectrum permeability at wavelength λ
$\Delta\lambda$ = measured wavelength interval [nm]

UPF indicate the ability of fabrics to protect the skin against sun burning saying how much longer a person can stay in the sun with the fabric covering the skin as compared with the uncovered skin to obtain same erythemal response.[3-20] According to the standards excellent protection is if UPF is higher 40 (Table 3). However, for the countries with UV index 7-10 as Mediterranean countries, Australia and USA, the UPF should be 15 times higher than UV index [17]. Therefore, it is recommended for people who spend eight hours in the open to use UV clothing with UPF between 105 and 150 if they want excellent UV protection.

Table 3. UV protection rating according to AS/NZS 4399:1996

UPF range	UPF rating	UV-R protection category	UV-R blocking [%]
< 14	0, 5, 10	non-rateable	<93,3
15-24	15, 20	good	93,3-95,8
25-39	25, 30, 35	very good	95,9-97,4
> 40	40, 45, 50, 50+	excellent	> 97,5

Remission spectrophotometer SF 600 PLUS CT (Datacolor) was used for measuring spectral characteristics of cotton and PES/cotton blend fabrics. CIE whiteness degree (W_{CIE}) was calculated automatically according to ISO 105-J02:1997 *Textiles - Tests for colour fastness - Part J02: Instrumental assessment of relative whiteness.* The discrepancy in wet state was determined through color differences of color coordinates according to:

$$\Delta E^*_{ab} = \left[(\Delta H^*)^2 + (\Delta L^*)^2 + (\Delta C^*)^2\right]^{\frac{1}{2}} \tag{2}$$

where ΔL* is change in lightness, ΔC* change in chroma and ΔH* change in hue.

The relative intensity of fluorescence (Φ_{rel}) was calculated from measured fluorescence on adapted spectrophotometer Specol SV (Carl Zeiss). Illuminant is high voltage Hg bulb (λ_{max} = 366 nm). Fluorescent Reference Standard (Datacolor) was used for $\Phi_{rel.\ standard}$ = 40, with amplifying of 200x.

RESULTS AND DISCUSSION

The UV protective properties of cotton and cotton/polyester blend fabrics achieved by light conversion of fluorescent compounds applied in textile finishing and care was researched in this chapter. For that purpose, three stilbene derivatives fluorescent compounds were selected: FWA for cellulosic materials – one commonly used in textile finishing and the other in detergent formulations; and UV absorber. UV protection was determined *in vitro* through Ultraviolet protection factor, UPF. Additionally the influence to fabric whiteness was researched. Main characteristics of fabrics are collected in Table 4.

Table 4. Main characteristics of cotton (C) and polyester/cotton blend (P/C) fabrics: Mean UPF, UV-A and UV-B transmission, UV protection rating according to AS/NZS 4399:1996, CIE whiteness (W_{CIE}), relative intensity of fluorescence (Φ_{rel}), maximum of remission (R_{max}) and wavelength (λ_{max})

Fabric	**Mean UPF**	τ_{UVA}	τ_{UVB}	**UPF rating**
C	7.276	16.714	11.969	5: Non-rateable
P/C	18.426	17.148	3.289	15: Good
Fabric	W_{CIE}	Φ_{rel}	R_{max} [%]	λ_{max} [nm]
C	74.3	0	86.51	700
P/C	70.7	0	85.34	700

In textile finishing process fluorescent compounds were applied by exhaustion procedure in wide concentration range. Since the fabric properties change in wet state, the discrepancy in whiteness and UV protection was research in distilled water as well as Adriatic Sea water. The UV protective properties of cotton and PES/cotton blend fabric achieved by light conversion of fluorescent compounds are presented in Tables 5-7. The discrepancy of UV protection in wet state by distilled (DW) and sea (SW) water is shown in Figures 3-8. Remission curves of cotton fabric treated with FWA - disodium 4.4'-bis[(4-anylino-6-morpholino-1.3.5-triazine-2-yl)amino]-stilbene-2.2'-disulphonate (F2) in wide concentration range as example of Stokes law are presented in Figure 9. CIE whiteness (W_{CIE}), relative intensity of fluorescence (Φ_{rel}), maximum of remission (R_{max}) and wavelength (λ_{max}), and the discrepancy of whiteness in wet state of cotton fabrics treated with all fluorescent compounds are collected in Tables 8-13.

Table 5. Mean UPF, UV-A and UV-B transmission, and UV protection rating according to AS/NZS 4399:1996 of cotton and PES/cotton fabrics treated with fluorescent whitening agent - bis(4,4'-triazinylamino)-stilbene-2,2'-disulfonic acid derivative (F1)

Sample	Mean UPF	τ_{UVA}	τ_{UVB}	UPF rating	
C-F1-0,004	9,502	9,472	12,219	5	Non-rateable
C-F1-0,006	9,605	9,407	12,738	5	Non-rateable
C-F1-0,0125	9,379	9,501	11,251	5	Non-rateable
C-F1-0,1	14,005	6,490	5,513	10	Non-rateable
C-F1-0,5	16,219	5,635	4,005	15	Good
C-F1-1	30,061	3,230	2,032	30	Very good
C-F1-10	125,094	0,776	0,439	50+	Excellent
C-F1-50	203,793	0,503	0,333	50+	Excellent
P/C -F1-0,004	35,797	1,366	11,160	30	Very good
P/C -F1-0,006	35,493	1,517	10,231	30	Very good
P/C -F1-0,0125	36,606	1,504	10,185	30	Very good
P/C -F1-0,1	38,589	1,221	9,901	35	Very good
P/C -F1-0,5	45,006	1,383	5,862	45	Excellent
P/C -F1-1	45,122	1,526	4,899	45	Excellent
P/C -F1-10	62,291	1,258	2,883	50+	Excellent
P/C -F1-50	88,355	0,842	1,926	50+	Excellent

Table 6. Mean UPF, UV-A and UV-B transmission, and UV protection rating according to AS/NZS 4399:1996 of cotton and PES/cotton fabrics treated with fluorescent whitening agent - disodium 4.4’-bis[(4-anylino-6-morpholino-1.3.5-triazine-2-yl) amino]-stilbene-2.2’-disulphonate (F2)

Sample	Mean UPF	τ_{UVA}	τ_{UVB}	UPF rating	
C-F2-0,004	9,245	9,776	10,985	5	Non-rateable
C-F2-0,006	9,459	9,600	9,901	5	Non-rateable
C-F2-0,0125	9,690	9,539	8,468	5	Non-rateable
C-F2-0,1	18,578	5,179	2,673	15	Good
C-F2-0,5	62,023	1,554	0,656	50+	Excellent
C-F2-1	63,339	1,589	0,585	50+	Excellent
C-F2-10	497,005	0,268	0,214	50+	Excellent
C-F2-50	548,558	0,208	0,158	50+	Excellent
P/C -F2-0,004	28,589	2,221	9,901	25	Very good
P/C -F2-0,006	31,578	1,833	10,012	30	Very good
P/C -F2-0,0125	32,950	1,552	11,193	30	Very good
P/C -F2-0,1	34,161	2,185	6,341	30	Very good
P/C -F2-0,5	66,276	1,607	0,651	40	Excellent
P/C -F2-1	180,311	0,660	0,291	50+	Excellent
P/C -F2-10	606,725	0,225	0,426	50+	Excellent
P/C -F2-50	98,540	0,836	1,408	50+	Excellent

Table 7. Mean UPF, UV-A and UV-B transmission, and UV protection rating according to AS/NZS 4399:1996 of cotton and PES/cotton fabrics treated with fluorescent UV absorber -stilbene disulphonic acid triazine derivative (F3)

Sample	Mean UPF	τ_{UVA}	τ_{UVB}	UPF rating	
C-F3-0,004	12,078	7,389	8,518	10	Non-rateable
C-F3-0,006	11,338	8,118	7,936	10	Non-rateable
C-F3-0,0125	11,022	8,151	9,663	10	Non-rateable
C-F3-0,1	37,246	2,649	2,667	20	Good
C-F3-0,5	90,434	1,057	0,984	50+	Excellent
C-F3-1	122,067	0,867	0,803	50+	Excellent
C-F3-10	424,074	0,260	0,285	50+	Excellent
C-F3-50	1000,000	0,100	0,100	50+	Excellent
P/C –F3-0,004	31,038	1,906	10,376	30	Very good
P/C –F3-0,006	33,758	1,714	9,321	30	Very good
P/C –F3-0,0125	34,136	1,679	9,896	30	Very good
P/C –F3-0,1	41,600	1,470	6,699	40	Excellent
P/C –F3-0,5	81,291	0,773	2,960	50+	Excellent
P/C –F3-1	70,671	1,040	2,671	50+	Excellent
P/C –F3-10	161,614	0,486	1,170	50+	Excellent
P/C –F3-50	160,207	0,536	1,105	50+	Excellent

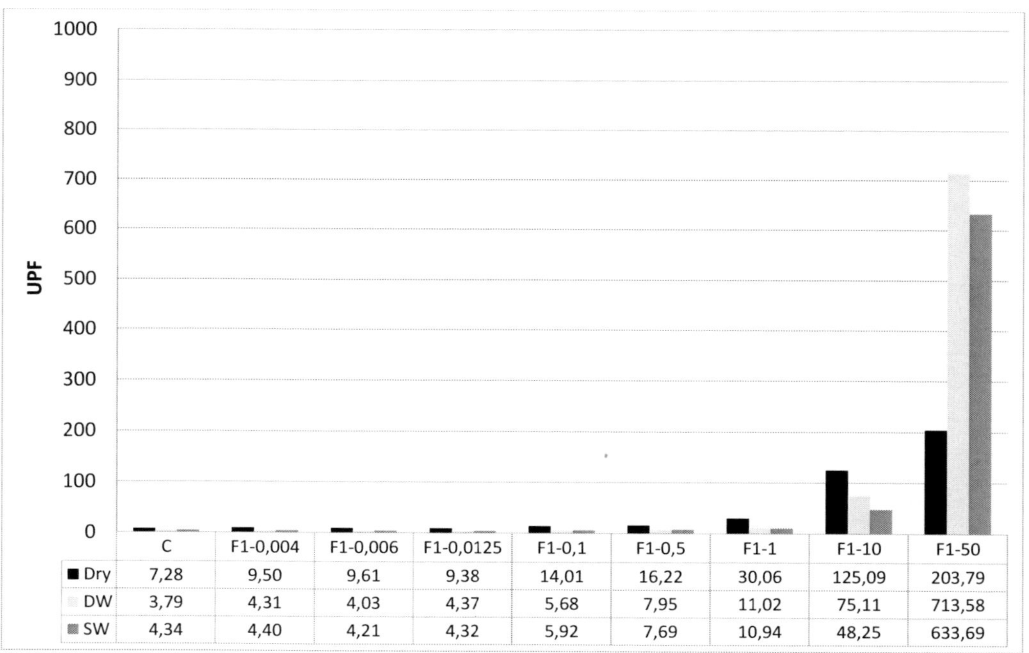

Figure 3. The discrepancy of UV protection in wet state by distilled (DW) and sea (SW) water of cotton fabric treated with FWA - bis(4,4'-triazinylamino)-stilbene-2,2'-disulfonic acid derivative (F1).

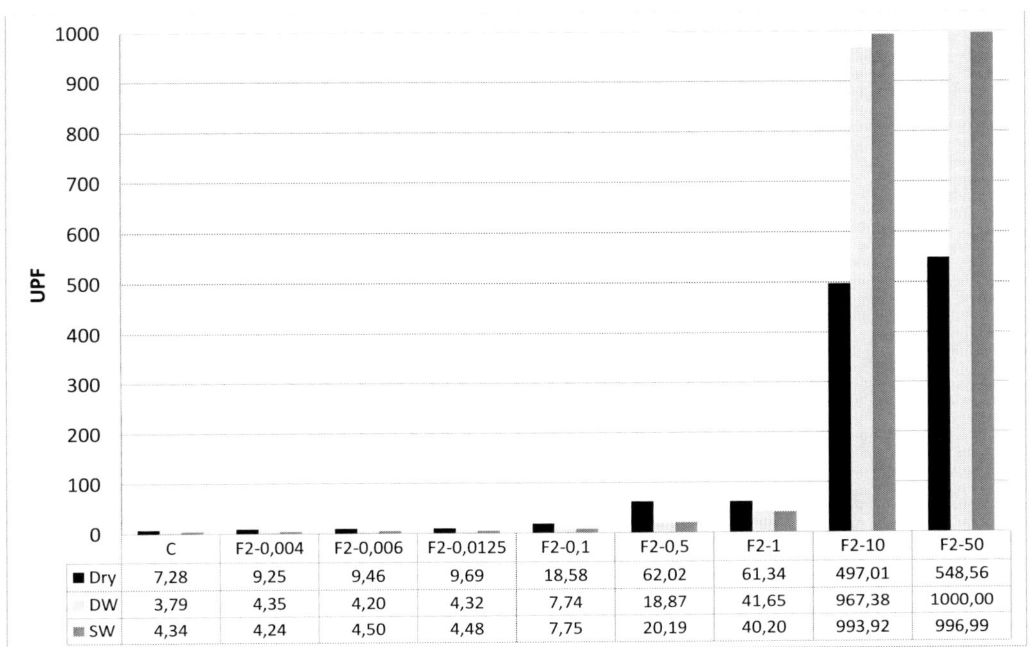

	C	F2-0,004	F2-0,006	F2-0,0125	F2-0,1	F2-0,5	F2-1	F2-10	F2-50
Dry	7,28	9,25	9,46	9,69	18,58	62,02	61,34	497,01	548,56
DW	3,79	4,35	4,20	4,32	7,74	18,87	41,65	967,38	1000,00
SW	4,34	4,24	4,50	4,48	7,75	20,19	40,20	993,92	996,99

Figure 4. The discrepancy of UV protection in wet state by distilled (DW) and sea (SW) water of cotton fabric treated with FWA - disodium 4.4'-bis[(4-anylino-6-morpholino-1.3.5-triazine-2-yl) amino]-stilbene-2.2'-disulphonate (F2).

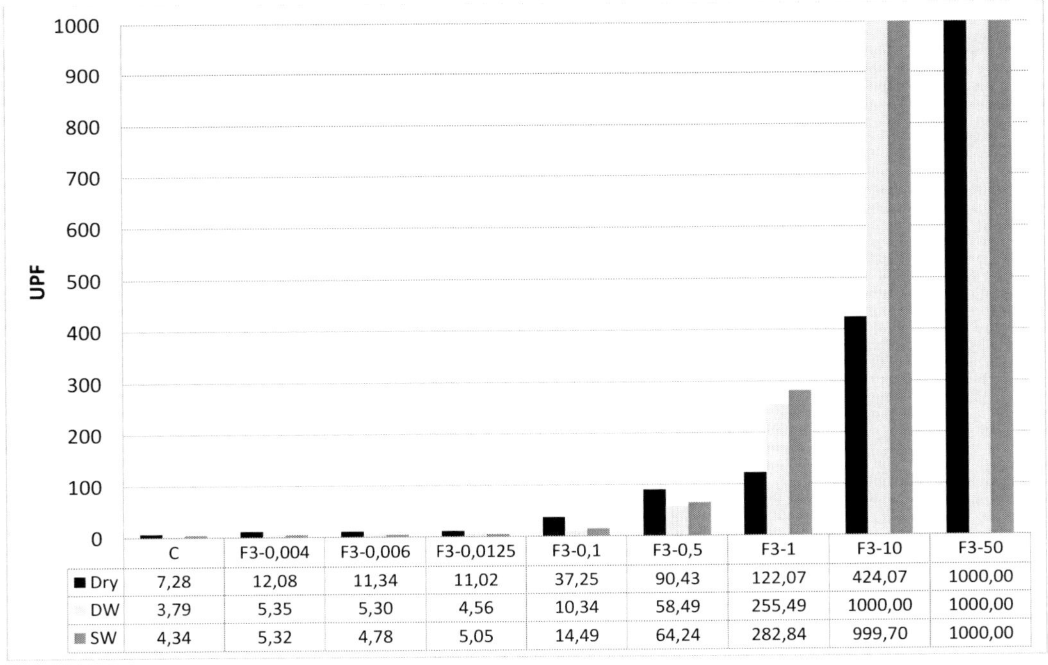

	C	F3-0,004	F3-0,006	F3-0,0125	F3-0,1	F3-0,5	F3-1	F3-10	F3-50
Dry	7,28	12,08	11,34	11,02	37,25	90,43	122,07	424,07	1000,00
DW	3,79	5,35	5,30	4,56	10,34	58,49	255,49	1000,00	1000,00
SW	4,34	5,32	4,78	5,05	14,49	64,24	282,84	999,70	1000,00

Figure 5. The discrepancy of UV protection in wet state by distilled (DW) and sea (SW) water of cotton fabric treated with UV absorber - stilbene disulphonic acid triazine derivative (F3).

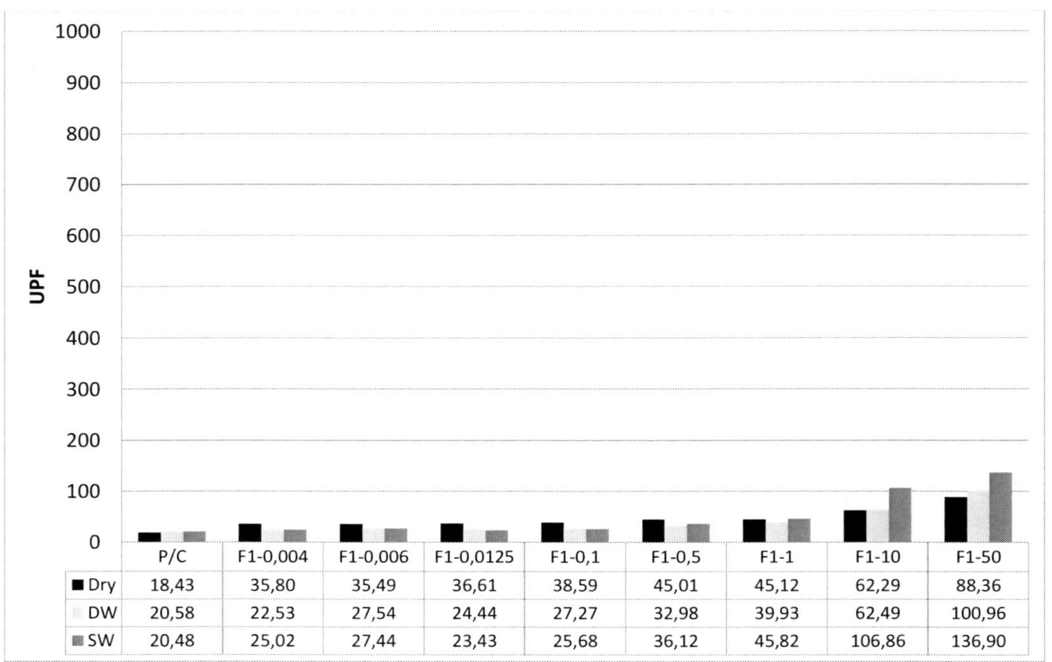

Figure 6. Discrepancy of UV protection in wet state – distilled (DW) and sea (SW) water of polyester/cotton blend fabric treated with fluorescent whitening agent - bis(4,4'-triazinylamino)-stilbene-2,2'-disulfonic acid derivative (F1).

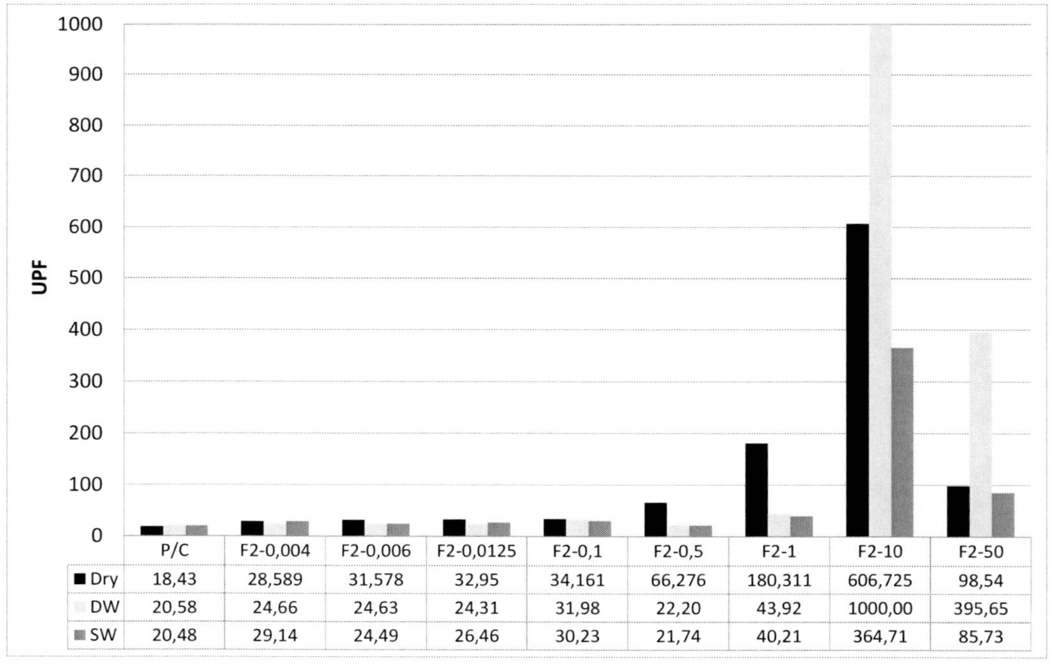

Figure 7. The discrepancy of UV protection in wet state by distilled (DW) and sea (SW) water of polyester/cotton fabric treated with FWA - disodium 4.4'-bis[(4-anylino-6-morpholino-1.3.5-triazine-2-yl) amino]-stilbene-2.2'-disulphonate (F2).

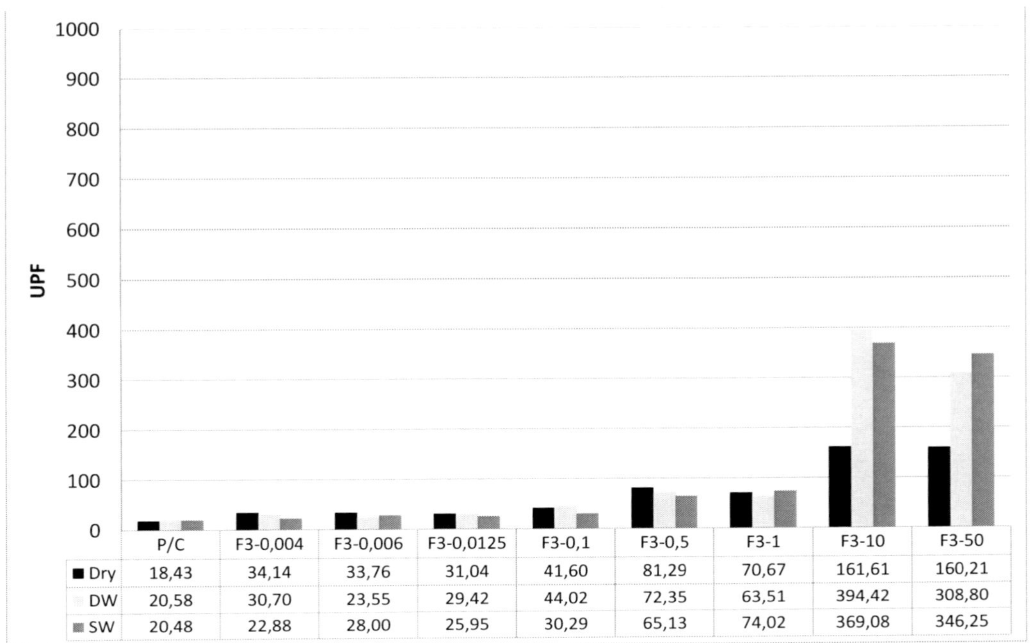

	P/C	F3-0,004	F3-0,006	F3-0,0125	F3-0,1	F3-0,5	F3-1	F3-10	F3-50
Dry	18,43	34,14	33,76	31,04	41,60	81,29	70,67	161,61	160,21
DW	20,58	30,70	23,55	29,42	44,02	72,35	63,51	394,42	308,80
SW	20,48	22,88	28,00	25,95	30,29	65,13	74,02	369,08	346,25

Figure 8. The discrepancy of UV protection in wet state by distilled (DW) and sea (SW) water of polyester/cotton fabric treated with UV absorber - stilbene disulphonic acid triazine derivative (F3).

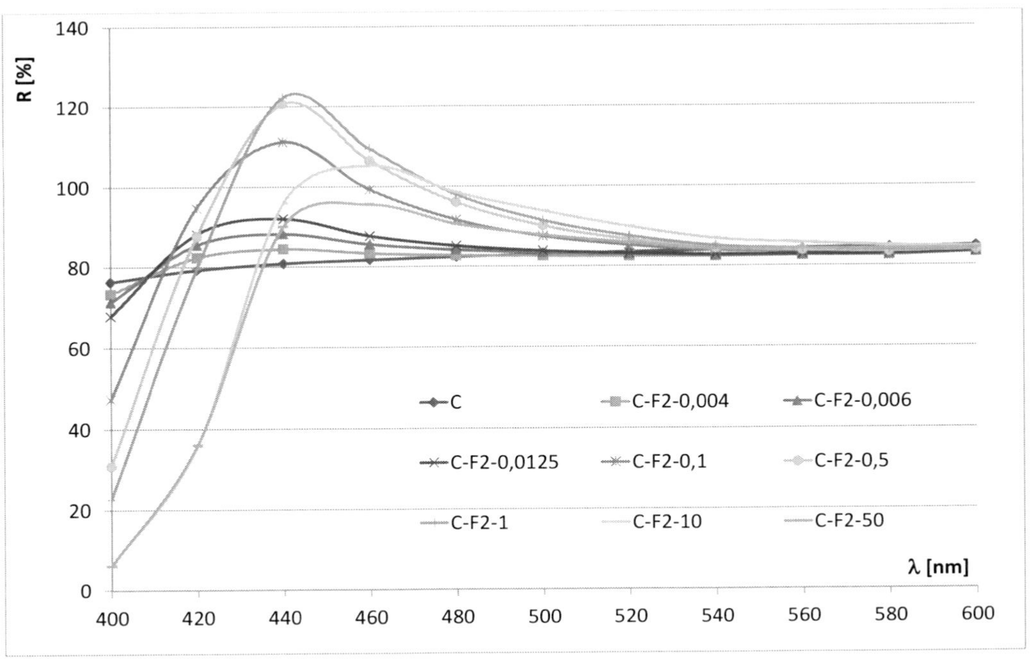

Figure 9. Remission curves of cotton fabric treated with FWA - disodium 4.4'-bis[(4-anylino-6-morpholino-1.3.5-triazine-2-yl) amino]-stilbene-2.2'-disulphonate (F2) in wide concentration range.

Table 8. CIE whiteness (W_{CIE}), relative intensity of fluorescence (Φ_{rel}), maximum of remission (R_{max}) and wavelength (λ_{max}), and the discrepancy of whiteness in wet state of cotton fabrics treated with FWA - bis(4,4'-triazinylamino)-stilbene-2,2'-disulfonic acid derivative (F1)

Fabric	W_{CIE}	Φ_{rel}	R_{max} [%]	λ_{max} [nm]	dE*	Discrepancy
C	74.3	0	86.51	700	-	-
C-DW	61.7	0	83.25	700	2.633	Darker yellow
C-SW	62.9	0	83.47	700	2.413	Darker yellow
C-F1-0.004	77.4	0	85.83	700	-	-
C-F1-0.004-DW	67.4	0	83.28	700	2.147	Darker yellow
C-F1-0.004-SW	66.7	0	82.95	700	2.428	Darker yellow
C-F1-0.006	79.0	4.56	85.95	700	-	-
C-F1-0.006-DW	69.8	4.23	83.32	700	2.072	Darker yellow
C-F1-0.006-SW	69.7	4.25	83.31	700	2.107	Darker yellow
C-F1-0.0125	83.4	8.85	85.88	700	-	-
C-F1-0.0125-DW	76.3	7.28	83.42	700	1.787	Darker less blue
C-F1-0.0125-SW	73.6	7.02	82.78	700	2.336	Darker redder less blue
C-F1-0.1	109.1	27.72	96.84	440	-	-
C-F1-0.1-DW	109.4	27.99	95.29	440	2.021	Darker redder bluer
C-F1-0.1-SW	109.4	27.90	95.45	440	1.855	Darker redder bluer
C-F1-0.5	127.1	38.18	106.37	440	-	-
C-F1-0.5-DW	127.6	37.80	105.35	440	1.895	Darker redder bluer
C-F1-0.5-SW	130.2	39.32	107.18	440	1.999	Darker redder bluer
C-F1-1	135.9	40.98	112.60	440	-	-
C-F1-1-DW	139.1	45.99	113.26	440	2.306	Darker redder bluer
C-F1-1-SW	138.8	45.31	113.43	440	2.146	Darker redder bluer
C-F1-10	143.4	51.53	118.55	440	-	-
C-F1-10-DW	146.0	55.15	120.55	440	1.598	Darker redder bluer
C-F1-10-SW	143.0	50.53	118.73	440	1.470	Darker bluer
C-F1-50	132.2	48.73	114.07	440	-	-
C-F1-50-DW	134.3	49.29	115.02	440	1.855	Darker redder bluer
C-F1-50-SW	126.7	43.37	110.89	440	1.689	Darker less red less blue

Table 9. CIE whiteness (W_{CIE}), relative intensity of fluorescence (Φ_{rel}), maximum of remission (R_{max}) and wavelength (λ_{max}), and the discrepancy of whiteness in wet state of cotton fabrics treated with FWA - disodium 4.4'-bis[(4-anylino-6-morpholino-1.3.5-triazine-2-yl) amino]-stilbene-2.2'-disulphonate (F2)

Fabric	W_{CIE}	Φ_{rel}	R_{max} [%]	λ_{max} [nm]	dE*	Discrepancy
C-F2-0.004	84.7	4.64	85.95	700		
C-F2-0.004-DW	77.5	4.22	83.47	700	1.798	Darker less blue
C-F2-0.004-SW	76.1	4.20	83.36	700	2.304	Darker redder less blue
C-F2-0.006	93.0	16.67	88.16	440	-	-
C-F2-0.006-DW	86.2	14.44	83.59	440	1.787	Darker redder bluer
C-F2-0.006-SW	84.4	12.98	83.55	700	1.576	Darker redder bluer

Fabric	W_{CIE}	Φ_{rel}	R_{max} [%]	λ_{max} [nm]	dE*	Discrepancy
C-F2-0.0125	100.5	27.22	91.95	440	-	-
C-F2-0.0125-DW	97.1	22.24	88.97	440	1.833	Darker redder bluer
C-F2-0.0125-SW	94.5	17.76	87.88	440	2.152	Darker redder bluer
C-F2-0.1	134.3	47.07	111.15	440	-	-
C-F2-0.1-DW	136.0	49.93	111.15	440	1.857	Darker less green bluer
C-F2-0.1-SW	134.6	46.74	110.27	440	1.450	Darker bluer
C-F2-0.5	147.4	60.66	120.68	440	-	-
C-F2-0.5-DW	148.7	62.75	121.00	440	1.756	Darker bluer
C-F2-0.5-SW	147.7	61.53	120.75	440	1.526	Darker less red bluer
C-F2-1	148.1	62.09	122.24	440	-	-
C-F2-1-DW	148.2	62.60	122.25	440	1.623	Darker bluer
C-F2-1-SW	147.9	58.87	122.35	440	2.500	Darker less red bluer
C-F2-10	98.4	39.68	105.29	460	-	-
C-F2-10-DW	104.6	42.32	105.75	460	2.924	Darker less green bluer
C-F2-10-SW	101.3	40.30	105.04	460	2.419	Darker less green bluer
C-F2-50	82.3	20.01	95.51	460	-	-
C-F2-50-DW	72.8	19.93	91.63	460	2.148	Darker less green yellow
C-F2-50-SW	60.0	14.78	87.41	460	4.283	Darker yellow

Table 10. CIE whiteness (W_{CIE}), relative intensity of fluorescence (Φ_{rel}), maximum of remission (R_{max}) and wavelength (λ_{max}), and the discrepancy of whiteness in wet state of cotton fabrics treated with UV absorber - stilbene disulphonic acid triazine derivative (F3)

Fabric	W_{CIE}	Φ_{rel}	R_{max} [%]	λ_{max} [nm]	dE*	Discrepancy
C-F3-0.004	93.1	12.20	88.73	440	-	-
C-F3-0.004-DW	91.7	11.61	86.49	440	1.916	Darker redder bluer
C-F3-0.004-SW	85.4	9.65	83.76	440	1.945	Darker less blue
C-F3-0.006	96.4	13.72	92.96	440	-	-
C-F3-0.006-DW	89.0	11.42	89.69	440	1.721	Darker redder
C-F3-0.006-SW	90.5	12.79	88.24	440	1.922	Darker redder less blue
C-F3-0.0125	102.0	17.27	90.17	440	-	-
C-F3-0.0125-DW	98.4	13.75	85.48	440	1.887	Darker redder bluer
C-F3-0.0125-SW	95.6	13.23	85.66	440	1.809	Darker redder bluer
C-F3-0.1	130.0	39.39	107.87	440	-	-
C-F3-0.1-DW	131.6	40.61	107.83	440	1.595	Darker redder bluer
C-F3-0.1-SW	131.5	40.60	107.87	440	1.697	Darker redder bluer
C-F3-0.5	146.9	56.95	120.13	440	-	-
C-F3-0.5-DW	147.0	58.68	120.21	440	1.411	Darker bluer
C-F3-0.5-SW	144.2	55.55	118.37	440	1.559	Darker less red
C-F3-1	149.2	62.49	122.80	440	-	-
C-F3-1-DW	147.1	59.66	121.67	440	1.385	Darker less red
C-F3-1-SW	144.9	56.55	120.59	440	1.579	Darker less red less blue
C-F3-10	99.9	24.20	105.67	460	-	-
C-F3-10-DW	66.3	17.44	96.41	460	6.897	Darker greener less blue
C-F3-10-SW	68.1	19.50	97.00	460	6.509	Darker greener less blue
C-F3-50	71.8	13.66	100.18	460	-	-
C-F3-50-DW	16.3	4.48	85.38	460	11.017	Darker greener yellow
C-F3-50-SW	15.3	3.83	84.91	460	11.173	Darker greener yellow

Table 11. CIE whiteness (W_{CIE}), relative intensity of fluorescence (Φ_{rel}), maximum of remission (R_{max}) and wavelength (λ_{max}), and the discrepancy of whiteness in wet state of polyester/cotton blend fabrics treated with FWA - bis(4,4'-triazinylamino)-stilbene-2,2'-disulfonic acid derivative (F1)

Fabric	W_{CIE}	Φ_{rel}	R_{max} [%]	λ_{max} [nm]	dE*	Discrepancy
P/C	70.7	0	85.34	700	-	-
P/C-DW	62.1	0	83.38	700	1.766	Darker yellow
P/C-SW	61.5	0	83.33	700	1.880	Darker greener yellow
P/C-F1-0.004	75.1	5.23	85.36	700	-	-
P/C-F1-0.004-DW	68.5	5.00	83.52	700	1.627	Darker less red yellow
P/C-F1-0.004-SW	67.9	4.93	83.30	700	1.743	Darker less red yellow
P/C-F1-0.006	76.4	6.86	85.28	700	-	-
P/C-F1-0.006-DW	67.4	5.55	83.29	700	1.928	Darker less red yellow
P/C-F1-0.006-SW	69.1	5.85	83.45	700	1.661	Darker yellow
P/C-F1-0.0125	77.8	7.65	85.47	700	-	-
P/C-F1-0.0125-DW	71.1	7.23	83.45	700	1.617	Darker yellow
P/C-F1-0.0125-SW	70.6	6.92	83.62	700	1.593	Darker yellow
P/C-F1-0.1	91.6	17.76	86.76	440	-	-
P/C-F1-0.1-DW	90.3	15.43	85.09	440	1.152	Darker redder bluer
P/C-F1-0.1-SW	89.3	15.09	84.92	440	0.935	Darker redder
P/C-F1-0.5	106.3	18.98	94.12	440	-	-
P/C-F1-0.5-DW	106.2	18.82	93.28	440	1.046	Darker redder bluer
P/C-F1-0.5-SW	107.5	19.54	93.45	440	1.524	Darker redder bluer
P/C-F1-1	112.6	20.48	98.07	440	-	-
P/C-F1-1-DW	115.1	25.74	98.51	440	1.438	Darker redder bluer
P/C-F1-1-SW	114.7	23.91	98.02	440	1.629	Darker redder bluer
P/C-F1-10	126.9	51.51	107.92	440	-	-
P/C-F1-10-DW	132.4	50.14	109.86	440	1.984	Darker redder bluer
P/C-F1-10-SW	132.5	49.53	110.28	440	1.937	Darker redder bluer
P/C-F1-50	124.7	48.73	107.95	440	-	-
P/C-F1-50-DW	130.7	49.29	111.29	440	2.196	Darker redder bluer
P/C-F1-50-SW	128.9	38.67	110.00	440	2.103	Darker redder bluer

Table 12. CIE whiteness (W_{CIE}), relative intensity of fluorescence (Φ_{rel}), maximum of remission (R_{max}) and wavelength (λ_{max}), and the discrepancy of whiteness in wet state of polyester/cotton blend fabrics treated with FWA - disodium 4.4'-bis[(4-anylino-6-morpholino-1.3.5-triazine-2-yl) amino]-stilbene-2.2'-disulphonate (F2)

Fabric	W_{CIE}	Φ_{rel}	R_{max} [%]	λ_{max} [nm]	dE*	Discrepancy
P/C-F2-0.004	78.3	4.44	85.30	700	-	-
P/C-F2-0.004-DW	72.4	4.01	83.57	700	1.401	Darker yellow
P/C-F2-0.004-SW	72.3	3.86	83.70	700	1.421	Darker yellow
P/C-F2-0.006	92.8	14.63	87.55	440	-	-
P/C-F2-0.006-DW	83.6	11.98	83.36	700	2.035	Darker less red less blue
P/C-F2-0.006-SW	86.2	12.78	83.32	440	1.743	Darker less red less blue

Fabric	W_{CIE}	Φ_{rel}	R_{max} [%]	λ_{max} [nm]	dE*	Discrepancy
P/C-F2-0.0125	98.2	17.65	85.40	440	-	-
P/C-F2-0.0125-DW	93.8	15.24	83.77	440	1.315	Darker less blue
P/C-F2-0.0125-SW	94.0	15.66	83.69	440	1.374	Darker less blue
P/C-F2-0.1	112.2	43.07	97.78	440	-	-
P/C-F2-0.1-DW	114.1	44.43	97.88	440	1.266	Darker redder bluer
P/C-F2-0.1-SW	113.1	45.01	97.31	440	1.290	Darker redder bluer
P/C-F2-0.5	148.7	60.52	121.66	440	-	-
P/C-F2-0.5-DW	148.5	59.74	121.14	440	1.626	Darker less red bluer
P/C-F2-0.5-SW	148.1	58.53	120.84	440	1.882	Darker less red bluer
P/C-F2-1	148.6	57.22	122.66	440	-	-
P/C-F2-1-DW	148.6	57.30	122.67	440	1.710	Darker bluer
P/C-F2-1-SW	147.2	53.77	121.92	440	1.623	Darker less red bluer
P/C-F2-10	97.1	49.68	101.34	460	-	-
P/C-F2-10-DW	100.3	42.02	104.18	460	1.915	Darker less green bluer
P/C-F2-10-SW	100.4	41.33	99.60	460	2.309	Darker less green bluer
P/C-F2-50	80.7	23.01	91.92	460	-	-
P/C-F2-50-DW	85.6	29.18	92.98	460	1.933	Darker less green less yellow
P/C-F2-50-SW	80.2	22.73	91.91	460	1.140	Darker less green less yellow

Table 13. CIE whiteness (W_{CIE}), relative intensity of fluorescence (Φ_{rel}), maximum of remission (R_{max}) and wavelength (λ_{max}), and the discrepancy of whiteness in wet state of polyester/cotton blend fabrics treated with UV absorber - stilbene disulphonic acid triazine derivative (F3)

Fabric	W_{CIE}	Φ_{rel}	R_{max} [%]	λ_{max} [nm]	dE*	Discrepancy
P/C-F3-0.004	82.2	11.00	85.19	700	-	-
P/C-F3-0.004-DW	75.5	9.63	83.29	700	1.552	Darker yellow
P/C-F3-0.004-SW	75.6	9.90	83.18	700	1.547	Darker yellow
P/C-F3-0.006	89.5	13.31	86.02	440	-	-
P/C-F3-0.006-DW	85.5	12.27	83.59	700	1.432	Darker redder less blue
P/C-F3-0.006-SW	86.3	12.75	83.66	700	1.244	Darker redder less blue
P/C-F3-0.0125	96.3	14.28	84.41	440	-	-
P/C-F3-0.0125-DW	90.3	13.35	83.85	700	1.321	Darker less blue
P/C-F3-0.0125-SW	91.7	13.86	83.58	700	1.392	Darker redder less blue
P/C-F3-0.1	107.6	22.38	95.51	440	-	-
P/C-F3-0.1-DW	106.9	20.64	94.39	440	1.170	Darker redder bluer
P/C-F3-0.1-SW	106.5	18.59	94.28	440	1.016	Darker redder bluer
P/C-F3-0.5	123.7	36.93	105.18	440	-	-
P/C-F3-0.5-DW	127.2	45.60	106.43	440	1.565	Darker redder bluer
P/C-F3-0.5-SW	125.7	43.59	106.21	440	1.297	Darker redder bluer
P/C-F3-1	126.5	47.42	107.63	440	-	-
P/C-F3-1-DW	129.4	46.44	109.47	440	1.317	Darker bluer
P/C-F3-1-SW	131.2	46.53	110.52	440	1.430	Darker bluer
P/C-F3-10	95.2	23.42	99.07	460	-	-
P/C-F3-10-DW	76.7	17.44	93.96	460	3.807	Darker greener less blue
P/C-F3-10-SW	67.0	15.43	92.22	460	5.810	Darker greener less blue
P/C-F3-50	74.6	16.66	95.52	460	-	-
P/C-F3-50-DW	39.9	7.83	87.61	460	7.130	Darker greener yellow
P/C-F3-50-SW	32.3	5.82	84.86	460	8.490	Darker greener yellow

Table 14. Mean UPF, UV-A and UV-B transmission of cotton fabrics treated with fluorescent compounds in laundering - 1st, 3rd, 6th and 9th washing cycle with ECE referent detergent

Sample	Mean UPF	τ_{UVA}	τ_{UVB}	Mean UPF	τ_{UVA}	τ_{UVB}
	1st			3rd		
C-ECE	7.134	17.056	12.270	7.441	15.515	11.754
C-F2-0.08	8.326	11.694	10.601	11.038	5.972	8.038
C-F2-0.12	8.929	9.575	10.054	14.078	3.978	6.369
C-F2-0.25	9.943	7.762	9.292	19.314	2.468	4.568
C-F3-0.2	14.674	8.196	5.955	41.424	2.380	2.057
C-F2-0.1+F3-0.1	11.498	8.356	7.539	30.264	2.382	2.845
	6th			9th		
C-ECE	7.135	15.660	12.253	6.970	15.750	12.765
C-F2-0.08	17.575	3.404	5.284	20.845	2.601	4.406
C-F2-0.12	22.768	2.178	3.772	29.965	1.437	2.959
C-F2-0.25	48.240	1.229	1.958	61.834	0.859	1.484
C-F3-0.2	89.895	1.450	0.982	124.911	0.823	0.652
C-F2-0.1+F3-0.1	57.638	1.484	1.474	85.133	0.935	1.093

Table 15. Mean UPF, UV-A and UV-B transmission of PES/cotton fabrics treated with fluorescent compounds in laundering - 1st, 3rd, 6th and 9th washing cycle with ECE reference detergent

Sample	Mean UPF	τ_{UVA}	τ_{UVB}	Mean UPF	τ_{UVA}	τ_{UVB}
	1st			3rd		
P/C-ECE	21.034	15.818	2.641	23.013	23.66	13.709
P/C-F2-0.08	27.411	10.643	2.336	39.416	5.812	1.717
P/C-F2-0.12	23.645	10.781	2.938	29.857	6.367	2.451
P/C-F2-0.25	27.319	8.069	2.515	48.332	3.522	1.558
P/C-F3-0.2	34.295	8.223	1.848	37.759	4.895	1.898
P/C-F2-0.1+F3-0.1	24.039	9.200	2.662	42.915	4.271	1.689
	6th			9th		
P/C-ECE	25.368	13.096	2.207	23.729	13.600	2.423
P/C-F2-0.08	45.893	4.579	1.558	43.958	4.100	1.704
P/C-F2-0.12	30.475	5.503	2.474	30.483	5.108	2.560
P/C-F2-0.25	50.035	3.401	1.542	51.041	2.961	1.601
P/C-F3-0.2	51.245	4.092	1.449	48.923	3.657	1.610
P/C-F2-0.1+F3-0.1	47.058	3.926	1.582	44.036	3.736	1.786

In textile care fluorescent compounds were added to ECE referent detergent or commercial detergent. It was applied separately or in combination through 9 washing cycles at 60°C. The achieved UV protections of cotton and PES/cotton blend fabric are presented through Mean UPF, UV-A and UV-B transmission in Tables 14-17. CIE whiteness (W_{CIE}), relative intensity of fluorescence (Φ_{rel}), maximum of remission (R_{max}) and wavelength (λ_{max}) achieved by repeated laundering are shown in Tables 18-21.

Table 16. Mean UPF, UV-A and UV-B transmission of cotton fabrics treated with fluorescent compounds in laundering - 1st, 3rd, 6th and 9th washing cycle with commercial detergent

Sample	Mean UPF	τ_{UVA}	τ_{UVB}	Mean UPF	τ_{UVA}	τ_{UVB}
	1st			3rd		
C-commerc.	9.742	12.351	8.893	10.914	8.708	8.236
C-F2-0.08	11.315	8.921	7.369	16.066	3.990	5.589
C-F2-0.12	10.342	8.923	8.249	16.677	3.415	5.416
C-F2-0.25	13.350	6.175	6.166	29.390	1.564	2.932
C-F3-0.2	18.551	7.473	4.627	49.628	2.042	1.610
C-F2-0.1+F3-0.1	13.189	7.980	6.527	57.378	1.488	1.576
	6th			9th		
C-commerc.	11.797	7.255	7.584	15.753	6.233	5.739
C-F2-0.08	25.343	2.038	3.704	35.565	2.348	2.562
C-F2-0.12	28.376	1.608	3.197	43.904	2.431	2.038
C-F2-0.25	55.566	0.768	1.601	95.917	1.630	0.926
C-F3-0.2	172.094	0.599	0.509	233.725	1.486	0.329
C-F2-0.1+F3-0.1	101.630	0.711	0.879	175.466	1.579	0.473

Table 17. Mean UPF, UV-A and UV-B transmission of PES/cotton fabrics treated with fluorescent compounds in laundering - 1st, 3rd, 6th and 9th washing cycle with commercial detergent

Sample	Mean UPF	τ_{UVA}	τ_{UVB}	Mean UPF	τ_{UVA}	τ_{UVB}
	1st			3rd		
P/C-commerc.	27.308	13.774	2.036	27.408	11.821	2.288
P/C-F2-0.08	26.200	11.901	2.156	32.072	7.495	1.995
P/C-F2-0.12	31.386	10.127	1.801	34.703	6.213	1.744
P/C-F2-0.25	35.318	7.956	1.844	34.593	5.138	2.033
P/C-F3-0.2	28.711	10.934	2.009	41.130.	5.320	1.629
P/C-F2-0.1+F3-0.1	22.038	11.623	2.802	30.837	6.508	2.492
	6th			9th		
P/C-commerc.	32.068	9.239	1.832	31.309	9.872	2.010
P/C-F2-0.08	40.072	4.893	1.743	40.819	6.003	1.827
P/C-F2-0.12	50.499	3.736	1.343	47.836	5.054	1.528
P/C-F2-0.25	42.789	3.462	1.746	46.379	4.433	1.660
P/C-F3-0.2	60.181	2.974	1.209	51.863	4.583	1.483
P/C-F2-0.1+F3-0.1	38.520	4.092	1.964	43.131	4.655	1.896

The impact of fluorescent compounds – FWAs and UV absorber on the UV protection of cotton and polyester/cotton blend fabrics was monitored by the UV-A and UV-B transmission and UPF. From Table 7 it is evident that high effects in textile cleaning of genetic and added impurities such are waxes, protein substances, pectin and other during scouring and bleaching in peroxide baths, where pigments are removed [42-44], leads to white cotton. On the other hand, it leads to low UV protection as well (Table 4). Therefore, chemically bleached cotton fabric (C) is non-rateable for UV protection since UPF is 7.28. Polyester/cotton blend (P/C) fabric gives off good UV protection (UPF=18.43 due to the present benzene ring in PES fibres that absorbs UV radiation.

Table 18. CIE whiteness (W_{CIE}), relative intensity of fluorescence (Φ_{rel}), maximum of remission (R_{max}) and wavelength (λ_{max}) of cotton fabrics treated with fluorescent compounds in laundering - 1st, 3rd, 6th and 9th washing cycle with ECE detergent

Sample	W_{CIE}	Φ_{rel}	R_{max} [%]	λ_{max} [nm]	W_{CIE}	Φ_{rel}	R_{max} [%]	λ_{max} [nm]
	1st				3rd			
C-ECE	80,00	-	82,71	700	81,39	-	82,49	700
C-F2-0,08	103,23	-	92,39	440	127,49	-	101,85	440
C-F2-0,12	115,32	-	95,03	440	135,94	-	105,17	440
C-F2-0,25	128,11	-	102,88	440	147,45	-	112,33	440
C-F3-0,2	116,75	-	98,65	440	142,34	-	110,13	440
C-F2-0,1+F3-0.1	124,05	-	99,55	440	145,22	-	111,54	440
	6th				9th			
C-ECE.	80,04	-	85,58	700	79,79	-	85,58	700
C-F2-0,08	138,28	-	115,59	440	146,86	-	122,07	440
C-F2-0,12	147,59	-	121,95	440	154,64	-	127,95	440
C-F2-0,25	156,35	-	129,59	440	160,66	-	134,63	440
C-F3-0,2	149,03	-	123,42	440	155,42	-	129,31	440
C-F2-0,1+F3-0.1	153,87	-	127,45	440	157,67	-	131,52	440

Table 19. CIE whiteness (W_{CIE}), relative intensity of fluorescence (Φ_{rel}), maximum of remission (R_{max}) and wavelength (λ_{max}) of polyester/cotton fabrics treated with fluorescent compounds in laundering - 1st, 3rd, 6th and 9th washing cycle with ECE detergent

Sample	W_{CIE}	Φ_{rel}	R_{max} [%]	λ_{max} [nm]	W_{CIE}	Φ_{rel}	R_{max} [%]	λ_{max} [nm]
	1st				3rd			
P/C-ECE	76,20	-	82,71	700	76,83	-	82,49	700
P/C-F2-0,08	101,41	-	92,39	440	117,12	-	101,85	440
P/C-F2-0,12	106,36	-	95,03	440	122,28	-	105,17	440
P/C-F2-0,25	119,11	-	102,88	440	131,97	-	112,33	440
P/C-F3-0,2	112,22	-	98,65	440	129,40	-	110,13	440
P/C-F2-0,1+F3-0.1	114,09	-	99,55	440	131,61	-	111,54	440
	6th				9th			
P/C-ECE	80,50	-	83,44	700	83,73	-	83,19	700
P/C-F2-0,08	125,37	-	106,77	440	129,06	-	109,45	440
P/C-F2-0,12	130,51	-	110,62	440	134,05	-	113,44	440
P/C-F2-0,25	136,24	-	115,58	440	136,88	-	116,52	440
P/C-F3-0,2	133,57	-	112,64	440	135,36	-	112,75	440
P/C-F2-0,1+F3-0.1	134,90	-	113,70	440	135,80	-	115,18	440

Table 20. CIE whiteness (W_{CIE}), relative intensity of fluorescence (Φ_{rel}), maximum of remission (R_{max}) and wavelength (λ_{max}) of cotton fabrics treated with fluorescent compounds in laundering - 1st, 3rd, 6th and 9th washing cycle with commercial detergent

Sample	W_{CIE}	Φ_{rel}	R_{max} [%]	λ_{max} [nm]	W_{CIE}	Φ_{rel}	R_{max} [%]	λ_{max} [nm]
	1st				3rd			
C-commerc.	95.36	0	86,32	700	103.80	0	86,04	700
C-F2-0,08	105.33	3,58	96,92	440	124.14	18,83	108,06	440
C-F2-0,12	110.91	8,60	99,93	440	129.88	24,60	111,66	440
C-F2-0,25	123.44	17,25	107,43	440	139.14	39,30	118,46	440
C-F3-0,2	112.33	13,99	100,36	440	136.64	28,16	115,86	440
C-F2-0,1+F3-0.1	110.83	17,99	99,84	440	138.50	32,59	117,95	440
	6th				9th			
C-commerc.	112.45	32,91	86,56	700	115.24	27,38	86,72	700
C-F2-0,08	140.66	65,63	116,47	440	143.88	45,22	120,53	440
C-F2-0,12	147.56	78,30	121,27	440	150.06	46,50	125,55	440
C-F2-0,25	153.36	89,43	126,91	440	154.34	51,64	130,55	440
C-F3-0,2	150.25	76,55	125,49	440	153.24	44,81	129,06	440
C-F2-0,1+F3-0.1	151.67	82,79	126,78	440	154.83	54,03	130,34	440

Table 21. CIE whiteness (W_{CIE}), relative intensity of fluorescence (Φ_{rel}), maximum of remission (R_{max}) and wavelength (λ_{max}) of polyester/cotton fabrics treated with fluorescent compounds in laundering - 1st, 3rd, 6th and 9th washing cycle with commercial detergent

Sample	W_{CIE}	Φ_{rel}	R_{max} [%]	λ_{max} [nm]	W_{CIE}	Φ_{rel}	R_{max} [%]	λ_{max} [nm]
	1st				3rd			
P/C-commerc.	85.85	0	85,51	700	96.83	0	85,19	700
P/C-F2-0,08	100.20	2.06	93,26	440	115.28	9,61	102,34	440
P/C-F2-0,12	103.79	2,14	95,21	440	118.81	12,56	104,37	440
P/C-F2-0,25	112.37	12,76	100,39	440	125.70	22,03	109,75	440
P/C-F3-0,2	102.39	4,15	97,39	440	121.77	16,82	105,85	440
P/C-F2-0,1+F3-0.1	105.22	4,62	94,57	440	122.91	18,83	106,53	440
	6th				9th			
P/C-commerc.	109.52	18,43	85,84	700	104.23	21,17	86,13	700
P/C-F2-0,08	136.60	49,08	108,71	440	129.32	34,23	111,80	440
P/C-F2-0,12	143.16	51,90	111,89	440	133.67	38,54	115,46	440
P/C-F2-0,25	149.62	63,29	116,25	440	135.73	40,06	118,91	440
P/C-F3-0,2	146.44	64,06	116,16	440	135.71	44,91	118,35	440
P/C-F2-0,1+F3-0.1	147.27	53,86	115,28	440	136.31	45,12	118,57	440

From the results in Tables 5 and 6 can be seen that fluorescent whitening agent applied even in small concentration leads to higher whiteness and higher UPF. By absorbing UV-A radiation optical brightened fabrics transform this radiation to blue fluorescence what leads to excellent UV protection in higher concentrations. Optical brightening due to its fluorescence contributes to the fabric high whiteness and beauty in optimal range of concentration. That is the concentration of fluorescent compound at which the maximum of Φ_{rel} or W_{CIE} are observed [16,39]. From the results of the whiteness and fluorescence of FWA treated cotton fabrics it can be seen that FWA concentration of 1% (up to 10% owf) in relation to mass of material is the optimum concentration for bis(4,4'-triazinylamino)-stilbene-2,2'-disulfonic acid derivative (F1), whilst for polyester/cotton blend fabric is 10% owf.

In the case of disodium 4.4'-bis[(4-anylino-6-morpholino-1.3.5-triazine-2-yl)amino]-stilbene-2.2'-disulphonate (F2) optimal concentration for cotton and polyester/cotton fabric is 0.5-1% owf. Since this UV absorber is fluorescent compound as well, having similar chemical composition (stilbene disulphonic acid derivative) as FWA, optimum concentration for UV absorber was determined as well, and it is 0.5-1% owf (Table 7). At the low concentrations of all fluorescent compounds – FWAs and UV absorber, blue fluorescence neutralizes the yellowness of bleached fabric giving the high luminosity and "most beautiful" white. Applied in the higher concentration than optimal one, from results of remission and wavelength maximums can be seen that the change in emission spectrum occurred. It is a consequence of well-known bathochromic shift of the remission spectrum (see Figure 9). It comes to a reduction of remission intensity with FWA and/or UV absorber's concentrations causing the extinction of fluorescence by quenching phenomenon, with a consequence of yellowness.

Cotton fabrics of the highest FWAs concentration have the highest UPF in dry state. Similar to the results of the cotton fabrics whiteness and fluorescence, at the optimal concentration of FWA excellent UV protection has been achieved. For bis(4,4'-triazinylamino)-stilbene-2,2'-disulfonic acid derivative (F1), UPF > 50 was achieved at concentration 10% owf ($UPF_{F1\text{-}0.5}$=125.094); whilst in the case of disodium 4.4'-bis[(4-anylino-6-morpholino-1.3.5-triazine-2-yl)amino]-stilbene-2.2'-disulphonate (F2) at 0.5% owf ($UPF_{F2\text{-}0.5}$=62.023). More benzene rings in the structure of the stilbene-type contribute to better UV protection. That confirms that FWA insures high protection of UV radiation.

By treating cotton fabric with an UV absorber in the wide concentration range protective effect is more enhanced. UV absorber offers excellent UV protection if applied in optimal concentration of 0.1% owf or higher. That is because UV absorbers absorb damaging UV-R range of 290 nm to 360 nm, and convert it into harmless heat energy. For difference of FWA's UV absorbers offer UV-B protection as well. However, the fabrics with the highest intensity of fluorescence do not show the highest UPF values. In dry state, UV protection increase with fluorescent compound concentration, regardless of quenching phenomenon.

Treatment of the polyester/cotton blend fabric with fluorescent compounds shows similar behavior as cotton ones. The presence of benzene ring in PES fibres results in good UV protection of polyester/cotton blend (P/C) fabric. For that reason, treatment of the polyester/cotton blend fabric results in very good UV protection for even smallest concentrations of fluorescent compounds applied. Since these applied fluorescent compounds are primary for the cellulosic fibers, only the cotton in the blend absorbed it. Therefore, in the higher concentrations of applied compounds, excellent UV protection has been achieved, but UPF value is lower than for cotton fabrics.

Washing fabrics with only the detergent, UPF stays mainly the same, and fabrics are non-rateable UV protection (Tables 14-17). Since commercial detergent contained the soap that fluorescence as well (can be seen after 6th cycle – Tables 20-21), UPF is little bit higher, but fabrics are still without UV protection.

UPF significantly grows when washed in a detergent containing fluorescent compounds. The influence of fluorescent whitening agent in initial launderings on the UPF shows that cotton fabrics are non-rateable for UV protection after the first laundering cycle regardless of applied detergent with fluorescent whitening agents added, and even when an UV absorber is added to the detergent as well. However, even small addition of disodium 4.4'-bis[(4-anylino-6-morpholino-1.3.5-triazine-2-yl)amino]-stilbene-2.2'-disulphonate (F2) increase UPF from 7.28 to UPF = 8.32 for ECE detergent and to UPF = 11.31 for commercial detergent. Application of UV absorber (F3) results in UPF of 14.67 for ECE detergent and to UPF = 18.55 for commercial one. To obtain better UV protection the treatment should be performed in the course of finishing. UV absorber offers excellent UV protection (UPF>40) after three laundering cycles regardless of applied detergent, whilst for achieving excellent UV protection with the fluorescent whitening agent six cycles are necessary.

Polyester/cotton blend fabric shows similar behaviour as cotton ones. The growth of UPF is not so much prominent as with cotton fabrics, as the fluorescent compounds used act on the cotton part of the PES/cotton blend only. However, very good UV protection can be achieved after 1 laundering cycle regardless of applied detergent. The excellent UV protection can be achieved applying stilbene type FWA (F2) after 6 laundering cycles and/or UV absorber (F3).

The obtained results confirm the well-known fact that fluorescent whitening agents applied in textile finishing or added into detergents in laundering manage to keep and even improve basic whiteness degree. This phenomenon is present even when lower concentration of fluorescent whitening agent is used than recommended. Obviously, whiteness degree grows with higher concentration. In the case of laundered samples with no fluorescent whitening agents, it can be seen that basic whiteness degree is somewhat higher, which is due to the perborate degradation of residual pigments on the cotton fabric. This occurs after the first laundering cycle already and is more prominent with every succeeding laundering cycle. It can be seen that higher remission is obtained after the 9th laundering cycle when higher concentration of fluorescent whitening agent is employed (0.25%), as compared to lower concentration (0.08%). High whiteness degrees are achieved in the combination of UV absorbers and fluorescent whitening agents. From the Tables 18-21 it can be seen that the wavelength of R_{max} did not changed after multiple laundering. Stilbene fluorescent whitening agent, as well as stilbene UV absorber, showed remission maximum at 440 nm. After repeated laundering and accumulation did not occur bathochromic shift, which confirmed that the whiteness and UV protective effects stay retain.

Somewhat lower degrees of whiteness are achieved on PES/cotton fabrics than on cotton fabric. The reason for that is in the fact that PES fibres cannot be optically brightened with applied FWAs. Since in this research stilbene derivatives were applied in laundering and finishing, PES fibres were not brightened, and the positive effects are achieved on the cotton component only. Therefore, the achieved effects on PES/cotton blend cannot compare to the ones achieved on 100% cotton fabric.

Considering the results of discrepancy of whiteness shown in Tables 9-11 it can be observed that all fabrics get darker when wet and in general bluer and redder. The reason for that is lower reflection of light from the fabric. In dry fabric, some of the photons of light are absorbed, but some are reflected and land on the eye's retina what gives the sensation of seeing a certain level of brightness. But when the fabric gets wet, the water fills in the interyarn spacing. When the light falls on the wet fabric, some of it enters the water at one angle and refracts at other because the light waves travel at a slower speed in water than it does in air. Fewer photons of light get back to the eyeball, and therefore the wet fabric "appears" darker than the dry one. When the water gradually evaporates, more and more light is reflected back to the eyeball, and can be seen brighter again. The amount of refraction, referred to as the refractive index, is affected by both the salinity and temperature of the water, and therefore there is a difference between fabrics treated with sea and distilled water. It is to point out that the salts in Sea water act as quenchers of fluorescence as well. Therefore, for the highest concentration of applied FWAs - disodium 4.4'-bis[(4-anylino-6-morpholino-1.3.5-triazine-2-yl)amino]-stilbene-2.2'-disulphonate (F2) 50% owf, degree of whiteness falls from 82.3 to 60.0. This phenomenon is even more evident for UV absorber applied in concentrations higher than optimal one. The whiteness for applied 10% owf decreases from 99.9 to 77.9, and for 50% owf from 71.8 to low 15.3.

Considering the different refractive index in water and in the air it is differently reflected from the surface as explained before. Because of higher and scattered reflection, transmission is lower for both water applied, distilled and sea water, resulting in higher UPF values (Figures 3-8). It can be said that in wet state cotton knit fabrics treated with fluorescent compounds give off better UV protection than in dry state regardless of the concentration and type of fluorescent compound applied. This phenomenon is more enhanced for Sea water, since the refractive index increases with salinity increment and decrease of temperature. That can be explained by that some of the Sun's radiant energy is reflected from the water surface; it is not absorbed, but additionally scattered by molecules suspended in the water, whilst the other part penetrates the water's surface, absorb and converse to other forms of energy, such as heat that warms or evaporates water, or is used by plants to fuel photosynthesis. Considering the applied concentrations, in general it can be said that higher concentration of fluorescent compound applied to cotton and polyester/cotton blend fabrics, better UV protection was achieved in wet state.

It was observed that for the concentrations lower than optimal one, UV protection in wet state is lower or similar, whilst for the higher concentrations it gets significantly higher. The achieved UV protection is excellent regardless of the drop and can even obey that request regarding UV index during the summer time in Mediterranean countries, as well as Australia and USA, which acquire UPF>UV index*15.

The concentration of 0.08% addition to detergent is the same amount as 0.004% owf applied in textile finishing, etc. The concentration of fluorescent compound accumulated in 9 laundering cycles is similar to the concentration of 0.1% owf in textile finishing. Therefore, the comparison of two procedures was done and it is shown in Figures 10 and 11.

As it can be seen in Figure 10, UV protection of cotton fabrics treated with fluorescent whitening agent - disodium 4.4'-bis[(4-anylino-6-morpholino-1.3.5-triazine-2-yl)amino]-stilbene-2.2'-disulphonate (F2) is similar regardless of procedure. However, if UV absorber was applied as addition to laundry detergent it is more efficient, than if applied in the same concentration in textile finishing. Considering 9x higher concentration and/or accumulation through 9 washing cycles it is evident that in accumulation UV protection gets significantly higher. It is to point out that application to commercial detergent resulted in higher UPF than if applied ECE reference detergent, as a result of fluorescence of the soap in commercial detergent composition.

On the other hand, the differences in UV protection of polyester/cotton blend fabrics (P/C), shown in Figure 11, are not so enhanced. The reason for that is in chemical composition of applied fluorescent compounds. All of them are stilbene derivatives, which are for application to cellulosic fibers, and therefore, only cotton absorbed it.

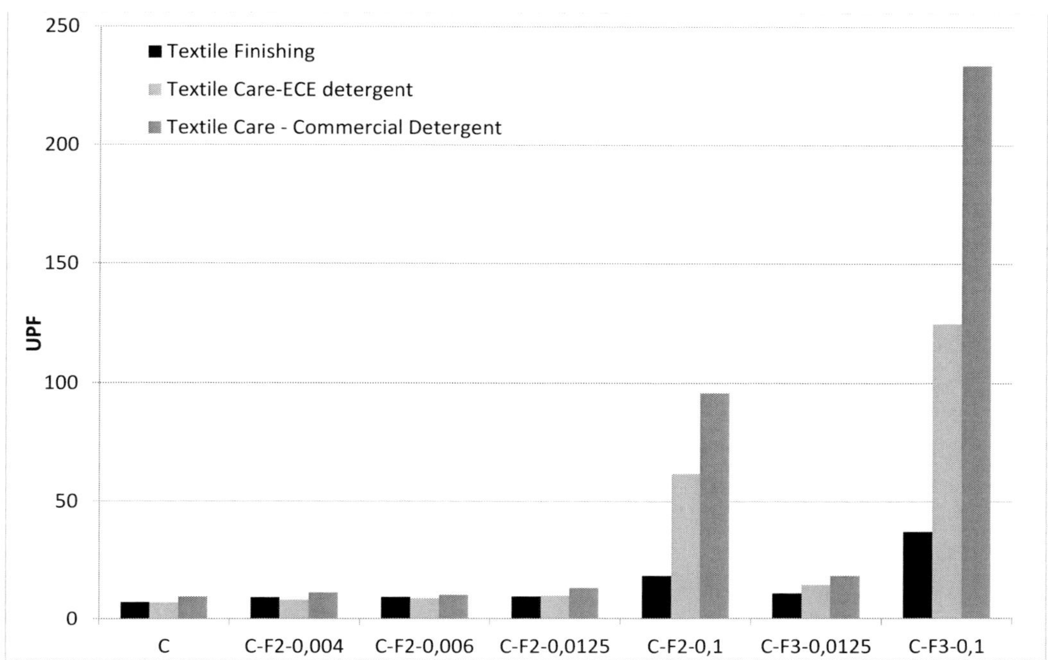

Figure 10. The differences in UV protection of cotton fabrics (C) as a result of different application of fluorescent compounds – FWA (F2) and UV absorber (F3) in textile finishing or textile care.

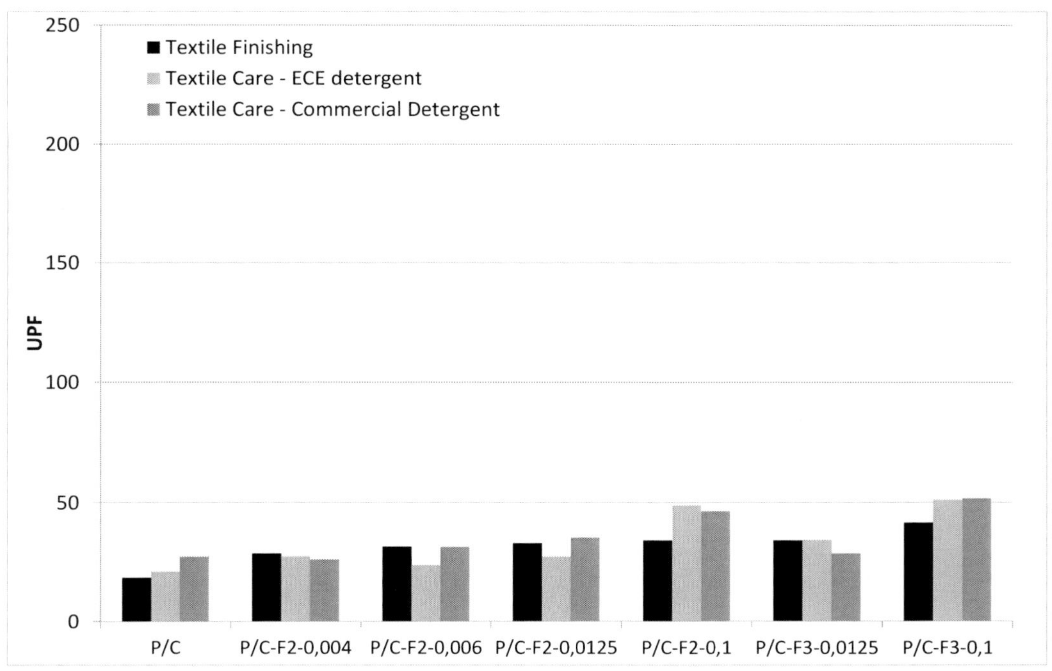

Figure 11. The differences in UV protection of polyester/cotton blend fabrics (P/C) as a result of different application of fluorescent compounds – FWA (F2) and UV absorber (F3) in textile finishing or textile care.

CONCLUSION

Primary prevention and early detection are essential regarding deduction of melanoma incidence. Considering prevention, especially in childhood and adolescence, it is necessary to apply sunscreening lotions and wear adequate clothing. Chemically bleached cotton and polyester/cotton blend fabrics are non-rateable for UV protection. Treatment with fluorescent compounds, FWA and UV absorber leads to its multifunctionality - high whiteness, neutralization of yellowness, giving to the fabric the high luminosity and protection against UV radiation. The fluorescence contributes to the high whiteness and beauty in optimal concentration. In the range of higher concentration quenching of fluorescence occurs, resulting in fabric yellowness. In wet state, regardless of applied water – sea or distilled, fabrics get darker, lowering its whiteness, but because of reflection from water, better UV protection is achieved. This phenomenon is more evident for Sea water, because of additional light scattering since it contains about 40% of inorganic salts. UV protection and optical effects of fabrics laundered in ECE and commercial detergent containing fluorescent compounds of stilbene type has been achieved by light conversion and cumulative addition through 9 washing cycles. For that reason, it is to suggest application of these compounds for prevention of skin cancer incidence, especially in commercial detergent formulation for protection of wider population.

ACKNOWLEDGMENTS

The authors would like to acknowledge the University of Zagreb for financial support to research “Optical and Protective Potential of Fluorescent Compounds in Cotton Material Finishing and Care” (KFPI 1, TP1.89).

REFERENCES

[1] Robins P, and Perez M. (1966). *Understanding melanoma*; *The Skin Cancer Foundation,* New York.

[2] Šitum M. (2012) Melanoma. Chapter 57 in Guidliness in common dermatoses and skin cancers diagnostics and treatments (in Croatian: Smjernice u dijagnostici i liječenju najčešćih dermatoza i tumora kože). Naklada Slap, Jastrebarsko.

[3] Tarbuk, A., Grancarić A. M., Šitum, M. and Martinis M: UV Clothing and Skin Cancer, *Collegium Antropologicum*. 34 (2010) 179-183.

[4] Armstrong, B. K., Kricker, A. (1993). How much melanoma is caused by sun exposure? *Melanoma Res* 3 (6), 395-401.

[5] Berwick, M., Armstrong, B. K., Ben-Porat, L., Fine, J., Kricker, A., Eberle, C., Barnhill, R. (2005) Sun exposure and mortality from melanoma. *J Natl Cancer Inst* 97(3), 195-199.

[6] Tarbuk, A., Grancarić A. M., and Šitum, M. (2014). Discrepancy of Whiteness and UV Protection in Wet State. *Collegium antropologicum*. 38, 4; 1110-1117.

[7] Lugović Mihić, L.; Bulat, V.; Šitum, M.; Čavka, V.; Krolo, I. (2008). Allergic hypersensitivity skin reactions following sun exposure. *Collegium antropologicum* 32 (suppl 2); 153-157.

[8] Šitum, M.; Buljan, M.; Čavka, V.; Bulat, V.; Krolo, I.; Lugović Mihić, L. (2008). Skin changes in the elderly people--how strong is the influence of the UV radiation on skin aging? *Collegium antropologicum* 32 (suppl 2); 9-13.

[9] Diffey, B. L. (1991). Solar ultraviolet radiation effects on biological systems. *Physics in Medicine and Biology* 36(3), 299-328.

[10] Eckhardt, C., H. Rohwer (2000). UV protector for cotton fabrics. *Textile Chemist and Colorist,* 32(4), 21-23.

[11] Hoffmann, K., Laperre, J., Avermaete, A., Altmeyer, P., Gambichler, T. (2001). Defined UV protection by apparel textiles, *Arch Dermatol.* 137(8),1089-1094.

[12] Gambichler, T., Rotterdam, S., Altmeyer, P., Hoffmann, K. (2001). Protection against ultraviolet radiation by commercial summer clothing: need for standardised testing and labelling, *BMC Dermatology* 1 (6).

[13] Reinert, G., Fuso, F., Hilfiker, R., Schmidt, E. (1997). UV-protecting properties of textile fabrics and their improvement. *Textile Chemist and Colorist* 29(12), 36-43.

[14] Gies, P. H., Roy, C. R., Toomey, S., Mclennan, A. (1998). Protection against solar ultraviolet radiation, *Mutation Research* 422, 15-22.

[15] Grancarić, A.M., Tarbuk, A., and Botteri, L. (2014). Light Conversion and Scattering in UV Protective Textiles. *AUTEX research journal.* 14 (4), 1-12.

[16] Grancarić, A. M., Tarbuk, A., Dumitrescu, I., Bišćan J. (2006). UV Protection of Pretreated Cotton – Influence of FWA's Fluorescence, *AATCC Review* 6(4), 44-48.

[17] Tarbuk, A., Grancarić, A.M., Jančijev, I., Sharma, S. (2006). Protection against UV radiation using a modified polyester fabric, *Tekstil* 55 (8), 383-394.

[18] Hilfiker, R., Kaufmann, W., Reinert, G., Schmidt, E. (1996). Improving sun protection factors of fabrics by applying UV- absorbers. *Text. Res. J.* 66(2), 61-70.

[19] Algaba, I., Riva, A., Crews, P. C. (2004). Influence of Fiber Type and Fabric Porosity on the UPF of Summer Fabrics, *AATCC Review*, 4(2), 26-31.

[20] Dobnik Dubrovski P., Dumitrescu J., Zabetakis A. (2004). Special Finishing Treatments and UPF improvement; in Book of Proceedings, 2nd International Textile, Clothing & Design conference – Magic World of Textiles, (Ed. Z. Dragčević), Dubrovnik, 3-6 October 2004, 340-346.

[21] Grancarić, A.M., Penava, Ž., Tarbuk, A. (2005) UV Protection of Cotton – the Influence of Weaving Structure, Hemijska industrija (*Serbian Society of Chemical Industry Journal*) 59(9-10), 230-234.

[22] Grancarić, A. M.; Tarbuk, A.; Marković, L. (2007). UV Protection with Zeolite Treated Cotton Knitted Fabric - The Influence of Yarn Linear Density; Buletinul Institutului Politehnic din Iasi. LIII (LVII) (5); 441-446.

[23] Grancarić, A. M., Tarbuk, A. (2009). EDA Modified PET Fabric Treated with Activated Natural Zeolite Nanoparticles, Materials Technology: *Advan. Performance Materials,* 24 (1); 58-63.

[24] Grancarić, A. M., Tarbuk, A., Kovaček, I. (2009). Nanoparticles of Activated Natural Zeolite on Textiles for Protection and Therapy, *Chem. Ind. & Chem. Engineering Quarterly.* 15(4), 203-210.

[25] Cox Crews P., Zhou Y. (2004). The effect of wetness on the UVR transmission of woven fabrics. *AATCC. Review*, 4(8), 41-43.

[26] Riva, A., Algaba, I., Prieto, R. (2007). Optical Brightening Agents Based on Stilbene and Distyryl Biphenyl for the Improvement of Ultraviolet Protection of Cotton Fabrics, *Tekstil* 56 (1), 1-6

[27] Saravanan, D.: UV protection textile materials, *AUTEX Research Journal* 7 (2007) 53-62

[28] Grancarić, A. M., Tarbuk, A. and McCall D. (2007). Surface Modification of Polyester Fabric with Tribomechanical-activated Natural Zeolite (TMAZ) Nanoparticles, *Polimeri* 28 (4); 219-224.

[29] Zhou Y., Cox Crews P., (1998). Effect of OBAs and repeated launderings on UVR transmission through fabrics. *Textile Chemist and Colorist* 30 (11), 19-24.

[30] Das, B. R. (2010) UV Radiation Protective Clothing. *The Open Textile Journal* 3, 14-21.

[31] Kim, J., Stone, J., Crews, P., Shelley, M. and Hatch, K. L. (2004). Improving Knit Fabric UPF Using Consumer Laundry Products: A Comparison of Results Using Two Instruments, *Family and Consumer Sciences Research Journal* 3, 141-158.

[32] Dekanić, T., Pušić, T., Soljačić I. Impact of artificial light on optical and protective effects of cotton after washing with detergent containing fluorescent compounds, *Tenside Surf. Det.* 51 (2014) 5, 451-459, doi: TS110329 – 16.7.14 dk/stm köthen

[33] Stanford, D. G., Georgouras, K. E. and Pailthorpe, M. T. (1995). The effect of laundering on the sun protection afforded by a summer weight garment, *Journal of the European Academy of Dermatology and Venereology* 5, 28-30.

[34] Tang, E., Cheng, G., Pang, X., Ma, X., Xing, F. (2006). Synthesis of nano-ZnO/poly(methyl methacrylate) composite microsphere through emulsion polymerization and its UV-shielding property, *Colloid and Polymer Science* 284 (4), 422-428.

[35] Farouk, A., Textor, T. Schollmeyer, E. Tarbuk, A. Grancarić, A. M. (2010). Sol-gel Derived Inorganic-organic Hybrid Polymers Filled with ZnO Nanoparticles as Ultraviolet Protection Finish for Textiles, *AUTEX research journal* 10 (8); 58-63.

[36] Sundaresan, K., Sivakumar A., Vigneswaran, C., Ramachandran, T. (2012). Influence of nano titanium dioxide finish, prepared by sol-gel technique, on the ultraviolet protection, antimicrobial, and self-cleaning characteristics of cotton fabrics, *Journal of Industrial Textiles* 41 (3), 259-277.

[37] Xin, J. H., Daoud, W. A., Kong, Y. Y. (2004). A new approach to UV-blocking treatment for cotton fabrics. *Text Res* J 74:97–10.

[38] Ranby, B., Rabek, J. F. (1975). *Photodegradation, Photo-oxidation and Photostabilization of Polymers,* John Wiley, (London, New York, Sydney and Toronto), 6-27.

[39] Grancarić A. M., Soljačić, I. (1980). Einflus der Konzentration optischer Aufheller auf Fluorescenz und Weissgrad von Baumwollgeweben, *Melliand Textilberichte* 61, 242-245.

[40] Lautenschlager, S., Wulf, H.. and Pittelkow, M. R.: Photoprotection, *The Lancet* 370 (2007) 528-537.

[41] Dekanić, T.; Pušić, T.; Soljačić, I. (2014). Light fastness of cotton optical and UV protection effects, *Book of Proceedings of the 7th International Textile*, Clothing &

Design Conference, Zagreb, University of Zagreb, *Faculty of Textile Technology*, 183-188.

[42] Pušić, T.; Tarbuk, A.; Dekanić, T. (2015). Bio-innovation in cotton scouring - acid and neutral pectinases. *Fibres & Textiles in Eastern Europe*. 23 (109), 1; 98-103.

[43] Tarbuk, A., Grancarić, A.M. Leskovac M. (2014). Novel cotton cellulose by cationisation during the mercerisation process - *Part 1: Chemical and morphological changes, Cellulose* 21 (3); 2167-2179.

[44] Tarbuk, A.; Pušić, T.; Jukić, M. Optimizing in cotton bioscouring with acid and neutral pectinases. *Tekstil* 62 (2013) 9-10; 353-360.

In: Encyclopedia of Dermatology (6 Volume Set)
Editor: Meghan Pratt

ISBN: 978-1-63483-326-4

Chapter 72

THE POTENTIAL OF MYCOSPORINE-LIKE AMINO ACIDS AS UV-SUNSCREENS

***Rajesh P. Rastogi*[1], *Ravi R Sonani*[1], *Datta Madamwar*[1] *and Aran Incharoensakdi*[2,*]**

[1]BRD School of Biosciences, Vadtal Road, Satellite Campus, Sardar Patel University, Anand, Gujarat, India
[2]Laboratory of Cyanobacterial Biotechnology, Department of Biochemistry, Faculty of Science, Chulalongkorn University, Bangkok, Thailand

ABSTRACT

Strong ultraviolet (UV) radiation is one of the most lethal and carcinogenic exogenous agents that can interact with and alter the normal life processes by means of its direct or indirect damaging effects. Mycosporine-like amino acids (MAAs) are important 'multipurpose' small biomolecules that provide protection from intense UV radiation without producing the reactive oxygen species (ROS). A number of MAAs have been reported from different taxonomic groups. MAAs have great potential in photoprotection and genome maintenance by minimizing the cellular damage from UV-induced ROS and thymine dimer formation. Moreover, due to strong UV-absorbing/screening function, photo-induction, strong antioxidant properties and resistance to abiotic stressors, MAAs are considered as natural photoprotectants that may be biotechnologically exploited in cosmetics and other pharmaceutical industries. In the present article, an attempt has been made to critically review and highlight the recent updates on various MAAs with respect to their function as potential UV-sunscreens.

Keywords: Mycosporine-like amino acids, UV radiation, oxidative stress, photoprotectants, sunscreens

* Corresponding author: Tel.: +66 2 218 5422; fax: +66 2 218 5418 (A. Incharoensakdi), E-mail: aran.i@chula.ac.th (A. Incharoensakdi).

1. INTRODUCTION

The increase in short wavelength solar ultraviolet (UV) radiation on the Earth's atmosphere due to anthropogenically increased ozone depleting substances has aroused tremendous concern about its negative impacts on living organisms in both aquatic as well as terrestrial ecosystems. UV radiation (280-400 nm) may affect several biochemical and physiological processes leading to loss of normal life functionality of photosynthetic and non-photosynthetic organisms including human beings (Rastogi and Sinha, 2011a). It has been established that solar UV-A radiation (315-400 nm) has less direct effects on living systems since native DNA of living organisms cannot absorb UV-A. However, UV-A can indirectly affect the cellular function by the generation of reactive oxygen species (ROS) via photosensitizing reactions. In contrast, UV-B (280-315 nm) radiation has direct effects on key cellular machinery such as proteins and nucleic acids (Rastogi et al., 2010a). The short wavelength solar UV radiation may cause protein modification, membrane disruption, enzyme inactivation, generation of DNA lesions, alteration of transcription and translation process, mutagenesis and several other external effects such as sunburn and skin cancer (Bruce and Brodland, 2000; Rastogi et al., 2010a).

Moreover, several defense mechanisms have been reported in diverse organisms to counteract the harmful effects of UV radiation (Rastogi and Sinha, 2011b). Biosynthesis of certain UV-absorbing/screening compounds in different organisms is considered as an effective mode of defense mechanisms to reduce the damaging effects of solar UV radiation (Karentz et al., 1991; Rastogi et al., 2010b; Carreto and Carignan, 2011). Mycosporine-like amino acids (MAAs) are considered as prominent photoprotectants that provide photoprotection against harmful UV radiation (Cockell and Knowland, 1999; Oren and Gunde-Cimerman, 2007). In the present chapter, we summarize the eco-biological importance of the biologically relevant molecules MAAs, with special emphasis on their UV-screening or photoprotective functions.

2. SOLAR ULTRAVIOLET RADIATION AND BIOLOGICAL EFFECTS

In the past few decades, loss in stratospheric ozone layer due to anthropogenically released ozone depleting substances such as chlorofluorocarbons (CFCs) and reactive nitrogen species such as nitrous oxide (N_2O) has generated tremendous concern about the increasing level of short wavelength UV radiations reaching the Earth's atmosphere (Ravishankara et al., 2009; Manney el., 2011; Cabrol et al., 2014; Williamson et al., 2014). In all the groups of UV radiation (280–400 nm), UV-B radiation produces more adverse effects on diverse habitats, despite the fact that most of the extraterrestrial UV-B is absorbed by the stratospheric ozone layer (McKenzie et al., 2003). It has been established that UV-C (100-280 nm) radiation is quantitatively absorbed by oxygen and ozone in the Earth's atmosphere, and does not show any harmful effects on our ecosystems. Furthermore, UV-A (315-400 nm) radiation has low efficacy in inducing the DNA damage, as it is not absorbed by native DNA molecules; however, it can damage DNA via indirect photosensitizing reactions by the formation of reactive oxygen species (Rastogi et al., 2010a). The data obtained from European Light Dosimeter Network (Eldonet) dosimeters (Häder et al., 1999) have revealed the extreme UV-B irradiance in different parts of the Earth (Jacovides et al., 2009; Cabrol et al., 2014). Several other environmental factors such as aerosols and various tropospheric pollutants, cloud cover, sun-angle and surface reflectants also affect the intensity of UV-B radiation reaching the Earth's surface to a certain extent (Madronich et al., 1998). UV radiation also induces single- and/or double-strand DNA breaks in various organisms (Rastogi et al., 2010a; Rastogi and Sinha, 2011a).

Moreover, the global climate change and increase in harmful short wavelength UV radiation can affect the normal life processes of all organisms inhabiting the aquatic or terrestrial habitats (Häder et al., 2014, 2015). In addition to UV effects on photosynthetic life (Rastogi et al., 2013; Rastogi et al., 2014a), a number of UV-induced effects such as occurrence of melanoma and non-melanoma skin cancer, sunburn, photo-allergy, eye disorders and immune suppression have also been reported in humans (McAteer et al., 1998; Lima-Bessa et al., 2008) (Figure 1). Solar UV-B radiation damages cellular DNA inducing mainly cyaclobutane purine/pyrimidine dimers (CPDs) and pyrimidine (6–4) pyrimidone photoproducts (6–4 PPs) and their Dewar isomers (Rastogi et al., 2010a). DNA double strand breaks (DSBs) may lead to loss of genetic information. Increased production of UV-induced ROS may alter the configuration of cell structure, lipids, proteins and DNA molecules, all of which are the cause of a number of human diseases (Valko et al., 2007). It has been shown that CPDs inhibit the progress of microbial and mammalian DNA polymerases (Britt, 1999). Moreover, UV-A-induced production of CPDs has also been observed in bacteria as well as in eukaryotic cells (Douki et al., 2003; Courdavault et al., 2004; Rastogi et al., 2014b). In response to detrimental effects of UV radiation, some organisms have developed certain defense mechanisms such as DNA repair and synthesis of UV-protective compounds to mitigate the harmful effects of short wavelength solar radiation (Rastogi et al., 2014c).

3. UV-Absorbing Compounds

A number of UV-absorbing/screening biomolecules such as mycosporines/mycosporine-like amino acids (MAAs), scytonemin, melanins, carotenoids, flavonoids, parietin and usnic acid, have been reported to be synthesized by diverse organisms (Figure 2) to counteract the detrimental effects of solar UV-B radiation (Rastogi et al., 2010b). There have been a number of reviews about diverse classes of photoprotective compounds from natural sources (Karsten et al., 2000; Bjerke et al., 2002; Gauslaa and McEvoy, 2005; Rastogi et al., 2010b; Rastogi and Incharoensakdi, 2013; 2014a, 2014b, 2014c); however, their application as photoprotectants and development of cosmeceutical products has only partially been elucidated. In the present review, we focus on the occurrence, biosynthesis and commercial application as potential sunscreens of the important UV-absorbing/screening compounds, MAAs from various sources.

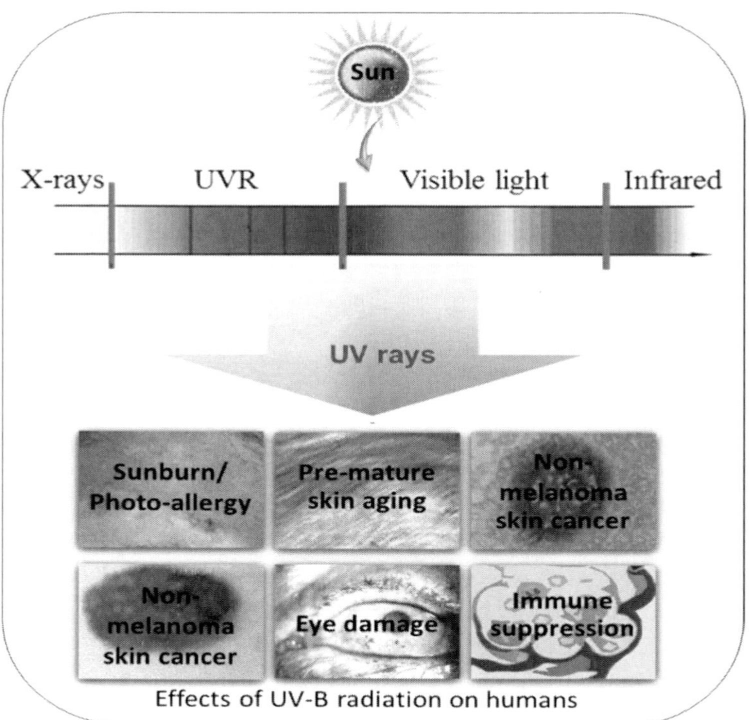

Figure 1. Effects of solar UV radiation on human health (details in text).

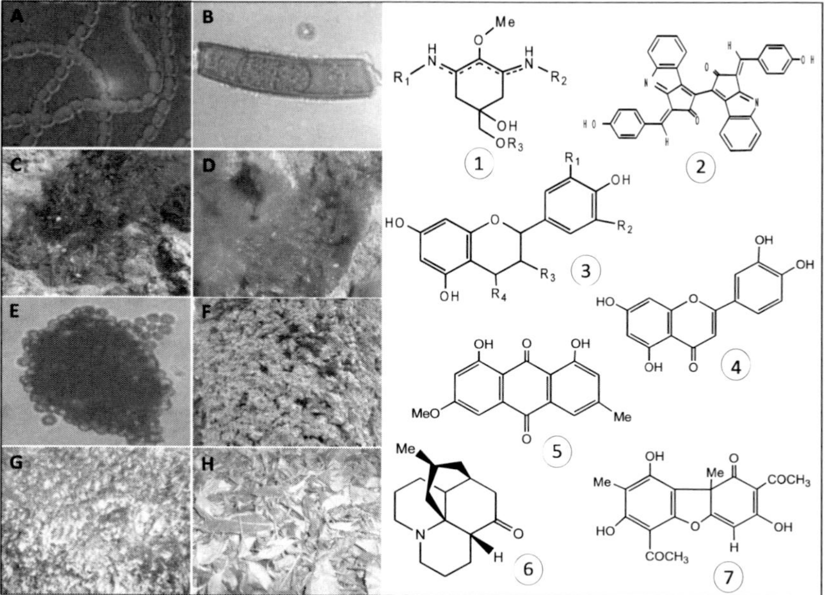

Figure 2. UV-absorbing/screening compounds (1 to 7) from different plant sources (A, B-The cyanobacterium *Anabaena* sp. and *Lynnbya* sp., respectively; C-Brown algae; D-Green algae; E-Fungi; F-Lichens; G-Bryophytes; H-tea leaves) [1 to 7: general structure of MAA, scytonemin, higher plant flavonoid, luteolin, parietin, lycopodine, and usnic acid, respectively].

3.1. Mycosporine-like Amino Acids

Mycosporine-like amino acids are small, colorless and highly hydrophilic compounds. They consist of cyclohexenone or cyclohexenimine chromophores, conjugated with the nitrogen substituent of an amino acid or its imino alcohol. The ring system of MAA includes a glycine subunit at the 3C atom, though some MAAs also contain sulfate esters or glycosidic linkages through the imine substituents (Wu Won et al., 1997). The UV absorption spectra of different MAAs differ due to variations in the attached side groups and nitrogen substituents (Böhm et al., 1995; Wu Won et al., 1997). Moreover, the precise stereostructure of MAAs (except palythine and palythene), including amino acids substituents is not completely elucidated. MAAs are extremely hydrophilic due to their zwitter ionic form derived from the amino acid substitution. Further hydrophilicity can also be increased by modification with sulfonic acids or sugar molecules (Böhm et al., 1995; Wu Won et al., 1997). Presently, more than 25 MAAs (Figure 3) have been reported from diverse organisms; however, a number of other UV-absorbing/screening compounds with potential application as UV photoprotectants remain to be explored from nature.

3.2. Occurrence and Distribution of MAAs

Among various UV-photoprotectant biomolecules, the biosynthesis of different MAAs has been reported from diverse taxonomic groups (Sinha et al., 2007; Rastogi et al., 2010b) (Table 1). Cyanobacteria are the most dominant photoautotrophs that can synthesize a range of different MAAs (Shibata, 1969). The MAAs shinorine and porphyra-334 have been found to be the most dominant MAAs in several species of terrestrial or fresh/marine water cyanobacteria (Karsten and Garcia-Pichel, 1996; Sinha et al., 2003; Volkmann et al., 2006; Rastogi et al., 2010b; Chuang et al., 2014; Rastogi et al., 2012). Rastogi and Incharoensakdi (2014a, b, c) have isolated and characterized some primary MAAs from different cyanobacteria inhabiting diverse habitats (Figure 4). Several MAAs were isolated from different species/strains of cyanobacteria inhabiting the hot springs (Rastogi et al., 2012). Two novel glycosylated MAAs such as a pentose-bound porphyra-334 derivative (MW 478 Da; UVλ_{max}: 335 nm) and other MAAs (MW1050 Da; UVλ_{max}: 312 and 340 nm) consisting of two distinct chromophores of 3-aminocyclohexen-1-one and 1,3-diaminocyclohexen and two pentose and hexose sugars were identified in *Nostoc commune* (Matsui et al., 2011). Recently, the glycosylated MAAs such as glycosylated porphyra-334 (MW 508 Da; UVλ_{max}: 334 nm) and palythine-threoninehave (MW 612 Da; UVλ_{max}: 322 nm) have also been reported in the cyanobacterium *Nostoc commune* (Nazifi et al., 2013).

Besides cyanobacteria, a range of MAAs have also been reported in cyanobacterial lichens (Coba et al., 2009), micro/macro algae and animals (Sinha et al., 2007) Table 1). A number of microalgae/phytoplankton such as diatoms (Riegger and Robinson, 1997; Hernando et al., 2002; Ingalls et al., 2010), dinoflagellates (Klisch and Häder, 2000; Banaszack and Trench, 2001; Laurion et al., 2004; Banaszak et al., 2006; Laurion and Roy, 2009), chlorophytes (Gröniger and Häder, 2002; Llewellyn and Airs, 2010; Rastogi and Incharoensakdi, 2013), and prymnesiophytes (Marchant et al., 1991; Riegger and Robinson, 1997; Hannach and Sigleo, 1998) have been found to produce different MAAs. Several species of macroalgae (Karsten et al., 1998a; Hoyer et al., 2002) belonging to chlorophyceae

(Han and Han, 2005), rhodophyceae (Kräbs et al., 2004; Coba et al., 2009; Yuan et al., 2009; Cardozo et al., 2011) and phaeophyceae have been reported to synthesize an array of MAAs and other UV-absorbing compounds.

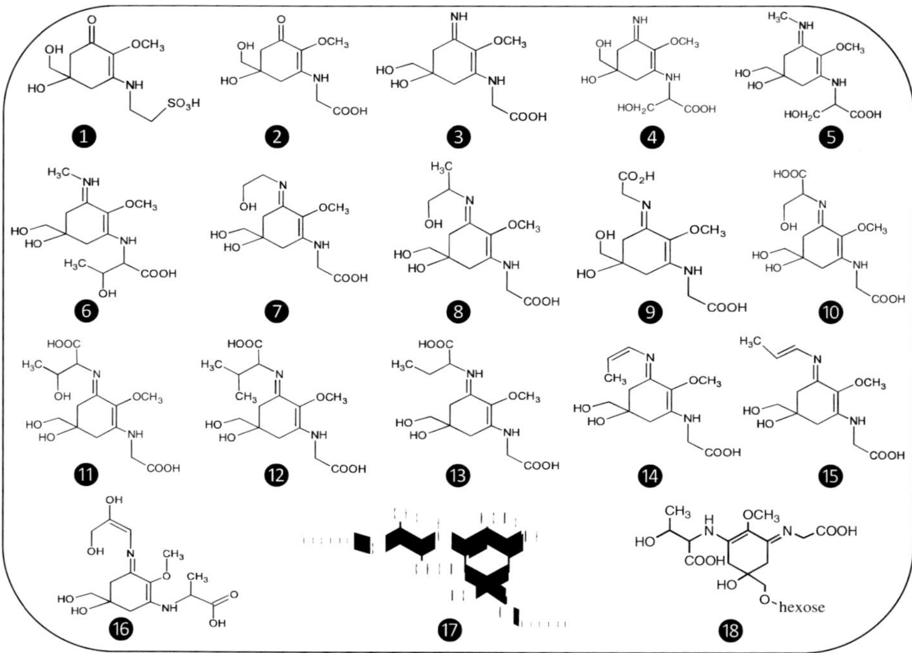

Figure 3. Chemical structure of some important MAAs found in different taxonomic groups. [1 to 18: Mycosporine-taurine, Mycosporine-glycine, Palythine, Palythine-serine, Mycosporine-methylamine-serine, Mycosporine-methylamine-threonine, Asterina-330, Palythinol, Mycosporine-2-glycine, Shinorine, Porphyra-334, Mycosporine-glycine-valine, Palythenic acid, Usujirene, Palythene, Euhalothece-362, Glycosylated palythine-threonine and Glycosylated porphyra-334, respectively].

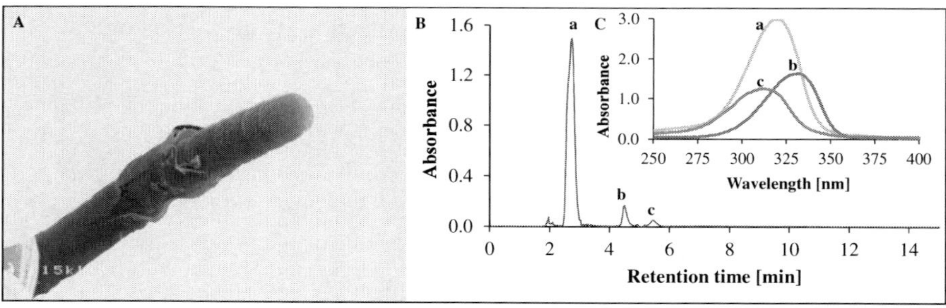

Figure 4. The cyanobacterium *Lyngbya* sp. (A) and high performance liquid chromatograph (B) showing the UV-absorption maxima (B-inset) of some MAAs such as palythine (a, UV λ_{max}: 320 nm), asterina-330 (b, UV λ_{max}: 330 nm) and an unknown MAA, M-312 (c, UV λ_{max}: 312) (Adapted from Rastogi and Incharoensakdi, 2014c).

Table 1. Occurrence and distribution of some common MAAs in different taxonomic groups

Taxonomic groups	Mycosporine-like amino acids												
	AS	**MG**	**M2G**	**MT**	**MGV**	**PE**	**PR**	**PL**	**PT**	**SH**	**US**	**DL**	**PS**
Cyanobacteria	+	+	+	+		+	+	+	+	+		+	
Green algae	+	+					+	+	+	+			
Brown algae	+	+					+	+	+	+			
Red algae	+	+				+	+	+	+	+			
Microalgae/phytoplankton	+	+	+	+	+	+	+	+	+	+	+		+
Copepods	+	+				+	+	+	+	+	+		
Corals	+	+	+			+	+	+	+	+			
Krill	+	+			+	+	+	+	+	+			
Amphipod	+	+			+	+	+	+	+	+			
Molluscs	+	+	+			+	+	+	+	+			
Fish	+	+			+	+	+	+	+	+			
Sea Anemones	+	+	+	+	+	+	+		+	+			
Sponge	+	+	+				+	+	+	+			

(For details please see the references, Sinha et al., 2007; Rastogi et al., 2014c; Rastogi et al., 2014 a, Rastogi et al., 2010b for details and references therein) [AS, asterina-330; MG,mycosporine-glycine; M2G, mycosporine-2-glycine; MT, mycosporine-taurine; MGV, mycosporineglycine-valine; PE, palythene; PR, porphyra-334; PL, palythinol; PT, palythine; SH, shinorine; US, usurijene; DL, dehydroxylusujirene; PS, palythine-serine]

The accumulation of several MAAs have also been reported in different animals such as arthropods, rotifers, molluscs, fishes, cnidarians, tunicates, eubacteriobionts, poriferans, nemertineans, echinodermates, platythelminthes, polychaetes, bryozoans and protozoans (Sinha et al., 2007). However, it has been thought that MAAs are not directly synthesized by animals, but rather accumulated in these animals as a result of dietary food acquisition (Carroll and Shick, 1996; Newman et al., 2000).

3.3. Regulation of MAAs Biosynthesis

The biosynthesis of MAAs in fungi and cyanobacteria are supposed to occur via the first part of the shikimate pathway, 3-dehydroquinate (DHQ) formed during the early part of the shikimate pathway. The DHQ molecule is assumed to act as a precursor for the synthesis of primary MAA, via gadusol or deoxygadusol (Portwich and Garcia-Pichel, 2003). Moreover, the main steps of the MAAs biosynthetic pathway and their genetic basis have recently been elucidated in *Anabaena variabilis* ATCC 29413 (Balskus and Walsh, 2010). A cluster of four genes (Ava_3858-3855) was found in the cyanobacterium *Anabaena variabilis*, responsible for the biosynthesis of a MAA shinorine using the common pentose-phosphate-pathway intermediate sedoheptulose-7-phosphate via 4-deoxygadusol (Balskus and Walsh, 2010; Spence et al., 2012). The dehydroquinate synthase homologue Ava_3858 and the O-methyltransferase Ava_3857 was found to convert the precursor into 4-deoxygadusol (4-DG), and the ATP-grasp homologue Ava_3856 converts the 4-DG as well as glycine into mycosporine-glycine (M-Gly) (Figure 5). The MAA M-Gly is converted into shinorine with addition of serine molecule catalyzed by a nonribosomal peptide synthetase (NRPS) encoded by Ava_3855 (Figure 5). Recently, the MAA biosynthetic gene cluster has also been reported in some other cyanobacteria such as *Nostoc punctiforme* (Gao and Garcia-Pichel, 2011) and *Aphanothece halophytica* (Waditee-Sirisattha et al., 2014). In *Nostoc punctiforme* ATCC 29133, the four gene cluster such as NpR5600, NpR5599, NpR5598, and NpF5597 was shown to catalyze the biosynthesis of M-Gly in a similar manner as was found in *A. variabilis*. However, the NpF5597 was found to encode D-Ala-D-Ala ligase and the direction of transcription of NpF5597 was opposite to those of NpR5600 and NpR5598 (Gao and Garcia-Pichel, 2011). In the halotolerant cyanobacterium *Aphanothece halophytica*, the MAA gene cluster was capable of synthesizing mycosporine-2-glycine. A unique MAA core 4-DG-synthesizing gene was separated from three other genes. The identified genes, Ap3857, Ap3856, and Ap3855, were homologous to Ava_ 3857/NpR5599, Ava_3856/NpR5598, and NpF5597, respectively. It was found that *A. halophytica* does not contain a gene homologous to Ava_3855 encoding NRPS, but contains a gene homologous to NpF5597 encoding D-Ala-D-Ala ligase (Waditee-Sirisattha et al., 2013).

3.4. MAA Biosynthesis under Different Abiotic Factors

A number of abiotic factors, such as short wavelength UV radiations, temperature, desiccation, light/dark periods, salt concentrations and various nutrients affect the biosynthesis of MAAs in cyanobacteria and other organisms (Rastogi et al., 2010b). Several studies have established the increased production of MAAs under different wavebands of UV radiation in cyanobacteria (Sinha et al., 2003; Singh et al., 2008a; Rastogi et al., 2010c; Rastogi and Incharoensakdi, 2014a, b, c; Rastogi and Incharoensakdi, 2013, 2015) and micro/macroalgae or phytoplanktons (Riegger and Robinson, 1997; Klisch and Häder, 2002). The production of MAAs in various organisms are highly responsive to UV-B radiation (Sinha et al., 2001; Singh et al., 2008a; Rastogi and Incharoensakdi, 2015; 2014a, c) (Figure 6); howevr, UV-A induced production of MAAs has also been reported in different organisms (Kräbs et al., 2004; Rastogi et al., 2010c). Korbee et al. (2005a) studied the accumulation of MAAs in *Porphyra leucosticte* and found the favorable role of blue light in the accumulation of porphyra-334, palythine and asterina-330 in contrast to the accumulation of shinorine which was observed under white, green, yellow or red light. Contrary to light period, the biosynthesis of MAAs was found to decrease under dark period (Rastogi et al., 2010c; Rastogi and Incharoensakdi, 2015), suggesting an energy-dependent process of MAA synthesis. The biosynthesis of MAAs is also affected under different nutrient conditions (Rastogi et al., 2010b). A remarkable decrease in MAA content was found under nitrogen limitations in the marine dinoflagellates (Litchman et al., 2002). Induction of some MAAs in *Anabaena variabilis* PCC 7937 was caused by salt and ammonium in a concentration-dependent manner (Singh et al., 2008b). Increased biosynthesis of certain photoprotective compounds under enriched ammonium concentrations was also found in the red alga *Porphyra* sp. (Korbee et al., 2005b, Peinado et al., 2004). Bio-conversion of a primary MAA into a secondary MAA was found under sulfur deficiency in *A. variabilis* PCC 7937 (Singh et al., 2010). High concentration of certain UV-absorbing compounds has also been reported under desiccation (Jiang et al., 2008) and warm temperature (Karsten et al., 1998) in the Rhodophytes *Chondrus crispus* and *Porphyra haitanensis*, respectively. Moreover, MAAs biosynthetic pathway may be regulated by multiple environmental signals.

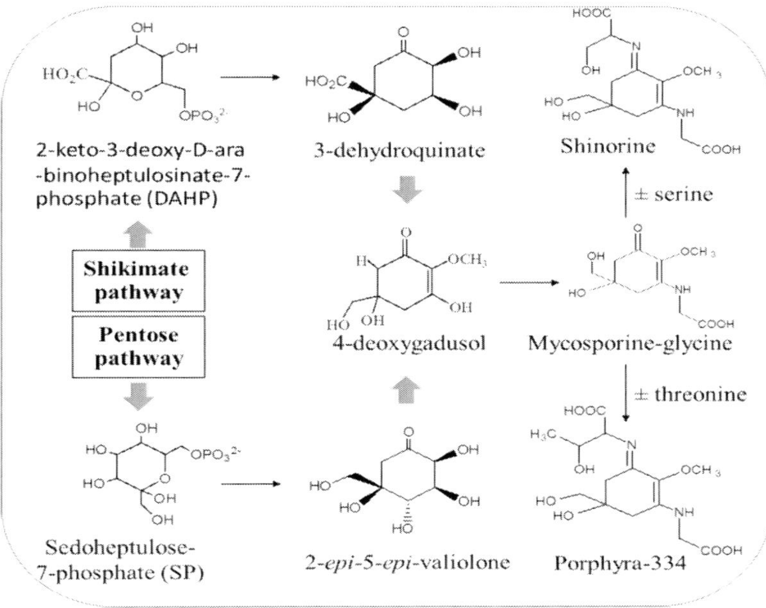

Figure 5. A proposed pathway of the biosynthesis of some primary MAAs (Adapted from Balskus and Walsh, Rastogi et al., 2010b, 2010; Spence et al., 2012) (details in text).

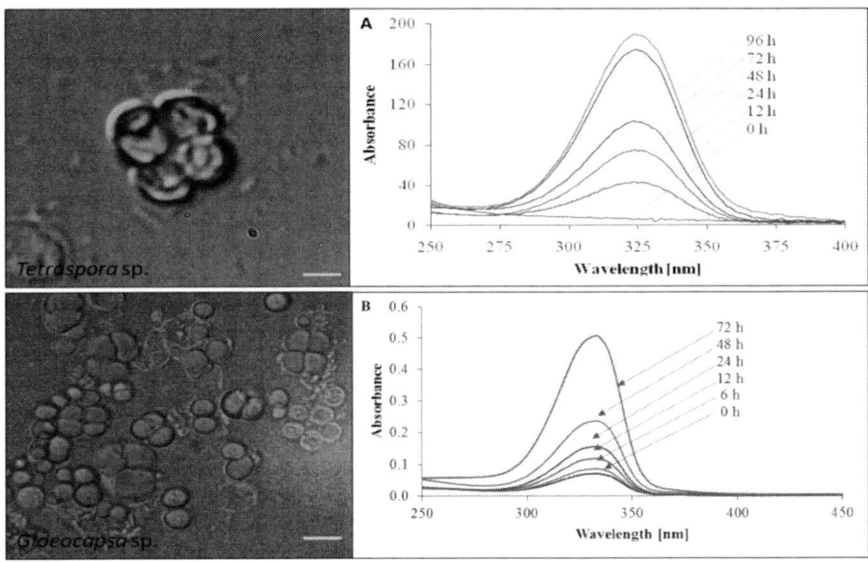

Figure 6. Induction of a 324 nm-MAA (A) and shinorine (B) after different durations of UV-B irradiation in the green alga *Tetraspora* sp. and Gloeocapsa sp. (Adapted from Rastogi and Incharoensakdi, 2013, 2014a).

4. MAAs As Sunscreens: Dominant Role in Photoprotection

Mycosporine-like amino acids (MAAs) are well-known UV-absorbing/screening compounds for their crucial role in photoprotection. Several properties such as strong UV-absorption maxima, high molar extinction coefficients, competence to dissipate absorbed radiation as heat without producing reactive oxygen species (ROS), UV-induction and stability under different physicochemical factors such as UV radiation, heat, pH, strong oxidizing agent and different organic solvents strongly support the MAAs as photoprotective compounds (Gröniger and Häder, 2000; Whitehead and Hedges, 2005; Conde et al., 2007; Rastogi and Incharoensakdi, 2014a, 2014c). It has been shown that MAAs provide protection from UV radiation not only to their producers, but also to primary and secondary consumers through the food chain (Helbling et al., 2002), and may be considered as a broad-spectrum UV absorbers/protectors. As discussed above, UV radiation can promote the occurrence of sunburn on skin cells; the application of UV-absorbing compound may provide protection against intense solar radiation or sunburns (Drolet and Connor, 1992). MAAs may protect the skin cells from UV-induced cell death. Recently, Rastogi and Incharoensakdi (2013) investigated for the first time the photoprotective activities of 324 nm-MAA and 322 nm-MAA isolated from a green microalga, *Tetraspora* sp., against UV radiation. It was found that the MAA porphyra-334 along with shinorine can suppress UV-induced aging in human skin (Daniel et al., 2004). The MAAs were found to protect eggs of the sea hare *Aplysia dactylomela* from UV radiation (Carefoot et al., 1998). The MAAs such as shinorine (SH), porphyra-334 (P-334) and mycosporine-glycine were found to protect the human fibroblast cells from UVR-induced cell death (Oyamada et al., 2008).

Some MAAs have been reported to have strong antioxidant or free radical scavenging capacity (Coba et al., 2007a, 2007b; Oren and Gunde-Cimerman, 2007) (Figure 7A). The MAA mycosporine-glycine (MG) was found to protect biological systems against photodynamic damage by quenching singlet oxygen with a high efficiency (Suh et al., 2003). Some MAAs such as porphyra-334 and shinorine showed high antioxidant activity against free radicals (Coba et al., 2007a, 2007b) generated from UV radiation (Oren and Gunde-Cimerman, 2007). The antioxidant activities of the MAAs M-gly and usujilene have also been reported to inhibit lipid peroxidation (Nakayama et al., 1999; Suh et al., 2003). The presence of the glycosylated MAAs with radical scavenging activity has been reported in the cyanobacterium *Nostoc commune* (Matsui et al., 2011). Recently, Rastogi and Incharoensakdi (2014a) have found the efficacy of MAAs (shinorine + M-307) from *Gloeocapsa* sp. as a potential sunscreen. The MAAs (palythine + asterina + M-312) isolated from *Lyngbya* sp. were found to act as strong radical scavenger (Rastogi and Incharoensakdi, 2014c).

Recently, some MAAs have been investigated for their potential role in genome maintainance (Rastogi, 2010). The UV-absorbing compound isolated from a red alga *Porphyra yezoensis* was found to block the production of thymine dimer (T<>T) (Misonou et al., 2003). Recently, Rastogi (2010) has also found the great efficacy of MAAs in reducing the most genotoxic and cytotoxic DNA lesions, CPD T<>T (Figure 7B). Moreover, some synthetic analogues of MAAs, such as tetrahydropyridine derivatives, have been developed for commercial application as suncare products (Bird et al., 1987; Chalmers et al., 1990; Coba et al., 2007b). Moreover, due to potent UV protecting capacity, MAAs can be a potential candidate for the commercial development of suncare products.

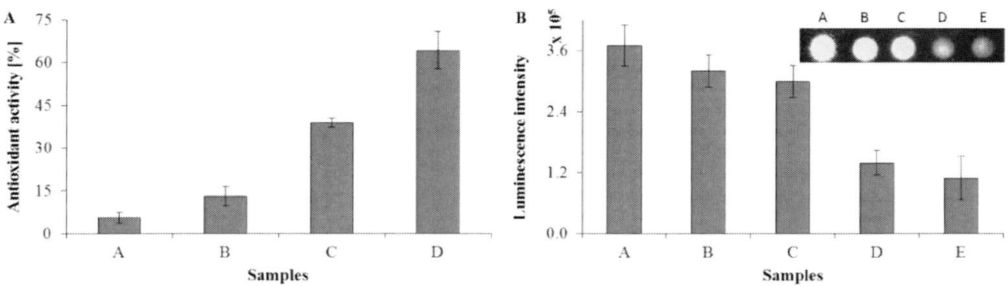

Figure 7. Free radical scavenging capacity of MAAs shinorine + M-307 (panel A) (adapted from Rastogi and Incharoensakdi, 2014a) and inhibition of thymine dimer formation (panel B: data not published). [in panel A; the samples contain 0.2(A), 0.4(B), 0.83(C) and 1.6 (D) mg/ml MAAs; in panel B; Control cells exposed to UV without (A) and with 0.05 (B), 0.1 (C), 0.25 (D) and 0.5 (E) mg/ml M-gly].

Conclusion

MAAs are multipurpose secondary compounds reported in a number of taxonomic groups. These compounds are highly stable against a number of physicochemical factors, act as strong antioxidants, and are able to prevent cellular as well as genomic damage resulting from UV-induced ROS. Several studies have established the anti-aging role of MAAs, minimizing the risk of skin cancer. Overall, MAAs can be considered as high value compounds that have great potential applications as natural photoprotectants and antioxidants that can be exploited in cosmetics and pharmaceutical industries for the development of novel *cosmeceuticals*.

Acknowledgments

Rajesh P. Rastogi is thankful to the University Grant Commission (UGC), New Delhi, India, for financial support in the form of Dr. D. S. Kothari Postdoctoral grant. Aran Incharoensakdi thanks Chulalongkorn University Ratchadaphiseksomphot Endowment Fund for financial support on the project "Value-added products and bioenergy from microalgae."

References

Balskus, EP; Walsh, CT. The genetic and molecular basis for sunscreen biosynthesis in cyanobacteria. *Science*, 2010, 329, 1653-1656.

Banaszack, AT; Trench, RK. Ultraviolet sunscreens in dinoflagellates. *Protist*, 2001, 152, 93-101.

Banaszak, AT; Santos, MG; LaJeunesse, TC; Lesser, MP. The distribution of mycosporine-like amino acids (MAAs) and the phylogenetic identity of symbiotic dinoflagellates in cnidarian hosts from the Mexican Caribbean. *J. Exp. Mar. Biol. Ecol.*, 2006, 337, 131-146.

Bird, G; Fitzmaurice, N; Dunlap, WC; Chalker, BE; Bandaranayake, WM. Sunscreen compositions and compounds for use therein. International patent application PCT/AU87/00330, publication no. WO 88/02251, 1987. Australian patent 595075. ICI Australia Operations Pty Ltd and Australian Institute of Marine Science, Townsville.

Bjerke, JW; Lerfall, K; Elvebakk, A. Effects of ultraviolet radiation and PAR on the content of usnic and divaricatic acids in two arctic-alpine lichens. *Photochem. Photobiol. Sci.*, 2002, 1, 678–685.

Böhm, GA; Pfleiderer, W; Böger, P; Scherer, S. Structure of a novel oligosaccharide-mycosporine-amino acid ultraviolet A/B sunscreen pigment from the terrestrial cyanobacterium *Nostoc* commune. *J. Biol. Chem.*, 1995, 270, 8536-8539.

Britt, AB. Molecular genetics of DNA repair in higher plants. *Trends Plant Sci.*, 1999, 4, 20-25.

Bruce, AJ; Brodland, DG. Overview of skin cancer detection and prevention for the primary care physician. *Mayo Clin. Ptoc.*, 2000, 75, 491-500.

Cabrol, NA; Feister, U; Häder, DP; Piazena, H; Grin, EA; Klein, A. Record solar UV irradiance in the Tropical Andes. *Environ. Toxicol.*, 2014, 2, 19.

Cardozo, KHM; Marques, LG; Carvalho VM; Carignan MO; Pinto E; Marinho-Soriano, E; Colepicolo, P. Analyses of photoprotective compounds in red algae from the Brazilian coast. *Braz. J. Pharmacogn.*, 2011, 21, 202-208.

Carefoot, TH; Harris, M; Taylor, BE; Donovan, D; Karentz, D. Mycosporine-like amino acids: possible UV protection in eggs of the sea hare *Aplysia dactylomela*. *Mar. Biol.*, 1998, 130, 389-396.

Carreto, JI; Carignan, MO. Mycosporine-Like amino acids: Relevant secondary metabolites. Chemical and ecological aspects. *Mar. Drugs*, 2011, 9, 387-446.

Carroll, AK; Shick, JM. Dietary accumulation of mycosporine-like amino acids (MAAs) by the green sea urchin (*Strongylocentrus droebachiensis*). *Mar. Biol.*, 1996, 124, 561–569.

Chalmers, PJ; Fitzmaurice, N; Rigg, DJ; Thang, SH; Bird, G. UV absorbing compounds and compositions. International Patent Application PCT/AU90/00078, publication no. WO 90/09995, 1990. Australian patent 653495. ICI Australia Operations Pty Ltd and Australian Institute of Marine Science, Townsville.

Chuang, LF; Chou, HN; Sung, PJ. Porphyra-334 isolated from the marine algae *Bangia atropurpurea*: Conformational performance for energy conversion. *Mar. drugs*, 2014 12, 4732-4740.

Coba, FDL; Aguilera, J; Figueroa, FL. Use of mycosporine-type amino acid porphyra-334 as an antioxidant. *Intl Patent WO2007/026035 A2* 2007a.

Coba, FDL; Aguilera, J; Figueroa, FL. Use of mycosporine-type aminoacid shinorine as an antioxidant. *Intl Patent WO2007/026038 A2* 2007b.

Coba, FDL; Aguilera, J; Figueroa, FL; de Gàlvez, MV; Herrera, E. Antioxidant activity of mycosporine-like amino acids isolated from three red macroalgae and one marine lichen. *J. Appl. Phycol.*, 2009, 21, 161-169.

Cockell, CS; Knowland, J. Ultraviolet radiation screening compounds. *Biol. Rev.*, 1999, 74, 311-345.

Conde, FR; Churio, MS; Previtali, CM. Experimental study of the excited-state properties and photostability of the mycosporine-like amino acid palythine in aqueous solution. *Photochem. Photobiol. Sci.*, 2007, 6, 669-674.

Courdavault, S; Baudouin, C; Charveron, M; Favier, A; Cadet, J; Douki, T. Larger yield of cyclobutane dimers than 8-oxo-7, 8-dihydroguanine in the DNA of UVA-irradiated human skin cells. *Mutation Res.*, 2004, 556, 135-142.

Daniel, S; Cornelia, S; Fred, Z. UV-A sunscreen from red algae for protection against premature skin aging. *Cosmet. Toilet. Manuf. Worldw.*, 2004, 139-143.

Douki, T; Reynaud-Angelin, A; Cadet, J; Sage, E. Bipyrimidine photoproducts rather than oxidative lesions are the main type of DNA damage involved in the genotoxic effects of solar UVA radiation. *Biochemistry*, 2003, 42, 9221-9226.

Drolet, BA; Connor, MJ. Sunscreens and the prevention of ultraviolet radiation-induced skin cancer. *J. Dermatol. Surg. Oncol.*, 1992, 18, 571-576.

Gao, Q; Garcia-Pichel, F. An ATP-grasp ligase involved in the last biosynthetic step of the iminomycosporine shinorine in *Nostoc punctiforme* ATCC 29133. *J. Bacteriol.*, 2011 193, 5923-5928.

Gauslaa, Y; McEvoy, M. Seasonal changes in solar radiation drive acclimation of the sun-screening compound parietin in the lichen *Xanthoria parietina*. *Basic. Appl. Ecol.*, 2005, 6, 75-82.

Gröniger, A; Häder, DP. Stability of mycosporine-like amino acids. *Recent Res. Devel. Photochem. Photobiol.*, 2000, 4, 247-252.

Gröniger, A; Häder, DP. Induction of the synthesis of an UVabsorbing substance in the green alga *Prasiola stipitata*. *J. Photochem. Photobiol. B.*, 2000, 66, 54-59.

Häder, DP; Williamson, CE; Wängberg, SÅ; Rautio, M; Rose, KC; Gao, K; Helbling, EW; Sinha RP; Worrest, R. Effects of UV radiation on aquatic ecosystems and interactions with other environmental factors. *Photochem. Photobiol. Sci.*, 2015, DOI: 10.1039/c4pp90035a.

Häder, DP; Villafañe, VE; Helbling, EW. Productivity of aquatic primary producers under global climate change. *Photochem. Photobiol. Sci.*, 2014, DOI: 10.1039/c3pp50418b.

Häder, DP; Lebert M; Marangoni R; Colombetti, G. ELDONET-European Light Dosimeter Network hardware and software. *J. Photochem. Photobiol. B.*, 1999, 52, 51-58.

Han, YS; Han, T. UV-B induction of UV-B protection in *Ulva pertusa* (chlorophyta). *J. Phycol.*, 2005, 41, 523-530.

Hannach, G; Sigleo, AC. Photoinduction of UV-absorbing compounds in six species of marine phytoplankton. *Mar. Ecol. Prog. Ser.*, 1998, 174, 207-222.

Helbling, EW; Menchi, CF; Villafañe, VE. Bioaccumulation and role of UV-absorbing compounds in two marine crustacean species from Patagonia, Argentina. *Photochem. Photobiol. Sci.*, 2002, 1, 820–825.

Hernando, M; Carreto, JI; Carignan, MO; Ferreyra, GA; Gross, C. Effects of solar radiation on growth and mycosporine-like amino acids content in *Thalassiosira* sp., an Antarctic diatom. *Polar Biol.*, 2002, 25, 12-20.

Hoyer, K; Karsten, U; Wiencke, C. Induction of sunscreen compounds in Antarctic macroalgae by different radiation conditions. *Mar. Biol.*, 2002, 141, 619-627.

Ingalls, AE; Whitehead, K; Bridoux, MC. Tinted windows: the presence of the UVabsorbing compounds called mycosporine-like amino acids embedded in the frustules of marine diatoms. *Geochim. Cosmochim. Acta*, 2010, 74, 104-115.

Jacovides, DO; Tymvios, FS; Asimakopoulos, DN; Kaltsounides, NA; Theoharatos, GA; Tsitouri, M. Solar global UVB (280-315 nm) and UVA (315-380nm) radiant fluxes and their relationships with broad- band global radiant flux at an eastern Mediterranean site. *Agr. Forest. Met.*, 2009, 149, 1188-1200.

Jiang, H; Gao, K; Helbling, EW. UV-absorbing compounds in *Porphyra haitanensis* (*Rhodophyta*) with special reference to effects of desiccation. *J. Appl. Phycol.*, 2008, 20, 387-395.

Karentz, D; McEuen, ES; Land, MC; Dunlap, WC. Survey of mycosporine-like amino acid compounds in Antarctic marine organisms: potential protection from ultraviolet exposure. *Mar. Biol.*, 1991, 108, 157-166.

Karsten, U; Garcia-Pichel, F. Carotenoids and mycosporine-like amino acid compounds in members of the genus *Microcoleus* (cyanobacteria): a chemosystematic study. *Syst. Appl. Microbiol.*, 1996, 19, 285-294.

Karsten, U; Sawall, T; West, J; Wiencke, C. Ultraviolet sunscreen compounds in epiphytic red algae from mangroves. *Hydrobiology*, 2000, 432, 159-171.

Karsten, U; Sawall, T; Wiencke, C. A survey of the distribution of UV absorbing substances in tropical macroalgae. *Phycol. Res.*, 1998a, 46, 271-279.

Klisch, M; Häder DP. Wavelength dependence of mycosporine-like amino acid synthesis in Gyrodinium dorsum. *J. Photochem. Photobiol. B.*, 2002, 66, 60-66.

Klisch, M; Häder, DP. Mycosporine-like amino acids in the marine dinoflagellate *Gyrodinium dorsum*: induction by ultraviolet irradiation. *J. Photochem. Photobiol. B.*, 2000, 55, 178-182.

Korbee, N; Figueroa, FL; Aguilera, FJ. Effect of light quality on the accumulation of photosynthetic pigments, proteins and mycosporine-like amino acids in the red alga *Porphyra leucosticta* (*Bangiales, Rhodophyta*). *J. Photochem. Photobiol. B.*, 2005a, 80, 71-78.

Korbee, N; Huovinen, P; Figueroa, FL; Aguilera, J; Karsten, U. Availability of ammonium influences photosynthesis and the accumulation of mycosporine-like amino acids in two *Porphyra* species (*Bangiales, Rhodophyta*). *Mar. Biol.*, 2005b, 146, 645-654.

Kräbs, G; Watanabe, M; Wiencke, C. A monochromatic action spectrum for the photoinduction of the UV-absorbing mycosporine-like amino acid shinorine in the red alga *Chondrus crispus*. *Photochem. Photobiol.*, 2004, 79, 515-519.

Laurion, I; Roy, S. Growth and photoprotection in three dinoflagellates (including two strains of *Alexandrium tamarense*) and one diatom exposed to four weeks of natural and enhanced UVB radiation. *J. Phycol.*, 2009, 45, 16-33.

Laurion, I; Blouin, F; Roy, S. Packaging of mycosporine-like amino acids in dinoflagellates. *Mar. Ecol. Prog. Ser.*, 2004, 279, 297-303.

Lima-Bessa, KMD; Armelini, MG; Chiganças, V; Jacysyn, JF; Amarante-Mendes, GP; Sarasin, A; Menck, CFM. CPDs and 6–4PPs play different roles in UV-induced cell death in normal and NER-deficient human cells. *DNA Repair*, 2008, 7, 303-312.

Litchman, E; Neale, PJ; Banaszak, AT. Increased sensitivity to ultraviolet radiation in nitrogen-limited dinoflagellates: photoprotection and repair. *Limnol. Oceanogr.*, 2002, 47, 86-94.

Llewellyn, CA; Airs, RL. Distribution and abundance of MAAs in 33 species of microalgae across 13 classes. *Mar. Drugs*, 2010, 8, 1273-1291.

Madronich, S; McKenzie, RL; Björn, LO; Caldwell, MM. Changes in biologically active ultraviolet radiation reaching the Earth's surface. *J. Photochem. Photobiol. B.*, 1998, 46, 5-19.

Manney, GL; Santee, ML; Rex, M; Livesey, NJ; Pitts, MC; Veefkind, P; et al. Unprecedented Arctic ozone loss in 2011, *Nature*, 2011, 478, 469-475.

Marchant, HJ; Davidson, AT; Kelly, GJ. UV-B protecting compounds in the marine alga *Phaeocystis pouchetii* from Antarctica. *Mar. Biol.*, 1991, 109, 391-395.

Matsui, K; Nazifi, E; Kunita, S; Wada, N; Matsugo, S; Sakamoto, T. Novel glycosylated mycosporine-like amino acids with radical scavenging activity from the cyanobacterium *Nostoc commune*. *J. Photochem. Photobiol. B.*, 2011, 105, 81-89.

McAteer, K; Jing, Y; Kao, J; Taylor, JS; Kennedy, MA. Solution-state structure of a DNA dodecamer duplex containing a cis-syn thymine cyclobutane dimer, the major UV photoproduct of DNA. *J. Mol. Biol.*, 1998, 282, 1013-1032.

McKenzie, RL; Aucamp, PJ; Bais, AF; Björn, LO; Ilyas, M. Changes in biologically active ultraviolet radiation reaching the Earth's surface. *Photochem. Photobiol. Sci.*, 2003, 2, 5-15.

Misonou, T; Saitoh, J; Oshiba, S; Tokitomo, Y; Maegawa, M; Inoue, Y; Hori, H; Sakurai, T; UV-absorbing substance in the red alga *Porphyra yezoensis* (Bangiales, Rhodophyta) block thymine dimer production. *Mar. Biotechnol.*, 2003, 5, 194-200.

Nakayama, R; Tamura, Y; Kikuzaki, H; Nakatani, N. Antioxidant effect of the constituents of susabinori (*Porphyra yezoensis*). *JAOCS*, 1999, 76, 649-653.

Nazifi, E; Wada, N; Yamaba, M; Asano, T; Nishiuchi, T; Matsugo, S; Sakamoto, T. Glycosylated porphyra-334 and palythine-threonine from the terrestrial cyanobacterium *Nostoc commune*. *Mar. Drugs*, 2013, 11, 3124-3154.

Newman, SJ; Dunlap, WC; Nicol, S; Ritz, D. Antarctic krill (*Euphausia superba*) acquire a UV-absorbing mycosporine-like amino acid from dietary algae. *J. Exper. Mar. Biol. Ecol.*, 2000, 255, 93-110.

Oren, A; Gunde-Cimerman, N. Mycosporines and mycosporine-like amino acids: UV protectants or multipurpose secondary metabolites? *FEMS Microbiol. Lett.*, 2007, 269, 1-10.

Oyamada, C; Kaneniwa, M; Ebitani, K; Murata, M; Ishihara, K. Mycosporine-like amino acids extracted from Scallop (*Patinopecten yessoensis*) ovaries: UV protection and growth stimulation activities on human cells. *Mar. Biotechnol.*, 2008, 10, 141-150.

Peinado, NK; Abdala Díaz, RT; Figueroa, FL; Helbling, EW. Ammonium and UV radiation stimulate the accumulation of mycosporine-like amino acids in *Porphyra columbina* (Rhodophyta) from Patagonia, Argentina. *J. Phycol.*, 2004, 40, 248-259.

Portwich, A; Garcia-Pichel, F. Biosynthetic pathway of mycosporines (mycosporine-like amino acids) in the cyanobacterium *Chlorogloeopsis* sp. strain PCC 6912. *Phycologia*, 2003, 42, 384-392.

Rastogi, RP. UV-B-induced DNA damage and repair in cyanobacteria, *PhD Thesis* 2010, Banaras Hindu University, Varanasi, India.

Rastogi, RP; Richa; Kumar, A; Tyagi, MB; Sinha, RP. Molecular mechanisms of ultraviolet radiation-induced DNA damage and repair. *J. Nucleic Acids*, 2010a. http://dx.doi.org/10.4061/2010/592980 (Article ID 592980).

Rastogi, RP; Richa; Sinha, RP; Singh, SP; Häder, DP. Photoprotective compounds from marine organisms. *J. Ind. Microbiol. Biotechnol.*, 2010b, 37, 537-558.

Rastogi, RP; Richa; Singh, SP; Häder, DP; Sinha, RP. Mycosporine-like amino acids profile and their activity under PAR and UVR in a hot-spring cyanobacterium *Scytonema* sp. HKAR-3. *Aust. J. Bot.*, 2010c, 58, 286-293.

Rastogi, RP; Sinha, RP. Genotoxin-Induced DNA Damage: Detection, Recovery and Influence on Human Health. In: Sinha RP, Sharma NK, Rai AK (eds). *Recent Advances in Life Sciences. India*: IK International Publishing House Pvt. Ltd., New Delhi, India, 2011a, pp. 275-309.

Rastogi, RP; Sinha, RP. Solar ultraviolet radiation-induced DNA damage and protection/repair strategies in cyanobacteria. *Inter. J. Phar. Bio Sci.*, 2011b, 2, B271–B288.

Rastogi, RP; Kumari, S; Richa; Han, T; Sinha, RP. Molecular characterization of hot spring cyanobacteria and evaluation of their photoprotective compounds. *Can. J. Microbiol.*, 2012, 58, 719-727.

Rastogi RP; Incharoensakdi A. UV radiation-induced accumulation of photoprotec-tive compounds in the green alga *Tetraspora* sp. CU2551. *Plant Physiol. Biochem.*, 2013, 70, 7-13.

Rastogi, RP; Incharoensakdi, A; Madamwar, D. Responses of a rice-field cyanobacterium *Anabaena siamensis* TISTR-8012 upon exposure to PAR and UV radiation. *J. Plant Physiol.*, 2014a, 171, 1545-1553.

Rastogi, RP; Singh, SP; Incharoensakdi, A; Häder, DP; Sinha, RP. Ultraviolet radiation-induced generation of reactive oxygen species, DNA damage and induction of UV-absorbing compounds in the cyanobacterium *Rivularia* sp. HKAR-4. *South Afr. J. Bot.*, 2014b, 90, 163-169.

Rastogi, RP; Madamwar, D; Incharoensakdi, A. Multiple defense systems in cyanobacteria in response to solar UV radiation. In: Davison D (ed). Cyanobacteria: Ecological Importance, Biotechnological Uses and Risk Management. USA: Nova Science Publishers 2014c, In Press.

Rastogi, RP; Incharoensakdi, A. UV radiation-induced biosynthesis, stability and antioxidant activity of mycosporine-like amino acids (MAAs) in a unicellular cyanobacterium *Gloeocapsa* sp. CU2556. *J. Photochem. Photobiol. B.*, 2014a, 130, 287-292.

Rastogi, RP; Incharoensakdi, A. Analysis of UV-absorbing photoprotectant mycosporine-like amino acid (MAA) in the cyanobacterium *Arthrospira* sp. CU2556. *Photochem. Photobiol. Sci.*, 2014b, 13, 1016-1024.

Rastogi, RP; Incharoensakdi, A. Characterization of UV-screening compounds, mycosporine-like amino acids, and scytonemin in the cyanobacterium *Lyngbya* sp. CU2555. *FEMS Microbiol. Ecol.*, 2014c, 87, 244-256.

Rastogi, RP; Incharoensakdi, A. Occurrence and induction of a ultraviolet-absorbing substance in the cyanobacterium *Fischerella muscicola* TISTR8215. *Phycol. Res.*, 2015. doi: 10.1111/pre.12069.

Ravishankara, AR; Daniel, JS; Portmann, RW. Nitrous oxide (N_2O): The dominant ozone-depleting substance emitted in the 21st century. *Science*, 2009, 326, 123-125.

Riegger, L; Robinson, D. Photoinduction of UV-absorbing compounds in Antarctic diatoms and *Phaeocystis Antarctica*. *Mar. Ecol. Prog. Ser.*, 1997, 160, 13-5.

Shibata, K. Pigments and a UVabsorbing substance in coral and a bluegreen alga living in the Great Barrier Reef. *Plant Cell Physiol.*, 1969, 10, 325-335.

Singh, SP; Sinha, RP; Klisch, M; Häder, DP. Mycosporinelike amino acids (MAAs) profile of a rice-field cyanobacterium *Anabaena doliolum* as influenced by PAR and UVR. *Planta*, 2008a, 229, 225-233.

Singh, SP; Klisch, M; Sinha, RP; Häder, D-P. Effects of abiotic stressors on synthesis of the mycosporine-like amino acid shinorine in the cyanobacterium *Anabaena variabilis* PCC 7937. *Photochem. Photobiol.*, 2008b, 84, 1500-1505.

Singh, SP; Klisch, M; Sinha, RP; Häder, DP. Sulfur deficiency changes mycosporine-like amino acid (MAA) composition of *Anabaena variabilis* PCC 7937: a possible role of sulfur in MAA bioconversion. *Photochem. Photobiol.*, 2010, 86, 862-870.

Sinha, RP; Klisch, M; Helbling, EW; Häder, D-P. Induction of mycosporine-like amino acids (MAAs) in cyanobacteria by solar ultraviolet-B radiation. *J. Photochem. Photobiol. B.*, 2001, 60, 129-135.

Sinha, RP; Ambasht, NK; Sinha, JP; Klisch, M; Häder, D-P. UVB-induced synthesis of mycosporine-like amino acids in three strains of *Nodularia* (cyanobacteria). *J. Photochem. Photobiol. B.*, 2003, 71, 51-58.

Sinha, RP; Singh, SP; Häder, D-P. Database on mycosporines and mycosporine-likeamino acids (MAAs) in fungi, cyanobacteria, macroalgae, phytoplankton and animals. *J. Photochem. Photobiol. B.*, 2007, 89, 29-35.

Spence, E; Dunlap, WC; Shick, JM; Long, PF. Redundant pathways of sunscreen biosynthesis in a cyanobacterium. *ChemBioChem.*, 2012, 13, 531-533.

Suh, HJ; Lee HW; Jung, J. Mycosporine glycine protects biological systems against photodynamic damage by quenching single oxygen with a high efficiency. *Photochem. Photobiol.*, 2003, 78, 109-113.

Valko, M; Leibfritz, D; Moncol, J; Cronin, MTD; Mazur, M; Telser, J. Free radicals and antioxidants in normal physiological functions and human disease. *Int. J. Biochem. Cell Biol.*, 2007, 39, 44-84.

Volkmann, M; Gorbushina, AA; Kedar, L; Oren, A. Structure of euhalothece-362, a novel red-shifted mycosporine-like amino acid, from a halophilic cyanobacterium (*Euhalothece* sp). *Microbiol. Lett.*, 2006, 258, 50-54.

Waditee-Sirisattha, R; Kageyama, H; Sopun, W; Tanaka, Y; Takabe, T. Identification and upregulation of biosynthetic genes required for accumulation of mycosporine-2-glycine under salt stress conditions in the halotolerant cyanobacterium *Aphanothece halophytica*. *App. Env. Microbiol.*, 2014, 80, 1763-1769.

Whitehead, K; Hedges, JI. Photodegradation and photosensitization of mycosporine-like amino acids. *J. Photochem. Photobiol.*, 2005, 80, 115-121.

Williamson, CE; Zepp, RG; Lucas, RM; Madronich, S; Austin, AT; Ballaré, CL; Norval, M; Sulzberger, B; Bais, AF; McKenzie, RL; Robinson, SA; Häder, D-P; Paul, ND; Bornman, JF. Solar ultraviolet radiation in a changing climate. *Nat. Clim. Change*, 2014, 4, 434-441.

Wu Won, JJ; Chalker, BE; Rideout, JA. Two new UVabsorbing compounds from Stylophora pistillata: sulfate esters of mycosporine-like amino acids. *Tetrahedron Lett.*, 1997, 38, 2525-2526.

Yuan, YV; Westcott, ND; Hu, C; Kitts, DD. Mycosporine-like amino acid composition of the edible red alga, *Palmaria palmata* (dulse) harvested from the west and east coasts of Grand Manan Island, New Brunswick. *Food Chem.*, 2009, 112, 321-328.

In: Encyclopedia of Dermatology (6 Volume Set)
Editor: Meghan Pratt

ISBN: 978-1-63483-326-4

Chapter 73

GUIDELINES FOR SCHOOL PROGRAMS TO PREVENT SKIN CANCER*

Karen Glanz, Mona Saraiya and Howell Wechsler

SUMMARY

Skin cancer is the most common type of cancer in the United States. Since 1973, new cases of the most serious form of skin cancer, melanoma, have increased approximately 150%. During the same period, deaths from melanoma have increased approximately 44%. Approximately 65%–90% of melanomas are caused by ultraviolet (UV) radiation. More than one half of a person's lifetime UV exposure occurs during childhood and adolescence because of more opportunities and time for exposure. Exposure to UV radiation during childhood plays a role in the future development of skin cancer. Persons with a history of ≥1 blistering sunburns during childhood or adolescence are two times as likely to develop melanoma than those who did not have such exposures. Studies indicate that protection from UV exposure during childhood and adolescence reduces the risk for skin cancer. These studies support the need to protect young persons from the sun beginning at an early age. School staff can play a major role in protecting children and adolescents from UV exposure and the future development of skin cancer by instituting policies, environmental changes, and educational programs that can reduce skin cancer risks among young persons.

This report reviews scientific literature regarding the rates, trends, causes, and prevention of skin cancer and presents guidelines for schools to implement a comprehensive approach to preventing skin cancer. Based on a review of research, theory, and current practice, these guidelines were developed by CDC in collaboration with specialists in dermatology, pediatrics, public health, and education; national, federal, state, and voluntary agencies; schools; and other organizations. Recommendations are included for schools to reduce skin cancer risks through policies; creation of physical, social, and organizational environments

* This is an edited, reformatted and augmented version of Morbidity and Mortality Weekly Report, April 26, 2002, Vol. 51, No. RR-4, issued by the Centers for Disease Control and Prevention.

that facilitate protection from UV rays; education of young persons; professional development of staff; involvement of families; health services; and program evaluation.

INTRODUCTION

Skin cancer is the most common type of cancer in the United States [1]. Since 1973, the number of new cases of melanoma, the skin cancer with the highest risk for mortality and one of the most common cancers among young adults, has increased. The incidence of melanoma has increased 150%, and melanoma mortality rates have increased by 44% [1]. Because a substantial percentage of lifetime sun exposure occurs before age 20 years [2, 3] and because ultraviolet (UV) radiation exposure during childhood and adolescence plays an important role in the development of skin cancer [2, 4], preventive behaviors can yield the most positive effects, if they are initiated early and established as healthy and consistent patterns throughout life. Children spend several hours at school on most weekdays, and some of that time is spent in outdoor activities. Schools, therefore, are in a position to teach and model healthy behaviors, and they can use health education activities involving families to encourage sun-safe behaviors at home. Thus, schools can play a vital role in preventing skin cancer.

This report is one of a series of guidelines produced by CDC to help schools improve the health of young persons by promoting behaviors to prevent the leading causes of illness and death [5–8]. The primary audience for this report includes state and local health and educational agencies and nongovernmental organizations concerned with improving the health of U.S. students. These agencies and organizations can translate the information in this report into materials and training programs for their constituents. In addition, CDC will develop and disseminate materials to help schools and school districts implement the guidelines. At the local level, teachers and other school personnel, community recreation program personnel, health service providers, community leaders, policymakers, and parents may use these guidelines and complementary materials to plan and implement skin cancer prevention policies and programs. In addition, faculty at institutions of higher education may use these guidelines to train professionals in education, public health, sports and recreation, school psychology, nursing, medicine, and other appropriate disciplines.

Although these skin cancer prevention guidelines are intended for schools, they can also guide child care facilities and other organizations that provide opportunities for children and adolescents to spend time in outdoor settings (e.g., camps; sports fields; playgrounds; swimming, tennis, and boating clubs; farms; and recreation and park facilities). These guidelines address children and adolescents of primary-and secondary-school age (approximately 5–18 years). The recommendations are based on scientific evidence, medical and behavioral knowledge, and consensus among specialists in education and skin cancer prevention. In 2003, CDC will publish a chapter on cancer in its *Community Guide to Preventive Services* [9], which will summarize information regarding the effectiveness of community-based interventions geared to-ward preventing skin cancer.

School-based programs can play an important role in achieving the following national Health Objectives for the Year 2010 related to skin cancer prevention: 1) increase the proportion of persons who use at least one of the following protective measures that might reduce the risk for skin cancer: avoid the sun between 10 a.m. and 4 p.m., wear sun-protective clothing when exposed to the sun, use sunscreen with a sun-protection factor (SPF) ≥15, and avoid artificial sources of UV light; and 2) reduce deaths from melanoma to <2.5 per 100,000 persons [10].

Burden of Skin Cancer

Skin cancer is the most common type of cancer in the United States [11]. The two most common kinds of skin cancer — basal cell carcinoma and squamous cell carcinoma — are highly curable. However, melanoma, the third most common type of skin cancer and one of the most common cancers among young adults, is more dangerous. In 2001, approximately 1.3 million new cases of basal cell or squamous cell carcinoma were diagnosed with approximately 2,000 deaths from basal cell and squamous cell carcinoma combined. Melanoma, by contrast, will be diagnosed in 53,600 persons and will account for 7,400 deaths, more than three fourths of all skin cancer deaths [12].

Basal cell carcinoma, which accounts for 75% of all skin cancers [11], rarely metastasizes to other organs. Squamous cell carcinoma, which accounts for 20% of all skin cancers, has a higher likelihood of spreading to the lymph nodes and internal organs and causing death [13], but these outcomes are also rare. Melanoma is nearly always curable in its early stages, but it is most likely to spread to other parts of the body if detected late. Melanoma most often appears on the trunk of men and the lower legs of women, although it also might be found on the head, neck, or elsewhere [14, 15].

In the United States, diagnoses of new melanomas are increasing, whereas diagnoses of the majority of other cancers are decreasing [16]. Since 1973, the annual incidence rate for melanoma (new cases diagnosed per 100,000 persons) has more than doubled, from 5.7 cases per 100,000 in that year to 14.3 per 100,000 in 1998 [1] (Figure). The rapid increase in annual incidence rates is likely a result of several factors, including increased exposure to UV radiation and possibly earlier detection of melanoma [17]. Since 1973, annual deaths per 100,000 persons from melanoma have increased by approximately 44%, from 1.6 to 2.3 (Figure). However, over the course of the 1990s, mortality rates have remained stable, particularly among women (16,18–19]. Although doctors must report other types of cancer (including melanomas) to cancer registries, they are not required to report squamous or basal cell cancer, which makes tracking trends in the incidence of these two cancers difficult. However, death rates for basal cell and squamous cell carcinoma have remained stable [12].

Risk Factors for Skin Cancer

Excessive Exposure to UV Radiation

Skin cancer is largely preventable by limiting exposure to the primary source of UV radiation, sunlight. Sunlamps and tanning beds are other sources. Persons with high levels of exposure to UV radiation are at an increased risk for all three major forms of skin cancer. Approximately 65%–90% of melanomas are caused by UV exposure [20]. The epidemiology implicating UV exposure as a cause of melanoma is further supported by biologic evidence that damage caused by UV radiation, particularly damage to DNA, plays a central role in the development of melanoma [4]. Total UV exposure depends on the intensity of the light, duration of skin exposure, and whether the skin was protected by sun-protective clothing and sunscreen. Severe, blistering sunburns are associated with an increased risk for both melanoma and basal cell carcinoma. For these cancers, intermittent intense exposures seem to carry higher risk than do lower level, chronic, or cumulative exposures, even if the total UV dose is the same. In contrast, the risk for squamous cell carcinoma is strongly associated with chronic UV exposure but not with intermittent exposure.

The two most important types of UV radiation, UV-A and UV-B radiation, have both been linked to the development of skin cancer. UV-A rays are not absorbed by the ozone layer, penetrate deeply into the skin, and cause premature aging and possibly suppression of the immune system [4, 21, 22]. Up to 90% of the visible changes commonly attributable to aging are caused by sun exposure. UV-B rays, which are partially absorbed by the ozone layer, tan and sometimes burn the skin. UV-B radiation has been linked to the development of cataracts [23–25] and skin cancer. Recommended skin cancer prevention measures protect against both UV-A and UV-B radiation.

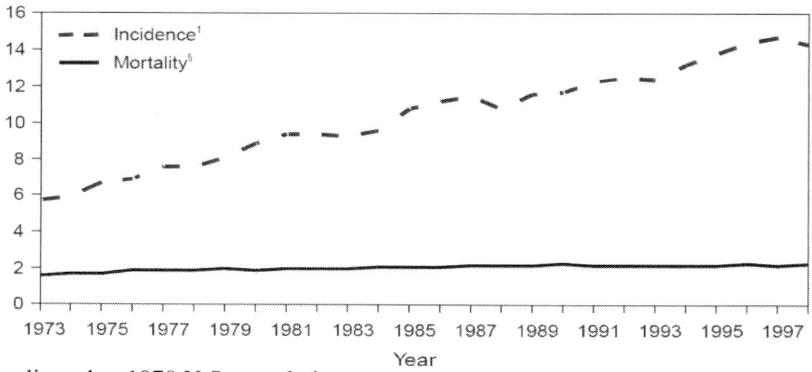

*Rate is age-adjusted to 1970 U.S. population.
†1973 Incidence rate: 5.7 per 100,000 persons; 1998 incidence rate: 14.3 per 100,000.
§1973 Mortality rate: 1.6 per 100,000; 1998 mortality rate: 2.3 per 100,000.
Source: Cancer Statistics Review, 1973–1998.

Figure. Melanoma of the skin (invasive): SEER incidence and U.S. mortality rates*, 1973–1998.

Childhood and Adolescent UV Exposure

Exposure to UV radiation during childhood and adolescence plays a role in the future development of both melanoma and basal cell cancer [26–32]. For example, the risk for developing melanoma is related strongly to a history of ≥1 sunburns (an indicator of intense UV exposure) in childhood or adolescence [27, 28, 33, 34). Similarly, sunburns during these periods have been demonstrated to increase the risk for basal cell carcinoma [30, 31].

Childhood is the most important time for developing moles, which is an important risk factor for skin cancer. Sun exposure in childhood might increase the risk for melanoma by increasing the number of moles [33]. A study supports the use of sun protection during childhood to reduce the risk for melanoma in adulthood [35].

Children and adolescents have more opportunities and time than adults to be exposed to sunlight [36–38] and thus more opportunities for development of skin cancer [4, 39, 40].

More than one half of a person's lifetime UV exposure occurs during childhood and adolescence [3, 41].

Skin Color and Ethnicity

Although anyone can get skin cancer, persons with certain characteristics are particularly at risk. For example, the incidence of melanoma among whites is approximately 20 times higher than among blacks [1]. Hispanics appear to be at less risk for melanoma than whites; a study conducted in Los Angeles, California, indicated that the incidence rates for Hispanics were 2–3 per 100,000, whereas the rate for non-Hispanic whites was 11 per 100,000 [42]. For basal cell and squamous cell carcinoma, rates among blacks are 1/80 of the rates among whites [43].

The ethnic differences in observed rates are attributable mostly to skin color. The color of the skin is determined by the amount of melanin produced by melanocytes, which also protect the skin from the damage produced by UV radiation. Although darkly pigmented persons develop skin cancer on sun-exposed sites at lower rates than lightly pigmented persons, UV exposure increases their risk for developing skin cancer [44]. The risk for skin cancer is higher among persons who sunburn readily and tan poorly [45], namely those with red or blond hair, and fair skin that freckles or burns easily [14, 46, 47].

Moles

The most measurable predictors of melanoma are having large numbers and unusual types of moles (nevi) [48,49]. Usually not present at birth, moles begin appearing during childhood and adolescence and are associated with sun exposure. Most moles are harmless but some undergo abnormal changes and become melanomas. A changing mole, particularly in an adult, is often indicative of the development of melanoma [45].

Family History

The risk for melanoma increases if a person has ≥1 first-degree relatives (i.e., mother, father, brother, and sister) with the disease. Depending on the number of affected relatives, the risk can be up to eight times that of persons without a family history of melanoma. Nonetheless, only approximately 10% of all persons with melanoma have a family history of melanoma [45, 50].

Age

The incidence of skin cancer increases exponentially with age because older persons have had more opportunities to be exposed to UV radiation and they have diminished capacity to repair the damage from UV radiation [4, 14, 43]. Approximately one half of all melanomas occur in persons aged <50 years. Melanoma is one of the most common cancers found in persons aged <30 years [14]; it is the most common cancer occurring among persons in the 25–29 age group and the third most common in the 20–24 age group [51].

Environmental Factors Affecting UV Radiation

Environmental factors that increase the amount of UV radiation exposure received by humans include a latitude closer to the equator; higher altitude; light cloud coverage (allows 80% of UV rays to go through the clouds); the presence of materials that reflect the sun (e.g., pavement, water, snow, and sand); being outside near noontime (UV-B radiation is highest in the middle of the day and varies more by time of day than does UV-A); and being outside during the spring or summer [21, 52]. Ozone depletion could potentially increase levels of solar radiation at the earth's surface [53, 54].

Artificial UV Radiation

In 2000, the National Institute of Environmental Health Sciences concluded that sunlamps and tanning beds are carcinogenic [55]. Although limited, epidemiologic evidence suggests that a causal relation exists between artificial UV radiation and melanoma [55, 56]. The type and amount of UV radiation emitted from some sunbeds appear to be similar to that of noontime summer sun, and in some cases, the amount is even higher than the sun would emit [57]. Artificial UV radiation can substantially damage the skin (i.e., cause sunburn) and has been linked to ocular melanoma [52, 58]. Sunlamps and tanning beds should be avoided.

Protective Behaviors

Options for skin cancer prevention (Box 1) include limiting or minimizing exposure to the sun during peak hours (10 a.m.–4 p.m.), especially the 1-hour period closest to the noon hour (11 a.m.–1:00 p.m. when the UV rays are the strongest), wearing sun-protective clothing, using sunscreens that have UV-A and UV-B protection, and avoiding sunlamps and tanning beds. Most medical and cancer organizations advocate the use of similar skin cancer prevention measures [59]. The American Cancer Society [60], the American Academy of Dermatology [61, 62], the American Academy of Pediatrics [63], the American Medical Association [64], and the National Cancer Institute [65] all recommend patient education on UV radiation avoidance and sunscreen use. The third U.S. Preventive Services Task Force is revising their guidelines on provider counseling for skin cancer prevention and sunscreen use.

BOX 1. SKIN CANCER PROTECTIVE BEHAVIORS

- Minimize exposure to the sun during peak hours (10 a.m.–4 p.m.).
- Seek shade from the midday sun (10 a.m.– 4 p.m.).
- Wear clothing, hats, and sunglasses that protect the skin.
- Use a broad-spectrum sunscreen (UV-A and UV-B protection) with a sun-protection factor of ≥15.
- Avoid sunlamps and tanning beds.

Avoiding the Sun and Wearing Proper Clothing and Sunglasses

Some forms of protection (e.g., avoiding the sun, seeking shade, and wearing sun-protective clothing) are the first approach toward preventing skin cancer. One study has demonstrated that wearing sun-protective clothing can decrease the number of moles [66]; another study demonstrated that the protective effect of clothing depends primarily on the construction of the fabric (a tighter weave permits less UV radiation to reach the skin) [67]. Other important factors include fiber type (natural cotton or Lycra™ transmits less UV radiation than bleached cotton) and color (darker colors transmit less UV radiation);

additional factors include whether the fabric is wet or stretched (transmission of UV radiation increases as the fabric becomes more wet and stretched) [68]. Wide-brimmed hats (>3-inch brim) and Legionnaire hats (baseball type of hat with attached ear and neck flaps) provide the best protection for the head, ears, nose, and cheeks [69]. In 2001, the Federal Trade Commission and the Consumer Safety Product Commission assisted in the development of voluntary industry standards in the United States for rating the UV protective value of different types of clothing and of shade structures [70]. These standards should help the public make informed decisions concerning protection against UV radiation [68, 71].

Sunglasses protect the eyes and surrounding areas from UV damage and skin cancer. Although no federal regulations exist for sunglasses, the American Academy of Ophthalmology recommends that sunglasses block 99% of UV-A and UV-B radiation. A chemical coating applied to the surface of the lens is the protective mechanism; protection does not correlate with the color or darkness of the lens [72]. Sunglasses can reduce UV radiation exposure to the eye by 80%, and when combined with a wide-brimmed hat or Legionnaire hat, UV exposure to the face is reduced by 65% [73].

Shade structures and trees can reduce direct UV radiation, but the protection offered is dependent on the direct and indirect UV radiation from the surrounding surface (e.g., sand and concrete) [74,75]. For example, umbrellas with more overhang provide more UV protection than those with less overhang.

Sunscreens

Sunscreens are an important adjunct to other types of protection against UV exposure. Using sunscreen is one of the most commonly practiced behaviors for preventing skin cancer.

During the previous decade, new studies have contributed to an increased understanding of the role of sunscreen in possibly preventing skin cancer. The U.S. Preventive Services Task Force is revising their recommendations on sunscreen use, but the International Agency for Research on Cancer has concluded that topical use of sunscreens probably prevents squamous cell carcinoma of the skin. The group drew no conclusions regarding whether the use of sunscreens reduces the incidence of basal cell carcinoma or melanoma [76] (Appendix A).

Clinical trials have demonstrated that sunscreens are effective in reducing the incidence of actinic keratoses, the precursors to squamous cell carcinoma [77, 78]. One randomized clinical trial demonstrated that sunscreens are effective in reducing squamous cell carcinoma itself [79]. Another randomized trial demonstrated that, among children who are at high risk for developing melanoma, sunscreens are effective in reducing moles, the precursors and strongest risk factor for melanoma [80]. Unfortunately, many persons use sunscreens if they intend to stay out in the sun longer, and they reduce the use of other forms of sun protection (e.g., clothing or hats), thereby, acquiring the same or even a higher amount of UV radiation exposure than they would have obtained with a shorter stay and no sunscreen [22, 76, 81].

The guidelines in this report recommend 1) using various methods (e.g., avoiding the sun, seeking shade, or wearing protective clothing) that reduce exposure to the full spectrum of UV radiation as the first line of protection against skin cancer and 2) using sunscreen as a complementary measure. In some instances, sunscreens might be the only responsible option. However, to be effective, sunscreens must be applied correctly (Appendix B). For example, users should apply sunscreen and allow it to dry before going outdoors and getting any UV exposure [82, 83]. Similarly, users should reapply sunscreen after leaving the water, sweating, or drying off with a towel. Use of insufficient quantities of sunscreen [84, 85] or use of a sunscreen with insufficient protection are other concerns. Manufacturers determine the SPF (a measure of protection from only UV-B radiation) by applying an adequate amount of sunscreen (1–2 ounces) on humans and testing under artificial light, which is usually not as strong as natural light [86]. No government standards measure how much protection sunscreens provide against UV-A rays.

Few studies have been conducted on sunscreens, despite their widespread use, which make it difficult to estimate the prevalence of allergies to sunscreens. Skin irritation, rather than an actual allergic reaction, is one of the more commonly reported adverse events [87]. Because the majority of the commercially available sunscreens are a combination of agents from various chemical groups, persons who might experience adverse effects should be aware of the active ingredients and try sunscreens with different ingredients. In previous years, the most commonly reported allergen was para-aminobenzoic acid (PABA) (rarely used today), whereas the current two most frequently cited allergens are benzophenone-3 and dibenzoyl methanes [22].

Prevalence of Behavioral Risk Factors, Sun-Safe Behaviors, and Attitudes Related to Sun Safety

In the United States, sunbathing and tanning habits were established during the early to mid-1900s [88, 89], most likely reflecting the increased availability of leisure time and fashion trends promoting tanned skin [89, 90]. In the late 1970s, the majority of the population had little knowledge concerning their personal susceptibility to skin cancer and believed that tanning enhanced appearance and was associated with better health [91]. More recent reports indicate that many Americans feel healthier with a tan and believe that suntanned skin is more attractive [36, 92, 93].

In 1992, 53% of U.S. adults were "very likely" to protect themselves from the sun by practicing at least one protective behavior (using sunscreen, seeking shade, or wearing sunprotective clothing) [94]. Among white adults, approximately one third used sunscreen (32%), sought shade (30%), and wore protective clothing (28%). Among black adults, 45% sought shade, 28% wore sun-protective clothing, and 9% used sunscreen [95]. Sun-protective behaviors were more common among the more sun sensitive, females, and older age groups among both whites and blacks.

Sun-safety behaviors might be most difficult to change among preadolescents and adolescents [96]. Teenagers spend a substantial amount of time outdoors, especially on weekends and during the summer [97, 98]. Many teenagers believe that a tan is desirable [92]; only teenagers who know persons with skin cancer or who perceive an increased personal susceptibility to skin cancer are more likely to use sunscreen [98]. However, teenagers who practice skin cancer prevention tend to only use sunscreen and to use it infrequently, inconsistently, and incorrectly [97, 98]. Girls tend to use sunscreen more than boys, but they also use tanning beds more frequently [97–101].

Sunscreen use by children is correlated positively with use by their parents [87, 102]. Some parents know the risks of skin cancer but do not realize that children are at risk [103, 104]. Some parents believe that a suntan is a sign of good health; others use sunscreen on their children as their only or preferred skin cancer prevention measure [36, 99, 105–107], even though other measures (e.g., using shade structures and wearing sunprotective clothing) are available. Sometimes parents apply sunscreen on their children incorrectly and inconsistently [22] (e.g., only after a child has experienced a painful sunburn) [97, 108].

Concerns Regarding Promoting Protection from UV Radiation

Sun-safety measures should not reduce student participation in physical activity. Regular physical activity reduces morbidity and mortality for multiple chronic diseases. Promoting lifelong physical activity in schools is a critically important public health and educational priority [8]. Schools might find it difficult to avoid scheduling outdoor physical activity programs around the midday hours. These schools can focus their efforts on other sun-safety measures (e.g., seeking shade; and wearing a hat, protective clothing, or sunscreen), which can be implemented without compromising physical activity while gradually making feasible scheduling changes.

In addition, because UV radiation plays a role in the synthesis of vitamin D, the limitation of UV exposure might be of some concern. This limitation might lead to a decrease in levels of vitamin D and increase the likelihood that rickets, a disorder involving a weakening of the bones, will develop in susceptible infants and children. However, the average age for presentation of rickets is 18 months, and the age groups of concern are typically infants and toddlers, not school-aged children between 5 and 18 years. Although the major source of vitamin D is through skin exposure to sunlight, supplementing the diet with foods (e.g., flesh of fatty fish, eggs from hens fed vitamin D, and vitamin D-fortified milk and breakfast cereal) can provide enough vitamin D to meet adequate intake requirements [109, 110]. The American Academy of Pediatrics [111] recommends vitamin D supplementation for breast-fed infants whose mothers are vitamin D deficient or for infants who are not exposed to adequate sunlight. Infants consuming at least 500ml of vitamin D-fortified formula per day and older children consuming at least 16 ounces of vitamin D-fortified milk per day will meet the adequate intake of vitamin D.

Guidelines for School Programs to Prevent Skin Cancer

Schools as Settings for Skin Cancer Prevention Efforts

Epidemiologic data suggest that several skin cancers can be prevented if children and adolescents are protected from UV radiation [26–32]. Schools can participate in reducing exposure of young persons to UV radiation from the sun during school-related activities by offering education and skill-building activities to reinforce the development of healthful behaviors. School-based efforts to prevent skin cancer can be more effective in the framework of a coordinated school health program [112, 113] that includes family and community participation [114] and builds on the context and current practices in the school and community. Coordinated school health programs aim to create and support environments where young persons can gain the knowledge, attitudes, and skills required to make and maintain healthy choices and habits. These programs integrate health education, a healthy school environment, physical education, nutrition services, health services, mental health and counseling services, health promotion programs for faculty and staff, and efforts to integrate school activities with family and community life [113].

Being aware of existing practices for sun exposure and sun protection among teachers, staff, and students might help define gaps in optimal sun-safety practices. Careful observations for a few days might also provide important information concerning students' use of shade areas and sunscreen at recess or lunch time, and staff's use of hats, shirts, and sunglasses. Discussions with students and staff who practice sun-safe behaviors might prove useful in planning and improving implementation of sun-safety practices.

Skin cancer prevention measures vary in both their ease of adoption and relevance. Schools should not allow an "all or nothing" approach to undermine the effectiveness of their skin cancer prevention efforts. For sun-safety protection, a shortsleeve shirt and cap might be better than no hat and a sleeveless top. Being flexible is important while moving in the direction of optimal skin cancer prevention environments, policies, and programs.

Skin Cancer Prevention Guidelines

These guidelines provide recommendations for skin cancer prevention activities within a coordinated school health program. In addition, these guidelines are based on scientific literature, national policy documents, current practice, and theories and principles of health behavioral change [115]. Schools and community organizations can work together to develop plans that are relevant and achievable. Sustained support from school staff, students, communities, state and local education and health agencies, families, institutions of higher education, and national organizations are necessary to ensure the effectiveness of school skin cancer prevention activities [116].

In this report, seven broad guidelines are included that school programs can use to reduce the risk for skin cancer among students: 1) policy, 2) environmental change, 3) education, 4) families, 5) professional development, 6) health services, and 7) evaluation (Box 2). Each guideline includes suggestions regarding key elements, steps for implementation, and realistic expectations for change.

Box 2. Recommendations for Skin Cancer Prevention in Schools

1. Establish **policies** that reduce exposure to ultraviolet radiation.
2. Provide an **environment** that supports sun-safety practices.
3. Provide health **education** to teach students the knowledge, attitudes, and behavioral skills they need to prevent skin cancer.
4. Involve **family** members in skin cancer prevention efforts.
5. Include skin cancer prevention with **professional development** of staff (e.g., preservice and in-service education).
6. Complement and support skin cancer prevention with school **health services**.
7. Periodically **evaluate** whether schools are implementing the guidelines on policies, environmental change, education, families, professional development, and health services.

- **Guideline 1: Policy** — Establish policies that reduce exposure to UV radiation.
- **Guideline 2: Environmental change** — Provide and maintain physical and social environments that support sun safety and that are consistent with the development of other healthful habits.
- **Guideline 3: Education** — Provide health education to teach students the knowledge, attitudes, and behavioral skills they need to prevent skin cancer. The education should be age-appropriate and linked to opportunities for practicing sun-safety behaviors.
- **Guideline 4: Family Involvement** — Involve family members in skin cancer prevention efforts.
- **Guideline 5: Professional development** — Include skin cancer prevention knowledge and skills in preservice and in-service education for school administrators, teachers, physical education teachers and coaches, school nurses, and others who work with students.
- **Guideline 6: Health services** — Complement and support skin cancer prevention education and sun-safety environments and policies with school health services.
- **Guideline 7: Evaluation** — Periodically evaluate whether schools are implementing the guidelines on policies, environmental change, education, families, professional development, and health services.

The recommendations represent the state-of-the-science in school-based skin cancer prevention. However, every recommendation is not appropriate or feasible for every school to implement nor should any school be expected to implement all recommendations. Schools should determine which recommendations have the highest priority based on the needs of the school and available resources. As more resources become available, schools could implement additional recommendations to support a coordinated approach to preventing skin cancer.

Guideline 1: Policy — Establish Policies that Reduce Exposure to UV Radiation

Policies can provide sun protection for all persons in a defined population (e.g., a school), not just those who are most motivated [117]. In addition, policies can involve formal organizational rules and standards or legal requirements and restrictions related to skin cancer prevention measures. Policies may be developed by a school, school board, or by other legal entities (e.g., municipal, state, and federal governments). To be effective, policies need to be communicated to school personnel, announced to affected constituents (e.g., students and their parents), managed and implemented, enforced and monitored, and reviewed periodically [118, 119].

Before establishing healthy skin cancer prevention policies, identify any existing policies that might deter skin cancer prevention. These existing policies might include outdoor activity schedules, prohibitions on wearing sunglasses or caps and hats at school, and rules that limit the use or provision of sunscreen at school (e.g., requiring parental permission, defining sunscreen as "medicine," and restricting teachers from applying sunscreen on children).

California enacted a law (effective January 2002) that requires their schools to allow students, when outdoors, to w ear school-site approved sun-protective hats and clothing. This legislation was deemed necessary because several school districts had banned hats because some styles or colors are connected with gang affiliation.

An effectively crafted skin cancer prevention policy provides a framework for implementing the other six guidelines. The policy demonstrates institutional commitment and guides school and community groups in planning, implementing, and evaluating skin cancer prevention activities. Such a policy creates a supportive environment for students to learn about and adopt sun-protection practices. Although a comprehensive policy is preferable, more limited policies addressing certain aspects of skin cancer prevention also can be useful.

Developing the Policy or Policies

Skin cancer prevention can be part of a larger school health policy. Although policies might be initiated by a person or small group, the most effective policies are developed with input from all relevant constituents. In schools, the constituents include students, teachers, parents, administrators, coaches, school nurses, health educators and other relevant personnel as well as community leaders and residents. Schools can also work with community partners (e.g., recreation and parks departments, health departments, after-school programs, camps, families, and youth advocacy groups) and others who organize outdoor activities for youth.

Policies require time for development and implementation and might not be as visible as educational programs [120]. Increased effort in the early stages of policy development might result in increased adoption [121]. In Australia, health and cancer prevention specialists developed a sun-protection policy kit for schools and a related staff development module [120]. Elementary schools were twice as likely to formally adopt a comprehensive sun-protection policy if they also received the staff development module (44% [kit and module] versus 21% [kit only]). However, few high schools adopted policies whether they received just the kit or the kit and the module (11% and 6%, respectively) [120]. Policy development requires a longterm commitment and sustained efforts and cooperation among all concerned parties.

Policy Options

Components of skin cancer prevention policies for a school or community to consider include 1) statement of purpose and goals; 2) schedule and physical environment policies; 3) policies related to personal protective clothing and sunglasses; 4) sunscreen policies; 5) education policies; 6) policies on outreach to families; and 7) policies on resource allocation and evaluation. When implementing a comprehensive policy (which would include all of these components) is not feasible, schools can start with some of these components and add others over time.

Policy 1: Statement of Purpose and Goals. Policies usually begin with a statement of purpose and goals that establish sun safety as a priority and highlight the importance of skin cancer prevention. In addition, the statement can 1) describe the influence of childhood sun exposure on the risk for developing skin cancer later in life; 2) identify actions that persons and institutions can take to reduce the risk for skin cancer; 3) highlight the importance of establishing a physical, social, and organizational environment that supports skin cancer prevention; and 4) specify dedicated financial and human resources for skin cancer prevention and for the other policy options described here.

Policy 2: Schedule and Structure Policies. Policies can provide the basis for across-the-board reduction of UV radiation exposure for children and adults in schools and communities by establishing 1) rules that encourage the scheduling of outdoor activities (including athletic and sporting events) during times when the sun is not at its peak intensity and 2) building and grounds codes to increase the availability of shade in frequently used outdoor spaces.

Eliminating the scheduling of outdoor activities during peak sun hours will be difficult, if not impossible, for many schools to do. For these schools, the best strategy might be to work toward a gradual shift in scheduling. School board policies could require architects to design new school buildings with adequate shade coverage adjacent to play and sports fields. Play and sports fields can be reviewed for existing and potential shade. School and community organization staff could evaluate frequently used spaces in the community for their UV protection status and add signs, reminders, or prompts to encourage sun safety. Finally, volunteer, business, health department, and political support can be secured by school and community organization staff to generate resources for improving the sun-safety environment, especially for providing sunscreen and shade.

Policy 3: Policies for Personal Protective Clothing and Sunglasses. Schools can develop policies that encourage or require students to wear protective clothing, hats, and sunglasses to prevent excessive sun exposure. These measures could be employed during physical education classes, recess, field trips, outdoor sports or band events, and camping or field trips. Some schools, especially in Australia, have a "no hat/no play" policy stating that students cannot play outdoors if they are not wearing hats [119]. Related policy initiatives could require the use of athletic, band, and physical education uniforms that reduce or minimize excessive sun exposure (e.g., long sleeves and broad-brimmed hats). Strategies that can be implemented to promote the adoption of these policies include gradually phasing-in new policies that involve students and sports teams designing new uniforms, securing business sponsorship for sun-safe uniforms, and conducting discussions that promote the use of hats and sunglasses.

Some schools might have policies that prohibit or discourage students and staff from wearing hats and sunglasses on school grounds (e.g., because they are associated with contraband or gang-related items). Possible transmission of head lice among younger children who share hats might also be a concern; however, policies can be implemented that address these concerns (e.g., prohibiting both sharing hats and wearing gang-related symbols).

Policy 4: Sunscreen Policies. Policies on sunscreen use at school or for after-school activities can range from encouraging parents to include sunscreen in required school-supply kits, using permission slips for students to be able to apply sunscreen at school [122], and establishing a sunscreen use routine before going outside. Policies also might require teachers and coaches to use sunscreen for outside activities and require that sunscreen be provided at official school-sponsored events that occur during midday. Necessary steps that might be implemented include modifying existing policies that restrict school-based sunscreen application [123], seeking support for purchasing sunscreen supplies, and supervising sunscreen use.

Policy 5: Education Policies. The ideal education policy should support planned and sequential health education to provide students with the knowledge, attitudes, and behavioral skills needed for skin cancer prevention (Guideline 3). Policies that require teaching skin cancer prevention within health education courses will need to be balanced with the overall educational mission of the school.

Policy 6: Policies for Outreach to Families. Schools and other organizations that serve youth have established methods of communicating with parents and other caregivers. Policies can ensure that these organizations routinely provide to their youth advice and information concerning skin cancer prevention. For example, information concerning skin cancer prevention might be distributed along with other health forms to parents at the beginning of the year or at parent and teacher visits.

Policy 7: Resource Allocation and Evaluation. Skin cancer prevention efforts will most likely be sustained if policies exist to guide the allocation of resources for skin cancer prevention. A funding policy usually includes accountability and ongoing evaluation, thus providing for periodic review and reconsideration of how effective the resources dedicated to skin cancer prevention are being used.

Guideline 2: Environmental Change — Provide and Maintain Physical and Social Environments that Support Sun Safety and that are Consistent with the Development of Other Healthful Habits

Policies can promote the provision of supportive resources for skin cancer prevention (e.g., shade, protective clothing and hats, sunscreen at a reduced price or free, and highly visible information and prompts for sun protection) in the physical and social environment. These policies help establish routine personal behaviors and social norms that promote skin cancer prevention in the context of organized group activities.

Physical Environments

The majority of schools in the United States were not designed with sun safety in mind. Sun protection should be considered in the design of new schools. The design of school buildings and adjacent grounds, and the availability of natural shade (e.g., trees and mountains) or constructed shade (e.g., awnings, pavilions, and tall buildings that cast a shadow) influence potential sun exposure. Students, teachers, and families can identify opportunities to extend or create new shaded areas. These areas can be temporary or permanent, natural or constructed. Students might participate in planting trees as part of their science instruction, in which they learn which trees provide good shade cover, how and where to plant them, and how long they will need to yield valuable protection. Existing structures can be modified by constructing roofs on dugouts, installing covers for bleachers, and using awnings and tarps. An increasing selection of portable or add-on shade structures are available that school groups can purchase and install. Major construction projects to build permanent pavilions and play areas can require substantial funding, but they might be the best option in some settings. School and community partnerships can support these endeavors.

School and community partnerships can facilitate provision of sunscreen that is at a reduced price or free for staff and students (through sunscreen manufacturers, pharmaceutical companies, local dermatologist offices, or hospitals) and can make sun safety more accessible during the school day or recreation period. An alternative school policy could encourage parents to apply sunscreen to their children in the morning and include it in their children's supply kits. In addition, schools and community organizations can provide hats and protective clothing (e.g., jackets) for persons who forget to bring their own on days with midday outdoor activity or field trips. Both hygiene, size, and acceptability are important considerations. However, if the school has a laundry facility for band and sports uniforms, a laundering system for emergency sun-safe protective clothing could be instituted.

Information and prompts or reminders can reinforce sun-safety awareness and serve as reminders to engage in skin cancer preventive practices. Both visual and audio messages (e.g., sun-safe posters or public address system announcements) can serve as cues to action for students as well as for families, teachers, and other professionals. After students have learned about the UV index (an indicator of the intensity of the sun's rays on a given day) [124], schools can post and announce the daily UV index to encourage students to practice sun-protection measures. Some schools and recreation settings also use signs that indicate the number of minutes a person can be in the sun before sustaining a sunburn.

Social Environments

A supportive social environment involves establishing social norms favoring skin cancer prevention and including personal preventive behaviors as a part of organized group activities. Program planners and advocates for skin cancer prevention should serve as role models, and adults should be invited to lead by example. Schools can also create a social environment that encourages sun-safety practices through existing peer education groups by having peer educators teach other students about sun safety and by using periodic recognition or a special designation to reward teachers, staff, or students who practice sun safety.

Guideline 3: Education — Provide Health Education to Teach Students the Knowledge, Attitudes, and Behavioral Skills They Need To Prevent Skin Cancer. The Education Should be Age-Appropriate and Linked to Opportunities for Practicing Sun-Safety Behavior

Health education that is designed effectively and implemented for youth can increase their health-related knowledge and contribute to the development of healthy changes in attitudes and behaviors [125]. Skin cancer prevention is likely to be most effective when it is taught as part of a comprehensive health education curriculum that focuses on understanding the relations between personal behavior and health [126] and that provides students with the knowledge and skills outlined by the National Health Education Standards [112].

The yearly timing of skin cancer prevention education can be tailored to the climate and linked with opportunities for sun exposure and sun protection. Therefore, in an area with high altitude where outdoor winter sports are common (e.g., Colorado), skin cancer prevention could be introduced before winter vacation. In northeastern coastal areas, skin cancer prevention might be most relevant before summer break. And during the school day, sun-safety lessons could directly precede recess or outdoor physical education, allowing the class session to be followed by an opportunity to practice positive sun-safety habits.

Skin cancer prevention can be included as part of a comprehensive health education curriculum because of the following characteristics:

- Behaviors that lead to UV radiation exposure might be related to other health risk factors;

- Skin cancer prevention shares many of the key goals of other health education content areas (e.g., increasing the value placed on health, taking responsibility for one's health, and increasing confidence in one's ability to make healthy behavioral changes); and
- Skin cancer prevention efforts can incorporate several of the social learning behavioral change techniques used in other health education domains [126].

In addition to health education classes, skin cancer prevention can be integrated into other subject areas. For example, a math exercise for students could be to calculate the length of safe-sun exposure when sunscreen is used at a certain SPF. In history or social studies classes, students could discuss the social value placed on tanning and fair skin and media portrayal of tanning. Science classes could explore the light spectrum and discuss how it relates to the risk for skin cancer, or discuss depletion of the ozone and its effect on UV exposure. This type of integrated approach requires collaborative planning and curriculum development among teachers to optimize skin cancer prevention education and to ensure consistency of messages and practices.

Scope and Sequence

Health education is most effective in promoting positive behavioral changes when it is repeated and reinforced over time [114]. Short-duration or single-presentation efforts can increase students' knowledge regarding sun safety and, in some cases, improve attitudes and sun-protection behavior immediately after the program. However, these changes are likely to be short-lived and cannot be expected to translate into sustained positive health behaviors [125]. Multiunit presentations have been more effective in achieving higher increases in knowledge and skill acquisition [125].

School-based health education to promote skin cancer prevention is most effective when it is provided consistently and sequentially and included periodically in every grade, from prekindergarten through 12th grade. Sequential instruction can build on information and skills learned previously. Resources for skin cancer prevention programs targeting youth are included in this report (Appendix C).

Active Learning and Behavioral Focus

In the previous decade, educational programs to encourage children to adopt sun-safety habits have been implemented and evaluated. Among the school-based studies reported, interventions have included one-time didactic formats and special events [97, 127, 128]; skin cancer prevention that is integrated into classroom curricula over time [126, 129, 130]; and peer-education programs [131, 132]. A majority of these studies have demonstrated that these interventions increased knowledge and favorable attitudes toward preventive behaviors. In addition, some of the programs that have multiple lessons and that occur over a longer period (e.g., 1 year) have yielded improvements in sun-protection behaviors [125]

Actively engaging children and adolescents in the learning process increases the likelihood for a positive effect. Youth are more likely to consider and adopt new or improved behaviors when they learn about them through fun, participatory activities rather than through lectures. For example, a recent study demonstrated increased improvement in knowledge of the effects of UV radiation among elementary school students who used an interactive computer-based program than among those who received the same information in a didactic format led by a teacher [133]. The students who completed the interactive CD-ROM program also exhibited significant positive changes in attitudes and a trend toward improvements in sun-safety behavioral scores [133]. The U.S. Environmental Protection Agency offers an Internet learning site where students can report and interpret daily measurements of UV radiation, relate the UV index information to their own community, and correspond with other participating schools [124, 134].

Health education activities should be tailored to the cognitive and behavioral level of the students [135]. For example, students in kindergarten through third grades might learn effectively through repetitious rhyming and learning the ABCs of skin cancer prevention. Games, puzzles, and contests make learning fun for students of most ages. More intellectually challenging activities might appeal to high school students, ranging from understanding the scientific basis of solar radiation and global climates, to making their own video to communicate sun-protection messages to their peers and communities. Teenagers can learn about media literacy and different cultures by analyzing images of models in popular magazines and discussing what sun exposure and a tan means to both white and non-white racial groups in the United States and worldwide.

School Programs in a Broader Context

The most important long-term objective of skin cancer prevention education in schools is the adoption and maintenance of sun-protection practices. Therefore, the transmission of detailed, factual information to students is the foundation of sun-safety practices. In addition, educational programs and curricula in schools are part of the broader mix of skin cancer prevention efforts and should not be expected to solely prevent skin cancer. Skin cancer prevention interventions in recreation, sports, and community settings can complement and reinforce efforts in the schools [120, 136–140]. Supportive policies, environments, teachers, and families are essential adjuncts to effectively planned and consistently implemented health education to prevent skin cancer.

Guideline 4. Family Involvement — Involve Family Members in Skin Cancer Prevention Efforts

The sun-safety practices of parents are the single most important determinant of the sun-protection behaviors of children [121, 141]. For younger children, adult family members can assist and provide sun-protection resources. For adolescents, the direct influence of parents might decrease and be subordinated by peer influence. Nonetheless, family support plays a key role in extending the desirable effects of school skin cancer prevention efforts.

Involving family members in skin cancer prevention efforts increases the likelihood that they will adopt and thus model healthful sun-protection behaviors, and also appears to favorably influence the sun-protection behaviors of students [122]. At a minimum, parents or guardians can be informed concerning school initiatives and policies and knowledgeable regarding how their cooperation is needed to ensure child health. Parents and guardians also can be encouraged to provide children with sun-protective clothing and sunglasses for outdoor activities. In addition, parents and guardians can serve as advocates for sun-protective policies and practices in schools and can also provide volunteer labor for health and recreation events. Their input and direct assistance can provide support for funding needed for environmental improvements and educational materials.

Guideline 5: Professional Development — Include Skin Cancer Prevention Knowledge and Skills in Preservice and In-service Education for School Administrators, Teachers, Physical Education Teachers and Coaches, School Nurses, and Others Who Work with Students

Even effectively designed skin cancer prevention programs cannot succeed if they are not implemented as designed. Therefore, appropriate and effective professional development efforts should be conducted for decision makers and caregivers at all levels. Professional development activities, including certification programs and in-service education, are provided routinely for teachers and other school staff (e.g., coaches and school nurses). Skin cancer prevention can be integrated into these activities.

All school staff should receive basic information concerning the importance of sun safety and key strategies for skin cancer prevention. The type of additional professional development needed will vary, depending on the responsibilities of the various caregivers. In-service education for principals might address policy implementation and monitoring, whereas school nurses might highlight proper sunscreen use. Classroom teachers who implement curricula should receive training that addresses both content areas and teaching strategies.

As principals, teachers, and other school staff adopt sun-protection behaviors, they can serve as role models for students. A brief training program, along with participation in conducting skin cancer prevention activities for children, can result in improved sun-protection practices among recreation leaders [142].

Guideline 6: Health Services — Complement and Support Skin Cancer Prevention Education and Sun-Safety Environments and Policies with School Health Services.

School health services provide an opportunity for nurses, health educators, and school health resource specialists to promote and reinforce skin cancer prevention practices. A child's school health record can include parental permission for the child to use sunscreen provided by the school as well as a list of possible allergies to sunscreens or their ingredients.

School health services staff also may conduct physical examinations for sports team eligibility, assist in managing and notifying parents concerning the long-term dangers of a severe sunburn, and prepare students for field trips. Each of these situations provides an opportunity to educate and remind students about skin cancer prevention.

Health professionals in the community, including pediatricians, primary care providers, nurses, pharmacists, and dermatologists are credible sources of information and guidance for skin cancer prevention. They can be advocates for skin cancer prevention policies, environmental changes, and programs, and support school programs through presentations, professional training, demonstrations, and classroom visits. During their consultation with children and parents, these health-care professionals can also assess sun-exposure patterns, reinforce sun-protective behaviors, and provide counseling to persons with sunburns [138, 143].

Guideline 7: Evaluation — Periodically Evaluate Whether Schools are Implementing the Guidelines on Policies, Environmental Change, Education, Families, Professional Development, and Health Services

Local school boards and administrators can use evaluation questions to determine whether their programs are consistent with CDC's *Guidelines for School Programs To Prevent Skin Cancer*. Personnel in federal, state, and local education and health agencies also can use these questions to 1) assess whether schools in their jurisdiction are providing effective education to prevent skin cancer and 2) identify schools that would benefit from additional training, resources, or technical assistance. The following questions can serve as a guide for assessing program effectiveness:

1. Do schools have a comprehensive policy on skin cancer prevention and is it implemented and enforced as written?
2. Does the skin cancer prevention program support physical and social environmental changes that promote sun safety and that are consistent with the development of other healthful habits?
3. Does the skin cancer prevention education program foster the necessary knowledge, attitudes, and skills to reduce UV exposure and prevent skin cancer?
4. Is education to reduce UV exposure provided, as planned, in prekindergarten through 12th grade?
5. Is in-service training provided, as planned, for education staff responsible for implementing skin cancer prevention programs?
6. Do school health services support skin cancer prevention?
7. Are parents or families, teachers, students, school health personnel, school administrators, and appropriate community representatives involved in planning, implementing, and assessing programs and policies to prevent skin cancer?
8. Does the skin cancer prevention program encourage and support sun-safety efforts by students and school staff?

CONCLUSION

Schools can play a substantial role in protecting students from unnecessary exposure to UV, thereby reducing their future risk for skin cancer. A comprehensive school approach to skin cancer prevention includes policies, environmental change, educational curricula, family involvement, professional development, integration with health services, and evaluation. The exposure of youth to harmful UV radiation today contributes to their risk for skin cancer later in life. Unlike many diseases, skin cancer is primarily preventable. Schools, in partnership with community groups and other national, federal, state, and voluntary agencies, can develop, implement, and promote initiatives that help protect youth from UV exposure [144, 145]. These guidelines serve as a framework for such initiatives.

Appendix A. Public Health Action Steps from the International Agency for Research on Cancer

1. Protection of the skin from solar damage ideally involves various actions that include wearing tightly woven protective clothing that adequately covers the arms, trunk, and legs and a hat that provides adequate shade to the whole of the head; seeking shade whenever possible; avoiding outdoor activities during periods of peak insolation; and using sunscreens. Sunscreens should not be used as the sole agent for protection against the sun.
2. Sunscreens should not be used as a means of extending the duration of solar exposure (e.g., prolonging sunbathing) and it should not be used as a substitute for clothing on sites that are usually unexposed (e.g., the trunk and buttocks).
3. Daily use of sunscreen with a high sun protection factor (>15) on exposed skin is recommended for residents of areas of high insolation who work outdoors or enjoy regular outdoor recreation. Daily use of a sunscreen can reduce the cumulative solar exposure that causes actinic keratoses and squamous cell carcinoma.
4. Adequate solar protection is more important during childhood than any other time in life, and parents and school managers should assiduously apply the first two recommendations.

Source: The International Agency for Research on Cancer Working Group on the Evaluation of Cancer-Preventive Agents. Sunscreens. In: IARC Handbooks of Cancer Prevention. Vol 5. Lyon, France: International Agency for Research on Cancer, 2001.

Appendix B. Sunscreen: How to Select, Apply, and Use It Correctly

When to Apply Sunscreen

- Apply sunscreen approximately 30 minutes before being in the sun (for best results) so that it can be absorbed by the skin and less likely to wash off when you perspire.
- Remember to reapply sunscreen after swimming or strenuous exercise.
- Apply sunscreen often throughout the day if you work outdoors, and wear hats and protective clothing.

How to Apply Sunscreen

- Shake well before use to mix particles that might be clumped up in the container. Consider using the new spray-on or stick types of sunscreen.

- Be sure to apply enough sunscreen. As a rule of thumb, use an ounce (a handful) to cover your entire body.
- Use on all parts of your skin exposed to the sun, including the ears, back, shoulders, and the back of the knees and legs.
- Apply thickly and thoroughly.
- Be careful when applying sunscreen around the eyes.

What to Look for When You Buy Sunscreen

- Pick a broad-spectrum sunscreen that protects against UV-A and UV-B rays and has a sun protection factor (SPF) of at least 15.
- Read product labels. Look for a waterproof brand if you will be sweating or swimming. Buy a nonstinging product or one specifically formulated for your face.
- Buy a brand that does not contain para-aminobenzoic acid (PABA) if you are sensitive to that ingredient.
- Try a sunscreen with different chemicals if your skin reacts badly to the one that you are using. Not all sunscreens have the same ingredients.
- Use a water-based sunscreen if you have oily skin or are prone to acne.
- Be aware that more expensive does not mean better. Although a costly brand might feel or smell better, it is not necessarily more effective than a cheaper product.
- Be aware of the expiration date because some sunscreen ingredients might degrade over time.

Appendix C. Skin Cancer Education Resources

Skin cancer information and resources are available from various governmental agencies, voluntary organizations, medical associations, and corporations. Information is often available in your state or local area. At the national level, information is available from the sources listed below. The Internet address links take you directly to each organization's skin cancer information section.

American Academy of Dermatology
930 North Meacham Road
P.O. Box 681069
Schaumburg, IL 60173-4965
Phone: 847-330-0230
http://www.aad.org/skincnrUpdates.html

AMC Cancer Research Center
Phone: 800-321-1557
http://www.amc.org/html/market/h_market_sunnydays.html
email: products@amc.org

American Cancer Society
1599 Clifton Road, N.E.
Atlanta, GA 30329
Phone: 800-227-2345
http://www3.cancer.org/cancerinfo

Anti-Cancer Council of Victoria
100 Drummond Street
Carlton Victoria 3053 Australia
Phone: 61-3-9635-5152
Fax: 61-3-9635-5260
http://www.sunsmart.com.au

CDC
National Center for Chronic Disease Prevention and Health Promotion
Division of Cancer Prevention and Control
4770 Buford Highway, N.E.; Mailstop K57

Atlanta, GA 30341-3724
Phone: 770-488-4751
http://www.cdc.gov/cancer/nscpep

National Cancer Institute
Cancer Information Service
Building 31, Room 10A16
31 Center Drive MSC-2580
Bethesda, MD 20892-2580
Phone: 800-422-6237
http://www.cancer.gov

National Council on Skin Cancer Prevention
http://www.skincancerprevention.org

Norris Cotton Cancer Center
The Sun Safe Project
Dartmouth Medical School
Department of Community and Family Medicine
7250 Strasenburgh
Hanover, NH 03755
Phone: 603-650-1566
http://www.dartmouth.edu/dms/sunsafe

U.S. Environmental Protection Agency
Sun Wise School Program
EPA Stratospheric Ozone Information
401 M Street SW (6205J)

Washington, DC 20460
Phone: 800-296-1996
http://www.epa.gov/sunwise

REFERENCES

[1] National Cancer Institute. SEER Cancer Statistics Review, 1973–1998. Available at http://seer.cancer.gov/Publications/CSR1973_1998/ melanoma.pdf.

[2] Weinstock, MA; Colditz, GA; Willett, WC; Stampfer, MJ; Bronstein, BR Jr; Speizer, FE. Nonfamilial cutaneous melanoma incidence in women associated with sun exposure before 20 years of age. *Pediatrics*, 1989, 84, 199–204.

[3] Stern, RS; Weinstein, MC,Baker, SG. Risk reduction for nonmelanoma skin cancer with childhood sunscreen use. *Arch Dermatol*, 1986, 122, 537–45.

[4] Gilchrest, BA; Eller, MS; Geller, AC; Yaar, M. The pathogenesis of melanoma induced by ultraviolet radiation. *N Engl J Med*, 1999, 340, 1341–8.

[5] CDC. Guidelines for effective school health education to prevent the spread of AIDS. *MMWR*, 1988, 37(S-2), 1–14.

[6] CDC. Guidelines for school health programs to prevent tobacco use and addiction. *MMWR*, 1994, 43(RR-2), 1–18.

[7] CDC. Guidelines for school health programs to promote lifelong healthy eating. *MMWR*, 1996, 45(RR-9), 1–41.

[8] CDC. Guidelines for school and community programs to promote lifelong physical activity among young people. *MMWR*, 1997, 46(RR-6), 1–36.

[9] CDC. Community guidelines. Available at http://www.thecommunity guide.org/ home_f.html.

[10] US Department of Health and Human Services. Objectives for Improving Health (Part A: Focus Areas 1–14), Cancer. In: Healthy people 2010 (conference ed, Vol 1). Washington, DC: US Department of Health and Human Services 2000, 3-18–3-19. Available at http://www.health.gov/healthypeople/Document/pdf/Volume1/03Cancer. pdf.

[11] Greenlee, RT; Murray, T; Bolden, S; Wingo, PA. Cancer statistics, 2000. *CA Cancer J Clin*, 2000, 50, 7–33.

[12] American Cancer Society. Cancer prevention and early detection— cancer facts & figures 2002. Atlanta, GA: American Cancer Society, 2002.

[13] Preston, DS; Stern, RS. Nonmelanoma cancers of the skin. *N Engl J Med*, 1992, 327, 1649–62.

[14] Armstrong, BK; English, DR. Cutaneous malignant melanoma. In: Schottenfeld D, Fraumeni JF, eds. Cancer epidemiology and prevention. 2nd ed. New York, NY: Oxford University Press, 1996.

[15] Green, A; MacLennan, R; Youl, P; Martin, N. Site distribution of cutaneous melanoma in Queensland. *Int J Cancer*, 1993, 53, 232–6.

[16] Ries, LA; Wingo, PA; Miller, DS; et al. The annual report to the nation on the status of cancer, 1973–1997, with a special section on colorectal cancer. *Cancer*, 2000, 88, 2398–424.

[17] Jemal, A; Devesa, SS; Hartge, P; Tucker, MA. Recent trends in cutaneous melanoma incidence among whites in the United States. *J Natl Cancer Inst*, 2001, 93, 678-83.
[18] Jemal, A; Devesa, SS; Fears, TR; Hartge, P. Changing patterns of cutaneous malignant melanoma mortality rates among whites in the United States. *J Natl Cancer Inst*, 2000, 92, 811–8.
[19] Hall, HI; Miller, DR; Rogers, JD; Bewerse, B. Update on the incidence and mortality from melanoma in the United States. *J Am Acad Dermatol*, 1999, 40, 35–42. Available at http://seer.cancer.gov/Publi cations/CSR1973_1998/melanoma.pdf.
[20] Armstrong, BK; Kricker, A. How much melanoma is caused by sun exposure?. *Melanoma Res*, 1993, 3, 395–401.
[21] Diffey, BL. Solar ultraviolet radiation effects on biological systems. *Phys Med Biol*, 1991, 36, 299–328.
[22] IARC Working Group on the Evaluation of Cancer-Preventive Agents. Sunscreens. In: IARC Handbooks of Cancer Prevention. Vol 5. Lyon, France: International Agency for Research on Cancer, 2001.
[23] Taylor, HR; West, SK; Rosenthal, FS; et al. Effect of ultraviolet radiation on cataract formation. *N Engl J Med*, 1988, 319, 1429–33.
[24] West, SK; Duncan, DD; Munoz, B, et al. Sunlight exposure and risk of lens opacities in a population-based study: the Salisbury Eye Evaluation project. *JAMA*, 1998, 280, 714–8.
[25] Rosmini, F; Stazi, MA; Milton, Rc; Sperduto, RD; Pasquini, P; Maraini, G. A dose-response effect between a sunlight index and age-related cataracts. Italian-American Cataract Study Group. *Ann Epidemiol*, 1994, 4, 266–70.
[26] Whiteman, DC; Whiteman, CA; Green, AC. Childhood sun exposure as a risk factor for melanoma: a systematic review of epidemiologic studies. *Cancer Causes Control*, 2001, 12, 69–82.
[27] Westerdahl, J; Olsson, H; Ingvar, C. At what age do sunburn episodes play a crucial role for the development of malignant melanoma. *Eur J Cancer*, 1994, 30A, 1647–54.
[28] Elwood, JM; Jopson, J. Melanoma and sun exposure: an overview of published studies. *Int J Cancer*, 1997, 73, 198–203.
[29] Kricker, A; Armstrong, BK; English, DR. Sun exposure and non- melanocytic skin cancer. *Cancer Causes Control*, 1994, 5, 367–92.
[30] Kricker, A; Armstrong, BK; English, DR; Heenan, PJ. Does intermittent sun exposure cause basal cell carcinoma? A case-control study in Western Australia. *Int J Cancer*, 1995, 60, 489–94.
[31] Gallagher, RP; Hill, GB; Bajdik, CD; et al. Sunlight exposure, pigmentary factors, and risk of nonmelanocytic skin cancer I. Basal cell carcinoma. *Arch Dermatol*, 1995, 131, 157–63.
[32] Gallagher RP. Sun exposure and non-melanocytic skin cancer. In: Grob JJ, Stern RS, MacKie RM, Weinstock WA, eds. Epidemiology, causes and prevention of skin diseases. 1st ed. London, England: Blackwell Science, 1997, 72–7.
[33] Armstrong, BK. Melanoma: childhood or lifelong sun exposure. In: Grob JJ, Stern RS, Mackie RM, Weinstock WA, eds. Epidemiology, causes and prevention of skin diseases. 1st ed. London, England: Blackwell Science, 1997, 63–6.
[34] Whiteman, D; Green, A. Melanoma and sunburn. *Cancer Causes Control*, 1994, 5, 564–72.

[35] Autier, P; Dore, JF; Cattaruzza, MS; et al. Sunscreen use, wearing clothes, and number of nevi in 6to 7-year-old European children. European Organization for Research and Treatment of Cancer Melanoma Cooperative Group. *J Nat Cancer Inst*, 1998, 90, 1873–80.

[36] Buller, DB; Callister, MA; Reichert, T. Skin cancer prevention by parents of young children: health information sources, skin cancer knowledge, and sun-protection practices. *Oncol Nurs Forum*, 1995, 22, 1559–66.

[37] Foltz, AT. Parental knowledge and practices of skin cancer prevention: a pilot study. *J Pediatr Health Care*, 1993, 7, 220–5.

[38] Hurwitz, S. The sun and sunscreen protection: recommendations for children. *J Dermatol Surg Oncol*, 1988, 14, 657–60.

[39] Taylor, CR; Stern, RS; Leyden, JJ; Gilchrest, BA. Photoaging/ photodamage and photoprotection. *J Am Acad Dermatol*, 1990, 22, 1–15.

[40] Autier, P; Dore, JF. Influence of sun exposures during childhood and during adulthood on melanoma risk. EPIMEL and EORTC Melanoma Cooperative Group. European Organization for Research and Treatment of Cancer. *Int J Cancer.*, 1998, 77, 533–7.

[41] Williams, ML; Pennella, R. Melanoma, melanocytic nevi, and other melanoma risk factors in children. *J Pediatr*, 1994, 124, 833–45.

[42] Parkin, DM; Muir, CS; Whelan, SL; Gao, YT; Ferlay, J; Powell, J. *Cancer incidence in five continents*. Vol 6. Lyon, France: International Agency for Research on Cancer, 1992.

[43] Scotto, J; Fears, TR; Freaumeni, JF, Jr. Incidence of nonmelanoma skin cancer in the United States. Washington, DC: US Department of Health and Human Services, Public Health Service, National Institutes of Health, National Cancer Institute, 1981: DHHS publication no. (NIH) 83-2433.

[44] Pennello, G; Devesa, S; Gail, M. Association of surface ultraviolet B radiation levels with melanoma and nonmelanoma skin cancer in United States blacks. *Cancer Epidemiol Biomarkers Prev*, 2000, 9, 291–7.

[45] Rhodes, AR; Weinstock, MA; Fitzpatrick, TB; Mihm, MC, Jr; Sober, AJ. Risk factors for cutaneous melanoma. A practical method of recognizing predisposed individuals. *JAMA*, 1987, 258, 3146–54.

[46] Scotto, J; Fears, TR; Kraemer, KH; Fraumeni, JF. Nonmelanoma skin cancer. In: Schottenfeld D, Fraumeni JF, eds. Cancer epidemiology and prevention. 2nd ed. New York, NY: Oxford University Press, 1996.

[47] Kricker, A; Armstrong, BK; English, DR; Heenan, PJ. Pigmentary and cutaneous risk factors for non-melanocytic skin cancer—a case-control study. *Int J Cancer*, 1991, 48, 650–62.

[48] Holly, EA; Kelly, JW; Shpall, SN; Chiu, SH. Number of melanocytic nevi as a major risk factor for malignant melanoma. *J Am Acad Dermatol*, 1987, 17, 459–68.

[49] Holly, EA; Kelly, JW; Ahn, DK; Shpall, SV; Rosen, JI. Risk of cutaneous melanoma by number of melanocytic nevi and correlation of nevi by anatomic site. In: Gallagher RP, Elwood JM, eds. Epidemiological aspects of cutaneous malignant melanoma. Boston, MA: Kluwer Academic Publishers, 1994, 159–72.

[50] Goldstein, AM; Tucker, MA. Genetic epidemiology of familial melanoma. *Dermatol Clin*, 1995, 35, 605–12.

[51] National Cancer Institute. *Canques.* Available at http://seer.cancer.gov/ScientificSystems/CanQues.

[52] International Agency for Research on Cancer. Solar and ultraviolet radiation. *IARC Monogr Eval Carcinog Risks Hum*, 1992, 55, 1–316.

[53] Koh, HK; Sinks, TH; Geller, AC; Miller, DR; Lew, RA. Etiology of melanoma. In: Nathanson L, ed. *Current research and clinical management of melanoma.* Boston, MA: Kluwer Academic Publishers, 1993, 1–27.

[54] Diffey, BL. Ozone Depletion and skin cancer. In: Grob JJ, Stern RS, Mackie RM, Weinstock WA, eds. Epidemiology, causes and prevention of skin diseases. 1st ed. London, England: Blackwell Science, 1997, 77–85.

[55] National Institute of Environmental Health Sciences. Report on carcinogens: solar UV radiation and exposure to sunbeds and sunlamps. 9th ed. Research Triangle Park, NC, 2000, 48–50.

[56] Swerdlow, AJ; Weinstock, MA. Do tanning lamps cause melanoma? An epidemiologic assessment. *J Am Acad Dermatol*, 1998, 38, 89–98.

[57] Miller, SA; Hamilton, SL; Wester, UG; Cyr, WH. An analysis of UVA emissions from sunlamps and the potential importance for melanoma. *Photochem Photobiol*, 1998, 68, 63–70.

[58] Spencer, JM; Amonette, RA. Indoor tanning: risks, benefits, and future trends. *J Am Acad Dermatol*, 1995, 33, 288–98.

[59] Saraiya, M; Frank, E; Elon, L; Baldwin, G; McAlpine, BE. Personal and clinical skin cancer prevention practices of U.S. women physicians. *Arch Derm*, 2000, 136, 633–42.

[60] McDonald, CJ. American Cancer Society perspective on the American College of Preventive Medicine's policy statements on skin cancer prevention and screening. *CA Cancer J Clin*, 1998, 48, 229–31.

[61] Committee on Guidelines of Care, American Academy of Dermatology. Guidelines of care for cutaneous squamous cell carcinoma. *J Am Acad Dermatol*, 1993, 28, 628–31.

[62] Committee on Guidelines of Care, American Academy of Dermatology. Guidelines of care for nevi I (nevocellular nevi and seborrheic keratoses). *J Am Acad Dermatol*, 1992, 26, 629–31.

[63] Committee on Environmental Health, American Academy of *Pediatrics*. Ultraviolet light: a hazard to children. *Pediatrics*, 1999, 104, 328–33.

[64] Council on Scientific Affairs. Harmful effects of ultraviolet radiation. *JAMA*, 1989, 262, 380–4.

[65] National Cancer Institute. Skin cancer (PDQ®): Prevention. Available at http://www.cancer.gov/cancer_information/doc_pdq.aspx?version=patient&viewid=dd7fa1a5-9c70-4625-9112-d2db13af013d.

[66] Autier, P; Dore, JF; Shifflers, E; et al. Melanoma and use of sunscreens: an EORTC case-control study in Germany, Belgium, and France. The EORTC Melanoma Cooperative Group. *Int J Cancer*, 1995, 61, 749–55.

[67] Welsh, C; Diffey, BL. The protection against solar actinic radiation afforded by common clothing fabrics. *Clinical Exp Dermatol*, 1981, 6, 577–82.

[68] Pailthorpe, M. Apparel textiles and sun protection: a marketing opportunity or a quality control nightmare? *Mutat Res*, 1998, 422, 175–83.

[69] Diffey, BL; Cheeseman, J. Sun protection with hats. *Br J Dermatol*, 1992, 127, 10–12.

[70] American Sun Protection Organization. Sun safety info: clothing. Available at http://www.americansun.org/pages/clothing.htm.

[71] Gies, HP; Roy, CR; Elliott, G; Zongli, W. Ultraviolet radiation protection factors for clothing. *Health Phys*, 1994, 67, 131–9.

[72] American Academy of Ophthalmology. Sunglasses. San Francisco, CA: American Academy of Ophthalmology, 1995.

[73] Gies, HP; Roy, CR; Elliot, G. Ultraviolet radiation protection factors for personal protection in both occupational and recreational situations. *Radiat Prot Aust*, 1992, 10, 59–66.

[74] Greenwood, JS; Soulos, GP; Thomas, ND. Under cover: guidelines for shade planning and design. Sydney, Australia: New South Wales Cancer Council and New South Wales Health Department, 1998.

[75] Parsons, PG; Neale, R; Wolski, P; Green, A. The shady side of solar protection. *Med J Aust*, 1998, 168, 327–30.

[76] Vainio, H; Miller, AB; Bianchini, F. An international evaluation of the cancer-preventive potential of sunscreens. *Int J Cancer*, 2000, 88, 838–42.

[77] Thompson, SC; Jolley, D; Marks, R. Reduction of solar keratoses by regular sunscreen use. *N Engl J Med*, 1993, 329, 1147–51.

[78] Naylor, MF; Boyd, A; Smith, DW; Cameron, GS; Hubbard, D; Neldner, KH. High sun protection factor sunscreens in the suppression of actinic neoplasia. *Arch Dermatol*, 1995, 131, 170–5.

[79] Green, A; Williams, G; Neale, R; et al. Daily sunscreen application and betacarotene supplementation in prevention of basal-cell and squamous-cell carcinomas of the skin: a randomised controlled trial. *Lancet*, 1999, 354, 723–9.

[80] Gallagher, RP; Rivers, JK; Lee, TK; Bajdik, CD; McLean, DI; Coldman, AJ. Broad-spectrum sunscreen use and the development of new nevi in white children: a randomized controlled trial. *JAMA*, 2000, 283, 2955–60.

[81] Weinstock, MA. Do sunscreens increase or decrease melanoma risk: an epidemiologic evaluation. *J Invest Dermatol Symp Proc*, 1999, 4, 97–100.

[82] McLean, DI; Gallagher, R. Sunscreens: use and misuse. *Dermatol Clin*, 1998, 16, 219–26.

[83] Odio, MR; Veres, DA; Goodman, JJ; et al. Comparative efficacy of sunscreen reapplication regimens in children exposed to ambient sunlight. *Photodermatol Photoimmunol Photomed*, 1994, 10, 118–25.

[84] Baade, PD; Balanda, KP; Lowe, JB. Changes in skin protection behaviors, attitudes, and sunburn: in a population with the highest incidence of skin cancer in the world. *Cancer Detect Prev*, 1996, 20, 566–75.

[85] Bech-Thomsen, N; Wulf, HC. Sunbathers' application of sunscreen is probably inadequate to obtain the sun protection factor assigned to the preparation. *Photodermatol Photoimmunol Photomed*, 1992–1993, 9, 242–44.

[86] Sayre, RM; Kollias, N; Ley, RD; Baqer, AH. Changing the risk spectrum of injury and the performance of sunscreen products throughout the day. *Photodermatol Photoimmnol Photomed*, 1994, 10, 148–53.

[87] Foley, P; Nixon, R; Marks, R; Frower, K; Thompson, S. The frequency of reactions to sunscreens: results of a longitudinal population-based study on the regular use of sunscreens in Australia. *Br J Dermatol*, 1993, 128, 512–8.

[88] Keesling, B,Friedman, HS. Psychosocial factors in sunbathing and sunscreen use. *Health Psychol*, 1987, 6, 477–93.
[89] Randle, HW. Suntanning: differences in perceptions throughout history. *Mayo Clinic Proc*, 1997, 72, 461–6.
[90] Chapman, S; Marks, R; King, M. Trends in tans and skin protection in Australian fashion magazines 1982 through 1991. *Am J Public Health*, 1992, 82, 1677–80.
[91] Johnson, EY; Lookingbill, DP. Sunscreen use and sun exposure: trends in a white population. *Arch Dermatol*, 1984, 120, 727–31.
[92] Banks, BA; Silverman, RA; Schwartz, RH; Tunnessen, WW, Jr. Attitudes of teenagers toward sun exposure and sunscreen use. *Pediatrics*, 1992, 89, 40–2.
[93] Lescano, CM; Rodrique, JR. Skin cancer prevention behaviors among parents of young children. *Children's Health Care*, 1997, 26, 107–14.
[94] Hall, HI; May, DS; Lew, RA; Koh, HK; Nadel, M. Sun protection behaviors of the U.S. white population. *Prev Med*, 1997, 26, 401–7.
[95] Hall, HI; Rogers, JD. Sun protection behaviors among African Americans. *Ethn Dis*, 1999, 9, 126–31.
[96] Marks, R. Role of childhood in the development of skin cancer. *Aust Paediatr J*, 1988, 24, 337–8.
[97] Mermelstein, RJ; Riesenberg, LA. Changing knowledge and attitudes about skin cancer risk factors in adolescents. *Health Psychol*, 1992, 11, 371–6.
[98] Reynolds, KD; Blaum, JM; Jester, PM; Weiss, H; Soong, SJ; Diclemente, RJ. Predictors of sun exposure in adolescents in southeastern U.S. population. *J Adolesc Health*, 1996, 19, 409–15.
[99] Robinson, JK; Rigel, DS; Amonette, RA. Trends in sun exposure knowledge, attitudes, and behaviors: 1986 to 1996. *J Am Acad Dermatol*, 1997, 37, 179–86.
[100] Jorgensen, CM; Wayman, J; Green, C; Gelb, CA. Using health communications for primary prevention of skin cancer: CDC's Choose Your Cover campaign. *J Womens Health Gend Based Med*, 2000, 9, 471–5.
[101] Hall, HI; Jones, SE; Saraiya, M. Prevalence and correlates of sunscreen use among US high school students. *J Sch Health*, 2001, 71, 453–7.
[102] Glanz, K; Lew, R; Song, V; Ah, Cook, VA. Factors associated with skin cancer prevention practices in a multiethnic population. *Health Educ Behav*, 1999, 26, 344–59.
[103] Maducdoc, LR; Wagner, RF, Jr; Wagner, KD. Parents' use of sunscreen on beach-going children: the burnt child dreads the fire. *Arch Dermatol*, 1982, 128, 628–9.
[104] Grob, JJ; Guglielmina, C; Gouvernet, J; Zarour, H; Noe, C; Bonerandi, JJ. Study of sunbathing habits in children and adolescents: application to the prevention of melanoma. *Dermatology*, 1993, 186, 94–8.
[105] Vail-Smith, K; Watson, CL; Felts, WM; Parrillo, AV; Knight, SM; Hughes JL. Childhood sun exposure: parental knowledge, attitudes, and behaviors. *J Health Educ*, 1997, 28, 149–55.
[106] Olson, AL; Dietrich, AJ; Sox, CH; Stevens, MM; Winchell, CW; Ahles, TA. Solar protection of children at the beach. *Pediatrics*, 1997, 99, E1.
[107] Hall, HI; McDavid, K; Jorgensen, CM; Kraft, JM. Factors associated with sunburn in white children aged 6 months to 11 years. Am J *Prev Med*, 2001, 20, 9–14.
[108] Robinson, JK; Rigel, DS; Amonette, RA. Summertime sun protection used by adults for their children. *J Am Acad Dermatol*, 2000, 42, 746–53.

[109] Standing Committee on the Scientific Evaluation of Dietary Reference Intakes, Institute of Medicine. Dietary reference intakes for calcium, phosphorus, magnesium, vitamin D, and fluoride. Washington, DC: National Academy Press, 1997.

[110] Vieth, R. Vitamin D supplementation, 25-hydroxyvitamin D concentrations and safety. *Am J Clin Nutr*, 1999, 69, 842–56.

[111] American Academy of Pediatrics. Vitamins: vitamin D. In: Kleinman RE, ed. Pediatric nutrition handbook, 4th ed. Elk Grove Village, IL: American Academy of Pediatrics, 1998, 275–7.

[112] Joint Committee on National Health Education Standards. National health education standards: achieving health literacy—an investment in the future. Atlanta, GA: American Cancer Society, 1995.

[113] McKenzie, FD; Richmond, JB. Linking health and learning: an overview of coordinated school health programs. In: Marx E, Wooley SF, eds. Health is academic: a guide to coordinated school health programs. New York, NY: Teachers College Press, 1998.

[114] Carlyon, P; Carlyon, W; McCarthy, AR. Family and community involvement in school health. In: Marx E, Wooley SF, eds. Health is academic: a guide to coordinated school health programs. New York, NY: Teachers College Press, 1998.

[115] Glanz, K; Lewis, FM; Rimer, BK; eds. Health behavior and health education: theory, research and practice. 2nd ed. San Francisco, CA: JosseyBass Inc, 1997.

[116] Henderson, A; Rowe, DE. *A healthy school environment*. In: Marx E, Wooley SF, eds. Health is academic: a guide to coordinated school health programs. New York, NY: Teachers College Press, 1998.

[117] Glanz, K; Lankenau, B; Foerster, S; Temple, S; Mullis, R; Schmid, T. Environmental and policy approaches to cardiovascular disease prevention through nutrition: opportunities for state and local action. *Health Educ Qtly*, 1995, 22, 512–27.

[118] Sallis, JF; Owen, N. Ecological models. In: Glanz K, Lewis FM, Rimer BK, eds. Health behavior and health education: theory, research and practice. 2nd ed. San Francisco, CA: Jossey-Bass Inc, 1997, 403–24.

[119] Queensland, Cancer, Fund. Working towards a SunSmart Queensland. Queensland, Australia: Queensland Cancer Fund, 1997.

[120] Schofield, MJ; Edwards, K; Pearce, R. Effectiveness of two strategies for dissemination of sun-protection policy in New South Wales primary and secondary schools. *Aust N Z J Public Health*, 1997, 21, 743–50.

[121] Glanz, K; Carbone, E; Song, V. Formative research for developing targeted skin cancer prevention programs for children in multiethnic Hawaii. *Health Education Research*, 1999, 14, 155–66.

[122] Glanz, K; Lew, RA; Song, V; Murakami-Akatsuka, L. Skin cancer prevention program in outdoor recreation settings: effects of the Hawaii SunSmart Program. *Effective Clinical Practice*, 2000, 3, 53–61.

[123] Wolf, SM; Swanson, LA; Manning, R. PROJECT SPF (Sun Safety, Protection and Fun): Arizona Department of Health Services Early Childhood Skin Cancer Prevention Education Program. *Health Educ Behav*, 1999, 26, 301–5.

[124] United States Environmental Protection Agency. The SunWise School Program Guide. Available at http://www.epa.gov/sunwise/guide.pdf.

[125] Buller, DB; Borland, R. Skin cancer prevention for children: a critical review. *Health Educ Behav*, 1999, 26, 317–43.

[126] Buller, MK; Loescher, LJ; Buller, DB. Sunshine and Skin Health: a curriculum for skin cancer prevention education. *J Cancer Educ*, 1994, 9, 155–62.
[127] Buller, MK; Goldberg, G; Buller, DB. Sun Smart Day: a pilot program for photoprotection education. Pediatric Dermatol, 1997, 14, 257–63.
[128] Thornton, CM; Piacquadio, DJ. Promoting sun awareness: evaluation of an educational children's book. *Pediatrics*, 1996, 98, 52–5.
[129] Buller, DB; Buller, MK; Beach, B; Ertl, G. Sunny days, healthy ways: evaluation of a skin cancer prevention curriculum for elementary schoolaged children. *J Am Acad Dermatol*, 1996, 35, 911–22.
[130] Girgis, A; Sanson-Fisher, RW; Tripodi, DA; Golding, T. Evaluation of interventions to improve solar protection in primary schools. *Health Educ Qtly*, 1993, 20, 275–87.
[131] Fork, HE; Wagner, RF; Wagner, KD. The Texas peer education sun awareness project for children: primary prevention of malignant melanoma and nonmelanocytic skin cancers. *Cutis*, 1992, 50, 363–4.
[132] Reding, DJ; Fischer, V; Gunderson, P; Lappe, K. Skin cancer prevention: a peer education model. *Wisc Med J*, 1995, 94, 75–9.
[133] Hornung, RL; Lennon, PA; Garrett, JM; DeVellis, RF; Weinberg PD, Strecher, VJ. Interactive computer technology for skin cancer prevention targeting children. *Amer J Prev Med*, 2000, 18, 69–76.
[134] Cantor, MA; Rosseel, K. The United States Environmental Protection Agency SunWise School Program. *Health Educ Behav*, 1999, 26, 303–4.
[135] Perry, CL. Creating health behavior change: how to develop community-wide programs for youth. *Thousand Oaks*, CA: Sage, 1999.
[136] Mayer, JA; Slymen, DJ; Eckhardt, L; et al. Reducing ultraviolet radiation exposure in children. *Prev Med*, 1997, 26, 516–22.
[137] Parrott, R; Duggan, A; Cremo, J; Eckles, A; Jones, K; Steiner, C. Communicating about youth's sun exposure risk to soccer coaches and parents: a pilot study in Georgia. *Health Educ Behav*, 1999, 26, 385–95.
[138] Dietrich, AJ; Olson, AL; Sox, CH; et al. A community-based randomized trial encouraging sun protection for children. *Pediatrics*, 1998, 102, E64.
[139] Dietrich, AJ; Olson, AL; Sox, CH; Tosteson, TD; Grant-Petersson, J. Persistent increase in children's sun protection in a randomized controlled community trial. *Prev Med*, 2000, 31, 569–74.
[140] Miller, DR; Geller, AC; Wood, MC; Lew, RA; Koh, HK. The Falmouth Safe Skin Project: evaluation of a community program to promote sun protection in youth. *Health Educ Behav*, 1999, 26, 369–84.
[141] Arthey, S; Clarke, VA. Suntanning and sun protection: a review of the psychological literature. *Soc Sci Med*, 1995, 40, 265–74.
[142] Glanz, K; Maddock, J; Lew, RA; Murakami-Akatsuka, L. A randomized trial of the Hawaii SunSmart program's impact on outdoor recreation staff. *J Am Acad Dermatol*, 2001, 44, 973–8.
[143] Easton, AN; Price, JH; Boehm, K; Telljohann, SK. Sun protection counseling by pediatricians. *Arch Pediatr Adolesc Med*, 1997, 151, 1133–8.
[144] Green, LW; Kreuter, MW. Health promotion planning: an educational and ecological approach. 3rd ed. Mountain View, CA: Mayfield Publishing, 1999.

[145] Hill, D; Dixon, H. Promoting sun protection in children: rationale and challenges. *Health Educ Behav*, 1999, 26, 409–17.

In: Encyclopedia of Dermatology (6 Volume Set)
Editor: Meghan Pratt
ISBN: 978-1-63483-326-4

Chapter 74

SHADE PLANNING FOR AMERICA'S SCHOOLS*

Centers for Disease Control and Prevention

WHAT IS THE PURPOSE OF THIS MANUAL?

In 2002, the Centers for Disease Control and Prevention (CDC) published the *Guidelines for School Programs to Prevent Skin Cancer*, which outlines steps that school communities can take to develop a comprehensive approach to reducing the risk for skin cancer among students, teachers, staff, and visitors. The guidelines include the following recommendations:

- Establish policies that reduce exposure to solar ultraviolet (UV) radiation.
- Provide and maintain physical and social environments that support sun safety.
- Provide opportunities for students to gain the knowledge, develop the attitudes, and practice the skills needed to prevent skin cancer.
- Involve family members in skin cancer prevention efforts.
- Provide pre-service and in-service skin cancer prevention education for school administrators, teachers, coaches, school nurses, and other professionals who work with students.
- Support sun-safety policies, sun-safe environments, and skin cancer prevention education with school health services.
- Evaluate the implementation of policies, environmental change, education, family involvement, professional development, and health services.

This manual has been created to support school communities in their implementation of the *Guidelines for School Programs to Prevent Skin Cancer* and, specifically, to help schools

---

* This is an edited, reformatted and augmented version of a report prepared under contract for the Centers for Disease Control and Prevention, National Center for Chronic Disease Prevention and Health, Division of Cancer Prevention and Control, 2008.

create and maintain a physical environment that supports sun safety by ensuring that school grounds have adequate shade.

Between 68% and 90% of all melanomas result from exposure to ultraviolet radiation.[1]

Why Should Schools Care About Skin Cancer?

Cancer of the skin is the most commonly diagnosed cancer in the United States and perhaps the most preventable. Melanoma and non-melanoma cancers, including basal cell cancer and squamous cell cancer, account for as much as 50% of all cancers. Because the reporting of non-melanoma cancers to cancer registries is not required, the exact number of non-melanoma cancer cases is not known. However, estimates indicate that as many as 1 million cases of basal cell and squamous cell skin cancer occur each year.[2] Melanoma, which accounts for only about 5% of skin cancer cases, also accounts for 79% of skin cancer deaths. From 1973 and through the early eighties, the incidence rate of melanoma among white men and women in the United States increased by about 6% per year. Since the early eighties, the increase has been around 3% annually. Approximately 55,100 new melanomas were diagnosed in the United States in 2004, and about 7,910 people died of melanoma that same year.[3]

Almost all of these cancers are preventable.[4] In most cases, exposure to solar UV radiation is the cause of the cancer. Using multiple methods for estimating the incidence of melanoma that might be attributable to exposure to the sun, Armstrong and Kricker, reporting in *Melanoma Research*, suggest that between 68% and 90% of all melanomas result from exposure to UV radiation.[5]

SOLAR RADIATION ADDED TO THE LIST OF "KNOWN" CARCINOGENS

The federal government's 11th edition of the Report on Carcinogens listed the sun and any other source of broad spectrum ultraviolet radiation as "known" causes of cancer.

"The report cites data indicating a cause-and-effect relationship between this radiation and skin cancer, cancer of the lip and melanoma of the eye. The report goes on to say that skin cancers are observed with increasing duration of exposure and for those who experience sunburn."

From National Institutes of Health News Release dated December 11, 2002

Why Shade?

There are many reasons that a school might want to improve the quality and increase the amount of accessible shade on school grounds. The most obvious and one of the most important reasons is that shade provides protection from solar UV radiation. Due to the scheduling complexities of physical education classes, sporting events, and other outdoor activities, students are often exposed to solar UV radiation during the peak sun hours of the day—between 10:00 a.m. and 4:00 p.m. For some schools and for some students, using sun protective methods, such as hats or sunscreen, or implementing policy changes could prove to be problematic. Providing shade in areas where students already participate in outdoor activities can afford passive protection from the sun's damaging rays.

What Are the Additional Benefits of Shade?

Extending the Classroom

Schools are often looking for ways to extend their classrooms. Two strategies for increasing shade on school grounds can also help schools create novel classroom experiences for their students. These strategies may be employed independently or in concert. The first is to modify existing structures or build new ones to provide shade where students play and socialize. The second calls for the strategic planting of additional shade-producing trees, vines, and shrubs. Structures built to provide shade can also be designed as covered outdoor learning areas, thereby extending the classroom beyond the school walls. Planting shade-producing vegetation affords schools the opportunity to create and maintain natural outdoor classrooms where students can enjoy hands-on experiences in the natural world. Both strategies could potentially provide teachers with new ideas for curricula and new reasons to take their students outdoors.

Extended Periods of Physical Activity

In adults, regular physical activity is linked to enhanced health and reduced risk for the development of many chronic diseases. Lifelong physical activity patterns are often developed in childhood and adolescence. In the section on preventing physical activity-related injuries in *CDC's Guidelines for School and Community Programs to Promote Lifelong Physical Activity Among Young People,* the use of shaded spaces or indoor facilities to reduce the incidence of heat-related illnesses is recommended. Not all schools have indoor facilities designed for active play; however, providing shade on existing outdoor play areas could reduce the temperature in those areas by as much as 10° to 20 °, increasing the period of time that students could engage in active outdoor play.

School Grounds Aesthetics

All too often, school grounds are an environment of concrete, asphalt, steel, turf grass, and chain link fences. In planning strategies to provide or increase shade on school grounds, schools have a second chance to improve the aesthetics of the school property, making the grounds more inviting to students, teachers, staff, parents, and visitors. A well-planned shade implementation project engages the entire school community in making the school a more pleasant place to learn.

Who Should Read This Manual?

A school includes not just the principal, teachers, students, and staff, but also key stakeholders and decision-makers that comprise the school community. In addition to school officials, the school community includes parents, neighbors, and members of the broader community, all of whom have a stake in helping to protect the community's children and adolescents from skin cancer. This manual was written as a reference tool for the entire school community, encompassing both the school district and the individual school.

How Can This Manual Be Used?

Section 1 School board members, superintendents, principals, and school health advisory councils can use this manual to acquaint themselves with issues relating to the damaging effects of solar UV radiation, skin cancer prevention, and planning for shade implementation at their schools. The first section gives information on both the short- and long-term effects of UV radiation on health and provides a rationale for developing sun-safe policies in schools.

Section 2 The second section addresses strategies for providing shade at schools and includes some of the advantages and disadvantages of each strategy. School board members, superintendents, principals, school health advisory councils, and school shade planning teams will find this information useful in determining the strategies that will work best at their school.

Section 3 The third section presents an overview of the process of planning a shade implementation project. School board members, superintendents, principals, and school health advisory councils can use it as a brief overview of the process. School shade planning teams can refer to this section for an introduction to the process and to sections 4 and 6 for more detailed information to guide them through the steps of shade planning.

Section 4 The fourth section presents information about schools and school districts that have engaged in shade planning projects and reveals some successful strategies. The needs of every school differ; there is no one-size-fits-all solution to providing shade at schools. This section offers a glimpse of shade strategies that others have employed.

Section 5 The fifth section gives the reader a basic introduction, or reintroduction, to solar geometry and the relationship between the Earth and Sun. Illustrations are included showing the effects of daily and seasonal changes in solar angles on the length and direction of shadows.

Section 6 The sixth section guides shade planning team members through the process of conducting a shade audit. The shade audit allows planning teams to consider the needs of the school in relation to the quantity and quality of shade already available to students, teachers, and staff.

SECTION 1. WHAT IS UV RADIATION?

Ultraviolet (UV) radiation is one component of a broad spectrum of electromagnetic radiation emitted by the sun. The spectrum also includes visible light, which we see, and infrared radiation, which we feel as heat.

The ultraviolet area of the spectrum can be further divided into three bands, ultraviolet A (UVA), ultraviolet B (UVB), and ultraviolet C (UVC). All UVC radiation and almost all UVB radiation are absorbed in the ozone layer of the atmosphere. UVA radiation penetrates the atmosphere unimpeded and, until recently, had been considered innocuous.

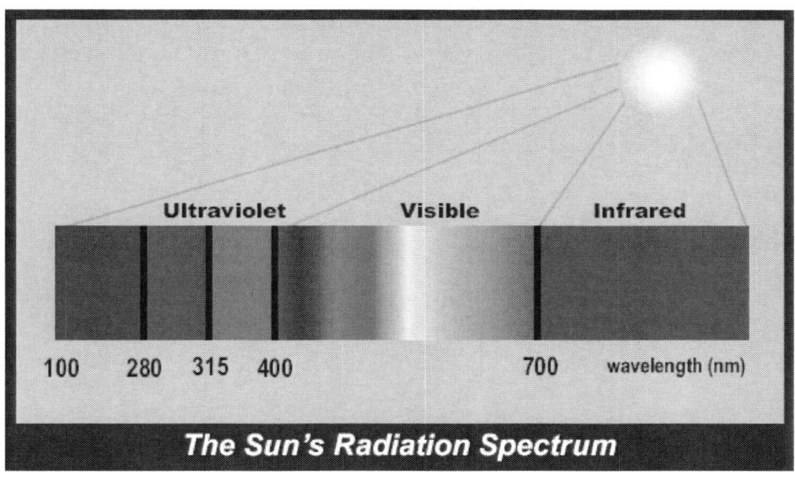

The Sun's Radiation Spectrum

What Are the Factors That Affect UV Radiation Levels?

Time of Day

At solar noon, the sun is at its highest point of the day. As much as 30% of total UV radiation is received in the hour before and the hour after solar noon, and as much as 75% is received during the 3 hours before and the 3 hours after solar noon.[6]

Time of Year

Because the angles of the sun change throughout the year, the intensity of UV radiation changes as well. In the northern hemisphere, UV radiation tends to be greater in the summer months.

SHADE PLANNING TOOLBOX

Q: What time is solar noon?

A: That depends on the day of the year, your latitude and longitude, and your location within your time zone.

On July 4, solar noon is at:
- 12:48 (EDT) in Boston
- 1:40 (EDT) in Knoxville
- 12:51 (CDT) in Nashville
- 12:53 (PDT) in San Diego

On February 1, solar noon is at:
- 11:57 (EST) in Boston
- 12:49 (EST) in Knoxville
- 12:00 (CST) in Nashville
- 12:02 (PST) in San Diego

To find out what time solar noon occurs on any day of the year at any location, visit the National Oceanic and Atmospheric Administration (NOAA) Surface Radiation Research Branch web site at http://www.srrb.noaa.gov/ highlights/sunrise/sunrise.html.

Geographical Latitude

UV radiation decreases as the distance from the equator increases.

Altitude

Because the atmosphere is thinner at higher altitudes and less able to absorb UVB, total UV radiation is greater at higher altitudes.

Weather Conditions

Although clouds reduce the full spectrum of solar radiation, they do not reduce UV radiation to the same extent that they reduce visible light and infrared radiation. Clouds may make us feel cooler and block our view of the sun, but they do not fully protect us from UV radiation.

Atmospheric Ozone

The stratosphere's ozone layer provides us with an enormous amount of protection against the damaging effects of UV radiation. Unfortunately, in certain areas, ozone has been depleted to a dangerous extent, primarily due to the release of chlorofluorocarbons (CFCs) and other ozone-depleting chemicals, such as carbon tetrachloride and methyl chloroform, into the atmosphere. Both carbon tetrachloride and methyl chloroform are solvents that have been used in industrial applications, and CFCs have, in the past, been used as refrigerants and aerosol propellants. The use of all three of these chemicals has since been restricted or prohibited.[7] Nonetheless, much of the damage that has been done remains.

What Are Direct and Indirect UV Radiation?

Direct UV radiation, or UV radiation that travels from the sun in a straight line, may pose the greatest risk to our health, but we are also at risk from exposure to indirect (scattered and reflected) UV radiation. Scattered UV radiation results from being bounced around by atmospheric dust and water droplets in clouds. Throughout the day, the level of indirect UV radiation varies, as does the level of direct UV radiation. In the early morning and late evening when the sun is low on the horizon, indirect UV radiation may exceed direct. Likewise, on a cloudy day, UV radiation scattered by atmospheric particles may result in greater exposure to indirect than to direct UV radiation.

UV radiation can also be reflected off buildings and the terrain. Smoother surfaces, such as concrete or asphalt, whether they are dark in color or not, typically result in greater reflectance of UV radiation than irregular surfaces. Surface irregularities, such as that found in grass or bark nuggets, reduce the level of reflectance, thereby reducing exposure to reflected UV radiation. One exception, however, is water. Smooth water absorbs almost all UV radiation, whereas the irregular surface of choppy water reflects a considerable amount of UV radiation. The following table lists surfaces and terrains commonly encountered on school grounds and their UV radiation reflectance. Materials with a lower reflectance are more desirable.

Ultraviolet Radiation Reflectance for School Grounds Surfaces

Surface	UV Radiation Reflectance[8,9,10]
Grass	1% – 4%
Still water	3% – 8%
Soil	4% – 6%
Asphalt	4% – 9%
Concrete	7% – 12%
Choppy water	8% – 13%
Dry sand	15% – 18%
Fresh snow	85% – 88%

How is UV Radiation Measured?

In the past, different countries measured and reported solar UV radiation intensity in different ways. One common way of reporting UV radiation intensity was in the form of estimated "burn time" or "time to burn," expressed as the number of minutes of solar exposure required for the reddening of a fair-skinned person's exposed skin, assuming a clear sky. Although there may be some advantages to this method of reporting UV radiation intensity, there are a number of disadvantages. In 1994, international agreement was reached on standardizing the measure of UV radiation intensity.

Revised by the World Health Organization in 2002 and adopted by the Environmental Protection Agency and the National Oceanic and Atmospheric Administration's National Weather Service in 2004, the UV Index is the internationally accepted system for reporting the intensity of UV radiation. Although the mathematical model developed to determine the UV Index might be complicated, the measurement is easy to understand. The UV Index is a measure of the amount of damaging UV radiation that reaches the earth's surface at noon on a given day and at a given location, expressed as a risk scale. It is predicted daily on a scale of 0 to 11+, where 0 represents a minimal risk of overexposure to UV radiation and any number higher than 11 represents an extreme risk of overexposure to UV radiation.

SHADE PLANNING TOOLBOX

Q: Where do I find the UV Index for tomorrow?

A: In most communities, the UV Index is reported in newspapers and on television with the daily weather forecast.

Every day at approximately 1:30 PM Eastern, the National Oceanic and Atmospheric Administration (NOAA) and the Environmental Protection Agency (EPA) post the UV Index for the next day at the EPA's Website, http://www.epa.gov/sunwise/ uvindex.html.

What Are the Health Effects of Exposure to UV Radiation?

Few people would dispute the beneficial effects of solar radiation. The sun warms the earth, fuels photosynthesis, and ensures the continued existence of life on earth. Many of us enjoy the warmth of the sun on our skin. But at some point in our lives, most of us have experienced the painful effect of too much sun exposure in the form of sunburn. Having experienced sunburn, many would agree that there must be some negative health effect to exposure to the sun. Although many different conditions occur as a normal response to exposure to UV radiation, they all fall into one of two classifications, acute or chronic. Acute effects of UV radiation exposure usually have a rapid onset and are of short duration, such as sunburn, tanning, and synthesis of vitamin D_3. Chronic effects of UV radiation exposure usually have a gradual onset and are of long duration, such as skin cancer and photoaging.

Sunburn

Sunburn is an acute injury resulting from excessive exposure to the sun. The redness associated with sunburn results from the dilation of superficial blood vessels in the skin. Redness usually appears within 4 hours of exposure, reaches a maximum within 12 hours, and fades after a few days. High doses of UV radiation can result in blistering and peeling.

Skin color, hair color, eye color, and freckles all are characteristics that help predict an individual's susceptibility to sunburn. Individuals are typically grouped into one of six sun-reactive types, ranging from those with blue or green eyes and very light skin that never tans to those with very dark hair and eyes and dark skin that almost never burns. Although sunburn is not as common among blacks, compared to whites, blacks are susceptible. Approximately 15% of the African American respondents to a national health survey reported experiencing mild to severe sunburns.[11] Differences also exist in the sun-sensitivity of different parts of the body. The face, neck, and trunk are two to four times more sensitive than the limbs.[12]

Tanning

Tanning, or melanin pigmentation, is a consequence of overexposure to the sun that many people find desirable. UVA exposure results in the skin's production of more melanin, the substance responsible for skin's pigmentation. There are two ways in which our skin can tan, by immediate tanning and by delayed tanning. Immediate tanning occurs as quickly as 5 to 10 minutes after exposure to the sun and will last as long as 2 hours. One's ability to exhibit immediate tanning is directly related to the genetically determined pigmentation of the skin. Delayed tanning, which is the more familiar form of tanning, is noticeable 1 to 2 days after exposure, increases for several days, and lasts for weeks or months. Although having a tan provides some degree of protection from UVB, melanin is not an effective sunscreen for Caucasian skin.[13]

Photosynthesis of Vitamin D_3

The only positive health effect associated with exposure to solar UV radiation is the synthesis of vitamin D_3. Without UVB, the body cannot synthesize vitamin D_3, which is essential for regulating calcium metabolism. Few studies have examined the effect of sun avoidance or the use of sunscreen on the production of vitamin D_3in children or adults. Therefore, the American Academy of Pediatrics has recommended that infants, children, and adolescents who do not consume at least 500 mL (16.9 oz) of vitamin D-fortified milk or formula daily should take one of the many available daily multivitamin supplements that contain 400 IU of vitamin D_3.[14]

Photoaging of the Skin

Exposure to UVA and UVB radiation, and perhaps to radiation in the infrared range as well,[13] causes photoaging, a process in which the skin's elastic fibers break down leading to wrinkled and leathery-looking skin. Dryness, deep wrinkles, sagging, loss of elasticity, and mottled pigmentation are all photoaging symptoms.

Eye Damage

Eye damage from solar radiation is a risk factor for developing a number of eye disorders including cataracts, skin cancer around the eyes and degeneration of the macula. Although the evidence is not conclusive, such damage appears to have a dose-response relationship and to be cumulative; that is, the more unprotected solar radiation exposure to the eyes over an entire lifetime, the greater one's risk for developing cataracts.[13, 15, 16]

Basal Cell Cancer

Typically occurring on the most sun-damaged parts of the body, basal cell carcinoma is a slow-growing cancer that begins as a raised lump on the skin and eventually breaks open to form an exposed sore. Although most of these types of cancers are colorless, some are dark in color. Like other skin cancers, basal cell cancer usually appears in middle age, as a result of UV radiation exposure during childhood or adolescence.

> **SUN PROTECTION IS THE KEY**
>
> The vast bulk of skin cancers in the U.S. are due to excessive skin exposure to UV radiation from the sun, so sun protection is the key to preventing the disease.
>
> Martin Weinstock, MD, PhD Director of Dermatoepidemiology at Brown University and Chair of the American Cancer Society (ACS) Skin Cancer Advisory Board

Squamous Cell Cancer preventing the disease.

Squamous cell cancer is a more aggressive form of skin cancer that ultimately basal cell cancer in appearance. It often follows a pre-cancerous condition called actinic keratosis, which is a dry and crusty area on the skin. Both basal cell and squamous cell carcinoma usually result from chronic exposure to UV radiation over a period of years.

Melanoma

By far, the most serious consequence of exposure to UV radiation is malignant melanoma. Unlike the other two types of skin cancer, basal cell and squamous cell, melanomas involve the dark pigmented cells of the skin, the melanocytes. A growing body of evidence indicates that intermittent sun exposure, as opposed to chronic sun exposure, causes this most deadly of skin cancers. Of particular concern, findings from certain studies point to childhood exposure to sunlight, especially severe childhood sunburn, as an indicator for melanoma as an adult.[17, 18, 19, 20]

Where Can I Find More Information?

Section 5, "The Earth-Sun Relationship," provides more information on seasonal sun angles and their effects on shade design. On the following pages are internet links to more information on skin cancer and its prevention as well as to sun-safety curricula.

Information on Skin Cancer and its Prevention

The Centers for Disease Control and Prevention	
www.cdc.gov/cancer/nscpep/skin.htm	CDC provides leadership for nationwide efforts to reduce illness and death caused by skin cancer. Although these efforts comprise a variety of approaches and strategies, their common focus is education and prevention. CDC's Web site describes programmatic approaches to skin cancer prevention and education.
The National Cancer Institute	
www.nci.nih.gov/cancertopics/types/ skin	The National Cancer Institute (NCI) is a component of the National Institutes of Health (NIH) and is the federal government's principal agency for cancer research and training. Articles related to the causes of cancer, diagnosis, prevention, treatment, and the most current cancer statistics are available at NCI's Web site.

The United States Environmental Protection Agency	
www.epa.gov/eb tpages/ humasunprotecti on.html	The Environmental Protection Agency's mission is to protect human health and to safeguard the natural environment. The agency's Web site contains information about the health risks posed by UV radiation and describes the steps people can take to protect themselves from overexposure to the sun.
The National Council on Skin Cancer Prevention	
www.skincancer prevention.org	The mission of the National Council on Skin Cancer Prevention is to facilitate national skin cancer awareness and prevention efforts through education and promotion of sun-safe behaviors. The council, comprising of 30 separate organizations, increases awareness and prevention behaviors among all populations by providing special programs addressing high-risk populations, including infants, children, young adults, parents, educators, outdoor workers, and athletes. Back issues of NEWSLINK, the council's quarterly electronic newsletter, are available at the ogranization's Web site.
The American Cancer Society	
www.cancer.org	The American Cancer Society is the nationwide community-based voluntary health organization dedicated to eliminating cancer as a major health problem by preventing cancer through research, education, advocacy, and service. The organization's Web site provides the latest research , information about activities and resources at the local level, and educational and advocacy materials.
The Skin Cancer Foundation	
www.skincancer. org	The Skin Cancer Foundation is the only national and international organization that is concerned exclusively with the world's most common malignancy—cancer of the skin. The foundation's Web site offers information on the three types of skin cancer; information on skin cancer prevention; news of local and national events; and public information posters, pamphlets, and brochures.

Sun Safety Curricula

National Safety Council—Environmental Health Center	
1025 Connecticut Avenue, NW Suite 1200 Washington, DC 20036 www.nsc.org/ehc/sunw ise/ activity.htm	The National Safety Council's Enviromental Health Center developed the Sun Safety Activity Guide for elementary school representatives who would like to incorporate sun safety into their school curricula. The guide includes cross-curriculum classroom activities and background information packaged as a 1-hour "core" sun-safety lesson. The core is divided into three 20-minute units, including the effects of UV, risk factors for overexposure to the sun, and sun protection habits. Included in the guide are developmentally appropriate activities for primary (grades K through 2) and intermediate (grades 3 through 6) learning levels.
Project S.A.F.E.T.Y.	
The University of Texas M. D. Anderson Cancer Center with Texas Cancer Council www.mdanderson.org/ departments/ projectsafety/	Project S.A.F.E.T.Y. (Sun Awareness for Educating Today's Youth) is a cross-curricular, multimedia skin cancer prevention program for grades 4 through 9. It is available free of charge to any school in Texas. It is also available to schools outside of Texas for a minimal cost.

(Continued)

The SHADE Foundation	
10510 N. 92nd Street Suite 100 Scottsdale, AZ 85258 www.shadefoundation.org	The mission of The SHADE Foundation, a non-profit organization, is to eradicate melanoma through the education of children and the community in the prevention and detection of skin cancer and the promotion of sun safety. In collaboration with the Environmental Protection Agency (EPA), the Foundation has developed partnerships with schools which implement the EPA SunWise School Program and, in turn, are awarded shade structures to the schools.
Sunny Days, Healthy Ways	
Klein Buendel, Inc. 14023 Denver West Parkway Suite No. 190 Golden, CO 80401 (877) 258-2915 www.info@sdhw.info/	Sunny Days, Healthy Ways is a sun-safety curriculum that uses a comprehensive, cross-curricular approach to teaching skin cancer prevention skills to children in grades K through 5. The curriculum provides an average of 8 hours of sun-safety instruction per grade that can be tailored to the teacher's time frame and needs. The curriculum includes prepared lesson plans, student activity sheets, experiment materials, story books, and assessments.
The SunSafe Project	
Norris Cotton Cancer Center Dartmouth Medical School One Medical Center Drive Lebanon, NH 03756 (603) 650-8254 http://sunsafe.dartmouth.edu	The SunSafe intervention aims to enhance and promote sun protection of children ages 2 to 9 years through the delivery of a multicomponent intervention in three settings: elementary schools and day care centers, town beach areas, and primary care practices. The school/day care component consists of an age-specific (2 to 9 years old) and grade-specific curriculum promoting sun protection. Child-care providers and elementary school teachers need 2 theme days or 2 class periods to deliver SunSafe materials. Ongoing reminder activities are suggested as a means for reinforcing the SunSafe message.
The United States Environmental Protection Agency	
SunWise School Program www.epa.gov/sunwise/	The SunWise School Program is an environmental and health education program that aims to teach children and their caregivers how to protect themselves from overexposure to the sun. Using classroom-based, school-based, and community-based components, the SunWise School Program seeks to develop sustained sun-safe behaviors in schoolchildren. The program's learning components build on a solid combination of traditional and innovative education practices already in use in many U.S. elementary and middle schools. Through the program, students and teachers will increase their awareness of simple steps that they can take to protect themselves from overexposure to the sun. Students will demonstrate the ability to practice health-enhancing behaviors and reduce health risks. Children also will acquire scientific knowledge and develop an understanding of environmental concepts related to sun protection. Currently, more than 12,000 schools are registered for the SunWise program, representing all 50 states, the District of Columbia, and Puerto Rico.

Commercial Products Disclaimer

The list of product manufacturers and retailers is provided for general information purposes only and does not represent an inclusive list of vendors.

Furthermore, reference to any specific commercial products or services by trade name, trademark, manufacturer, or otherwise, does not constitute or imply its endorsement, recommendation or favoring by the Centers for Disease Control and Prevention (CDC).
The list of product manufacturers and retailers contains URL addresses to Web sites and information created and maintained by private organizations. These links are provided for convenience of reference only. CDC does not control or guarantee the accuracy, relevance, timeliness, or completeness of this outside information. The inclusion of URL addresses to particular Web sites is not intended to reflect their importance, nor is it intended to endorse any views expressed or products or services offered by the author of the site or by the organization operating the server on which the site is maintained.

SECTION 2. STRATEGIES FOR PROVIDING SHADE

A number of strategies for providing shade on school grounds are available; however, no single approach is best for all schools. This section introduces three strategies for providing shade on school grounds: solid roof structures, shade cloth structures, and natural shade. Some of the advantages and disadvantages of each approach are discussed. This information will assist schools in determining how best to provide shade for their students, teachers, staff, and visitors. Regional differences in vegetation, the need for winter warmth, playground usage patterns, and seasonal weather threats to playground structures factor into the decision process of determining the best approach for each school. For many schools, a combination of strategies that capitalizes on the advantages of several approaches will be the most effective.

Solid Roof Structures

Solid roof structures are permanent structures that provide protection from the sun's harmful rays and can be designed to serve a multitude of purposes. Typically, the structures are designed to be open on at least three sides and often include furniture that can be moved around. To maximize flexibility, the design can include lighting and plumbing.

Advantages

- Provides "all-weather" protection.
- Provides additional classroom space.
- Provides exercise space during inclement weather.
- Provides flexibility of design.
- Can be used as a lunch or picnic area.
- Has a long life span.

Disadvantages

- Requires drainage and guttering.
- Can be more expensive than other strategies.

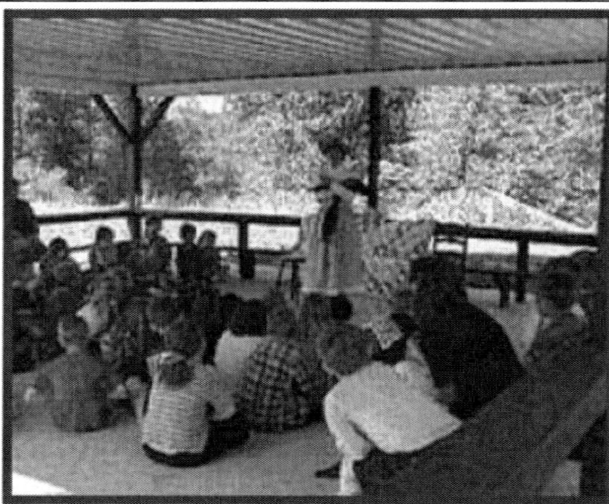

Outdoor classroom at Poplar Creek Elementary School—Siler, Kentucky.

With little more than a few hundred dollars, the support of local businesses, and a State environmental education grant, Principal Tom Shelly and the teachers at Poplar Creek Elementary School, along with the students and their parents, were able to fund the construction of this outdoor classroom and nature trail on their school grounds that otherwise would have cost as much as $30,000.

Considerations

- Schools considering any type of construction project will need to determine which of their local building codes and fire codes are applicable to their project.
- Careful planning will result in the positioning of the structure so that it creates shade at the right place, at the right time of day, throughout the year.
- Schools located in areas that experience heavy snowfall will need to consider the snow load when designing the roof of the structure.
- Likewise, schools located in areas that experience high winds will need to design accordingly.
- Exposed roof supports may be attractive nesting sites for birds. Strategies to deter this should be incorporated into the building's design.
- Lighting will allow for evening use of the building.
- To provide additional light during daytime hours, polycarbonate panels can be incorporated into the roof design and provide a great deal of light while blocking up to 99% of ultraviolet (UV) radiation.

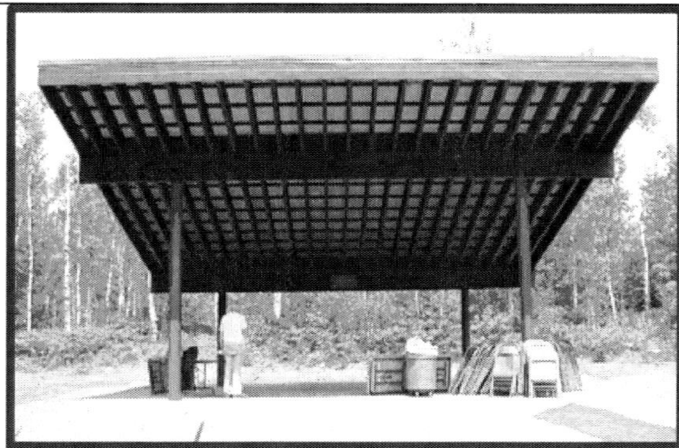

Outdoor classroom at Hermantown School Duluth, Minnesota.

Constructed by the Duluth Skyline Rotary Club as a gift to the Hermantown School District, the outdoor classroom is directly behind the Hermantown Elementary School. Besides serving as an outdoor classroom, the building is accessible to elementary school students during recess periods. According to Fred Majeski, the Superintendent of the Hermantown School District, the building, with its metal framing and roof and concrete floor, would have cost the school well over $25,000 to build, had it not been donated by the Rotary Club.

- No matter what type of design is selected, all buildings require maintenance. A maintenance schedule and estimated costs should factor into the design selection process.
- In the design of the structure, efforts should be made to close off the view of the sky by extending the eaves as far as possible. If the sky can be seen by people under the structure, they are at risk for exposure to indirect UV radiation.
- The design of any structure should ensure access for people with disabilities.
- If the structure is to be used as a classroom or meeting room, the acoustics of the building should also be addressed.

Shade Cloth Structures

Another strategy for providing shade on school grounds is the use of shade cloth or structural fabric supported by a framework or poles. This strategy often is used when the goal is to cover large play areas without employing extensive structural support. Shade cloth is typically a knitted or woven fabric that is rated as to how much sun is blocked. Transmission of the sun's rays through the fabric depends on the tightness of the weave or knit, with more densely woven or knitted fabric blocking out more of the sun's radiation. Fabrics with a looser weave transmit between 50% and 80% of the sun's harmful rays and are typically designed for horticultural applications.

Shade cloth that blocks 80% of solar radiation provides the approximate protective equivalent of sunscreen with a sun protection factor (SPF) of 6.7, whereas shade cloth that blocks 94% of solar radiation provides the approximate protective equivalent of sunscreen with an SPF rating of 15. Shade cloth rated to block 94% of solar radiation is the minimum that schools should consider.

Sun Protection Factor (SPF)

Advantages

- Can be relatively inexpensive to construct.
- Generally requires minimal upkeep.

Disadvantages

- Provides varying UV radiation protection.
- Can be susceptible to weather damage.
- Has a shorter life span than solid roof structures.

Considerations

- Because the UV protection qualities of shade cloth and other structural fabrics vary widely, care should be taken in determining the most appropriate fabric.
- Care must be taken in the positioning of supporting posts so that they do not create a danger to children at play.
- As with any other structure, one of shade cloth should be positioned for maximum sun protection.
- The structural integrity of a fabric structure is related to its curvature and positioning. Structures must be designed to withstand the snow and wind loads that can be expected in their locations.
- The design and installation of these structures should be left to specialists. Names and contact information of organizations that design and install fabric shade structures can be found at the end of this section.

What Does SPF Mean?

The common interpretation is how much longer skin covered with sunscreen takes to burn as compared to unprotected skin. Sunscreens can be rated for their protective factor against either UVA or UVB radiation or both. The thickness and thoroughness of application, the type of sunscreen, and the frequency of reapplication factor into whether or not sunscreen delivers the protection for which it is rated.

Natural Shade

Incorporating natural shade into the overall design offers several advantages. The best approach to creating shade is one that provides protection from the sun's harmful radiation during the spring, summer, and fall, yet does not completely block the sun's warmth during winter months. Incorporating deciduous trees, shrubs, and vines into the design provides the seasonal variation in protection that structures alone cannot provide. Likewise, evergreen trees, vines, and shrubs planted alongside structures can serve to block wind in the winter and provide protection from scattered UV radiation during the rest of the year.

Advantages

- Reduces the ambient temperature more so than structures.
- Provides seasonal sun protection.
- Provides low-cost alternatives.
- Improves the aesthetics of the school grounds.
- Provides an opportunity for students to learn about nature.

Disadvantages

- Vegetation takes time to grow.
- Trees can create litter, such as leaves, nuts, and fruits.

Considerations

- There are regional differences in vegetation. Plants native to a particular region have evolved to thrive in the conditions prevalent there. Whenever possible, locally grown native varieties of trees, shrubs, and vines should be used in the design. The United States Department of Agriculture (USDA) Cooperative Extension Service agent in your area can help determine the best species for your design.
- The effectiveness of trees and vines in providing UV radiation protection is directly related to the density of the plant's foliage.
- As a rule of thumb, trees should be planted to the south and west of where you want to shade so they can provide it during the midday and afternoon hours. Section 5, "The Earth-Sun Relationship," gives information on creating shade in the right place at the right time.
- Some plants are poisonous or cause allergic reactions. Other plants can attract bees or have dangerous spikes or thorns. One needs to become familiar with the possible harmful effects of the species that are being considered.
- Trees may interfere with a school's electrical service, plumbing, and drainage systems. Care should be taken that vegetation is not planted where it might later present a threat to the school's utility systems.
- Many trees will not tolerate root compaction, which occurs when foot traffic compacts the soil around the roots of a maturing tree. Several strategies will prevent

it, including a temporary fence around the maturing tree or specially designed pavers to absorb the impact of busy feet.

- A short-term or transitional structure can be built to provide shade while the vegetation is maturing.
- The first year after planting vegetation is the most important for ensuring the survival of trees, shrubs, and vines. Plants must be watered at regular intervals if rainfall is inadequate. The USDA Cooperative Extension Service agent in your area can help you determine an appropriate watering schedule.
- Some communities have restrictions on water use that might affect decisions on which plants would be most appropriate.

Where Can I Find More Information?

Section 5, "The Earth-Sun Relationship," gives more information on providing shade at the right place, at the right time, throughout the year. The following pages contain links to information about selecting trees, vines, and shrubs; sources for plants and products related to natural shade strategies; information on creating natural wildlife habitats; organizations that manufacture and install fabric shade structures; and contact information for the USDA's Cooperative Extension Service.

WILDLIFE HABITAT CREATION

American Forests: A Tree for Every Child	
www.americanforests.org/resources /kids/a_tree_ for_every_child	The "A Tree for Every Child" project is a hands-on, flexible environmental education program that allows students to see how practical action can create a better world. The project allows schools to teach students the benefits and rewards of planting trees as part of American Forests' Global ReLeaf 2000 campaign to plant 20 million trees for the new millennium.
Acorn Naturalists	
P.O. Box 2423 Tustin, CA 92781-2423 Toll Free: (800) 422-8886 http://acornnaturalists.com/store	This organization offers resources for science and environmental educators. Offerings include educator guides, interpretative tools, and books on nature and the environment. An online catalog is available.
Cornell Lab of Ornithology	
159 Sapsucker Woods Road Ithaca, NY 14850-1999 Toll Free: (800) 843-2473 http://birds.cornell.edu	This site describes classroom projects and provides educational materials that support habitat development. Projects include the Great Backyard Bird Count (which is held every February) and the Classroom Feeder Watch. The curriculum description for the Classroom Feeder Watch can be found at http://www.birds.cornell.edu/cfw/index.html
Project Wild	
555 Morningside Drive, Suite 212 Houston, TX 77005 Phone: (713) 520-1936 www.projectwild.org	Project Wild provides instructional materials that can be adapted for academic disciplines ranging from science and environmental education to social studies, math, and language arts. Numerous education materials, Web links, and guidebooks are available at this site, including the publication *Wild School Sites: A Guide to Preparing for Habitat Improvement Projects on School Grounds.*

Kidsgardening.com	
National Gardening Association 1100 Dorset Street South Burlington, VT 05403 Toll Free: (800) 538-7476 www.kidsgardening. com	This site is an online source of information and materials for environmental science in the classroom. A keyword-searchable resources directory provides links to regional resources.

RESOURCES FOR NATURAL SHADE SOLUTIONS

United States Department of Agriculture ***Cooperative State Research, Education, and Extension Service***	
www.csrees.usda.gov/qlinks/ partners/state_partners. html	This site provides links to the county offices of the Cooperative Extension Services system in each state. The Cooperative Extension Services system has field agents assigned to each county. That agent will be able to answer your questions regarding the best species to plant for the application that you are considering; provide you with sources for the trees, shrubs and vines; and offer detailed instructions on the proper way to plant and care for them.
United States Department of Agriculture ***U.S. Forest Service/Urban and Community Forestry***	
www.fs.fed.us/ucf/	The goal of the USDA Forest Service Urban and Community Forestry Program is to provide technical and financial assistance to help improve the livability of cities and communities by managing urban forest resources to promote a healthy ecosystem. This Web site provides links to the regional coordinators.

U.S. Department of Agriculture ***Natural Resources Conservation Service***	
www.plants.usda.gov	The PLANTS Database provides standardized information about plants of the United States and its territories. The databse includes names, distributional data, species abstracts, characteristics, images, and links to related Web sites with information on the region-specific culture for each species.
Treelink	
www.treelink.org	This Web site provides information, research, and networking for people who work in urban and community forestry. Tips on grant writing and fund-raising are also included.
The National Arbor Day Foundation	
www.arborday.org	The National Arbor Day Foundation helps individuals and groups plant and care for trees and encourages the celebration of Arbor Day to advance global environmental stewardship for the benefit of this and future generations.
The International Society of Arboriculture	
www.treesaregood.com	The International Society of Arboriculture is a worldwide professional organization dedicated to fostering a greater appreciation for trees. The Web site was created to provide the public with quality tree care-related information.

(Continued)

U.S. Environmental Protection Agency *Landscaping with Native Plants*	
Ariel Rios Building 1200 Pennsylvania Avenue, N.W. Washington, DC 20460 Phone: (202) 272-0167 www.epa.gov/glnpo/greenacres/ nativeplants/factsht.html	This Environmental Protection Agency site promotes landscaping with native plants and discusses the environmental benefits of using native plant material. Topics discussed include attracting birds and butterflies and being considerate of local weed laws. *The Wild Ones Handbook* is a compendium of practical information for landscaping with native plants.

SECTION 3. PLANNING FOR SHADE

Planning for shade requires the completion of a series of interrelated tasks. These include convening a planning team, conducting a site audit to determine whether the existing level of shade is adequate, determining the most appropriate strategies if more shade is required; and developing a plan to increase the amount of shade accessible to students, teachers, staff, and visitors. The process can be lengthy, taking as long as 1 year. This section briefly describes each step. In section 6, "How to Conduct a Shade Audit," the reader will find more detailed information on the steps for shade planning.

The Shade Planning Team

It is important for any school undertaking a shade planning project to first identify the stakeholder groups that may have an interest in, or be affected by, the resulting plan. Representatives of these groups should be included on the planning team. For most schools, the stakeholder list would include school administrators, the school nurse, coaches, teachers, students, parents, groups that use the school grounds after hours, and neighbors living adjacent to the school. In addition to stakeholder representatives, the planning team may need to call on professions with expertise in horticulture, landscaping, and architecture. Although it may not be necessary to include such individuals on the planning team, taking the time to identify and recruit them during the earliest stages of the planning process will keep the project moving when their expertise is required.

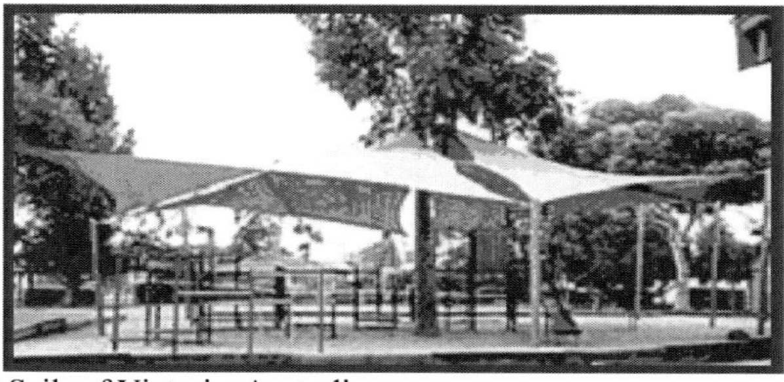

Designed by Shade 'n' Sails of Victoria, Australia.

Transitional shade.

The process will be well served if the goals of the team, the roles and responsibilities of its members, and a method for decision making are determined at the outset. In the course of developing and proposing a shade plan, many decisions will need to be made. One method for decision making that lends itself to a participatory process is decision by consensus.

The Shade Audit

Once a planning team has been assembled and its roles, goals, and procedures determined, the group's first major task will be to conduct a shade audit. The audit will help the planning team determine how much shade is currently accessible on the school grounds and if more is needed. The audit consists of a series of user interviews, behavioral observations, and environmental observations. All of the information collected through the audit will be used by the planning group to develop their recommendations.

Interviews

Although members of the planning team may be very familiar with their school, their expertise may not be comprehensive. Any shade planning endeavor should begin by interviewing several members of each of the identified stakeholder groups. In those interviews, the planning team can collect important background information regarding:

- When and where outdoor activities occur.
- Which areas of the school grounds are off-limits.
- Any long-term plans for the school grounds, including new construction.
- Opinions regarding the adequacy of existing shade.
- Expectations regarding the plans for additional shade.

Section 6, "How to Conduct a Shade Audit," contains sample interview questions for school principals, teachers, and students. Planning teams will need to tailor interview questions to issues and concerns specific to their school.

Prior to conducting stakeholder interviews, the planning team should secure a site plan. This is a drawing of the school grounds and buildings that has been drafted to scale. Often site plans are prepared by surveyors or architects, and may be available from the school's principal or the office of the superintendent of the school district. With a site plan, interviewees can refer to activities in relation to the zones and features of the school grounds and interviewers can record the information directly onto the plan.

Behavioral Observations

The next step in the planning process involves collecting data at the school site. Adequate data collection will require several visits to the school. Initial visits will be to observe outdoor activities conducted on the school grounds and document the usage patterns of students, teachers, and staff. Knowing in advance at what times the students can be expected to be outdoors will facilitate the process. Observers will want to document the types of activities taking place, the location in which they are occurring, the number of students participating, and their duration. Once again, it will be helpful for observers to have a site plan on which to make notes regarding outdoor student and teacher activities.

Environmental Observations

Other visits to the site are recommended in order to take measurements on school grounds without interfering with the school's day-to-day activities. On these visits, an accurate site plan will be essential. If none is available, the planning team will need to draw a freehand plan of the site, recording the distances between the various buildings and play equipment. It might be helpful to name different zones if they do not already have names, such as queuing area or passive play area. It is also important to document any significant topographical features, such as low spots, slopes, or ravines, as these will influence decisions about which shade planning strategies will be most appropriate. The site plan should indicate the boundaries of the school's property, which direction is north, and whether it is magnetic north or true north. Often there is an appreciable difference between the two. Determining true north will be important to ensure that shade is cast in the right place, at the right time of day, at the right time of year.

It may also be important to mark the locations of important features outside of the school boundaries, such as the neighboring homes or businesses.

Because ground and building surfaces can reflect ultraviolet (UV) radiation, the planning team should make notes regarding the surfaces and finishes of each building and play area on the school grounds.

It will be important for the planning team to also consider the school's sports areas, such as baseball diamonds, soccer fields, and basketball courts. In thinking about these features of the school grounds, the planning team should take into account the shade needs of the students and coaches who are participating and those of the spectators.

The next task will require some degree of horticultural expertise. The planning team should inventory each tree and planted area on the school grounds. Trees should be numbered on the site plan, and a separate set of notes should record the team's findings for each tree, including the following:

SHADE PLANNING TOOLBOX

When Is North Not Really North?

The short answer is "Almost always!" There is almost always a difference between true north and magnetic north. Fluid motion in the outer core, which is the molten metallic region of Earth, causes the magnetic field to change unpredictably both over time and by location.

Magnetic declination is the measurement of the angle between magnetic north and true north. For example, on July 4, 1955, the magnetic declination for Washington, D.C., was 6 degrees west of true north. On the same day in 2003, the magnetic declination was 10 degrees west of true north.

To find out more about magnetic declination, visit The National Geophysical Data Center at: http://www.ngdc.noaa.gov/seg/potfld/declination.shtml

- Species.
- Estimated height.
- Trunk diameter.
- Condition (e.g., broken branches, dead limbs), paying particular attention to any that appear to be unhealthy.
- Estimated diameter of the tree's canopy, that is, the upper part which includes the branches and leaves.
- Density of the tree's canopy.

Notes should also be made on the predominant vegetation for areas of densely planted mixed species.

The final task of the shade audit is to estimate the amount of existing shade on the school grounds. Measurements should be taken of all of the shade, regardless of whether it is in an off-limits area. There are two methods for measuring shade, one of which is highly technical and requires a detailed knowledge of sun projection techniques. The second method requires only that the planning team mark the shade patterns on the ground at the times of day that students are outdoors. The ground can be marked with chalk, rope, or baking flour, then measured and marked to scale on the site plan. Measurements will need to be taken at several times during the day and throughout the school year to ensure that seasonal changes in the shade patterns are recorded.

Assessing the Findings

Having completed interviews with representatives of stakeholder groups, observed usage patterns, and plotted the seasonal shade patterns at the school, the next step in the planning process is to analyze the quantity and quality of shade that is accessible on school grounds, and determine if and where additional shade is needed. The following questions will guide the analysis:

- Will future growth of existing trees result in additional accessible shade?
- Are any areas currently off-limits that could provide additional shade if they were accessible?
- Are any areas protected from direct UV radiation, but not protected from indirect (reflected or diffuse) UV radiation?
- Are there future building plans that might be modified to provide additional shade?

Shade Design

Based on the shade audit, the planning team should present its recommendations in text and graphic format. Recommendations should clearly state the shade goals for each specific zone of the school property, such as bus queuing area, sports venues, active play areas, or informal social gathering places, along with strategies for achieving those goals. The team should consider the range of options at the same time that it is considering the nature of the shade to be provided. Questions that the planning team should take into account when developing a shade plan include:

- Is there a need for protection from rain?
- What are the initial costs for each strategy considered?
- What are the long-term maintenance costs associated with each strategy?
- Is the strategy safe, considering the local weather conditions?
- Is there risk of vandalism, and how can that risk be minimized?

Consulting with knowledgeable architects, landscape architects, or horticulturists is advisable at this point. Not only will they know the species of vegetation that will meet the shade requirements for natural applications and the local building codes for any structural applications, they also can advise the planning team on the potentially complicated tasks of obtaining local building permits and contracting with builders and landscapers.

Funding

At the same time that the planning team is finalizing the shade design, team members can explore potential funding sources and volunteer resources for the project. Several potential sources for funding and hands-on participation are discussed further in section 4, "Case Studies" and in the appendices of this manual. Some possibilities include:

- Contributions from local and national corporations, including in-kind contributions.
- State and federal grants.
- Volunteers and financial contributions from community service organizations.
- Local fund-raisers.
- Support from environmental organizations.
- Advice from local master gardeners associations and programs.
- Volunteer project work for Boy Scout or Girl Scout troops.
- Student class projects.

Where Can I Find More Information?

Section 6, "How to Conduct a Shade Audit," provides more detailed information on the steps of conducting such an audit, including examples of questions that would be appropriate for interviews with stakeholders. On the following pages are resources for facilitating participatory decision-making processes, funding, and working with volunteers.

Resources for Shade Planning Teams

Facilitators Guide to Participatory Decision-Making (1996)	
Sam Kaner, with Lenny Lind, Catherine Toldi, Sarah Fisk, and Duane Berger New Society Publishers Gabriola Island, BC	This guide is designed to help groups increase participation and collaboration; promote mutual understanding; honor diversity; and make effective, inclusive, and participatory decisions.

Evergreen	
355 Adelaide Street West, Fifth Floor Toronto, Ontario M5V 1S2 Phone: (416) 596-1495 www.evergreen.ca	Evergreen is a Canadian non-profit environmental organization with a mandate to bring nature to Canadian cities through naturalization projects. Evergreen motivates people to create and sustain healthy, natural outdoor spaces and gives them the practical tools to be successful. Following are several publications available from Evergreen that should be of interest to shade planning teams. ***Hands for Nature: A Volunteer Management*** *Handbook* This booklet provides practical tips and ideas for working effectively with volunteers to create and sustain greening projects. It includes many insights and helpful statistics from the Community Greening Volunteerism 2002 Survey as well as generous input and discussions with experienced volunteer coordinators and greening participants. ***Design Ideas for the Outdoor Classroom: Dig it, Plant it, Build it, Paint it!*** This booklet is a collection of ideas and techniques for creating native plant and vegetable gardens, and includes a whole range of built and artistic features for your school grounds. ***All Hands in the Dirt: A Guide to Designing and Creating Natural School Grounds*** This manual will guide you through the planning process, providing tips and templates for designing a site that reflects your local natural environment and the ideas of all involved. ***Nature Nurtures: Investigating the Potential of School Grounds*** This report is a comprehensive review of the literature pertaining to school ground naturalization. It examines the work of some of the most advanced thinkers in the fields of child development, education, and environmental psychology, and it explores the web of benefits that results when an entire school community participates in creating more nurturing and diverse environments for learning on the school grounds.

SECTION 4. CASE STUDIES

Schools and school districts across the United States have already begun the process of shade planning. This section introduces three case studies. The first, Collier County, Florida, demonstrates the power of a single individual to motivate a school board to erect shade canopies over the playgrounds of all of the school district's elementary schools. The second case study, Pinellas County, Florida, demonstrates the fund-raising capacity of schools' parent-teacher organizations (PTOs) and the effect that they can have on decisions of local school boards. Lastly, the story of the collaboration between Shonda Schilling SHADE Foundation and the United States Environmental Protection Agency's SunWise School Program demonstrates the great potential for partnerships that exists for schools and organizations concerned with preventing skin cancer.

Collier County, Florida

Located in Southwest Florida, Collier County encompasses 2,025 square miles and is home to 296,678 residents, according to the U.S. Census Bureau (2004). The January average high temperature is 77.6°, which is also the lowest average high throughout the year. The county's per capita income for the year 1999 was just over $31,000, approximately $3,000 above the U.S. average for that year, and 10.3% of the county's population lived below the U.S. Department of Health and Human Service's poverty guidelines.

One reason for the county's higher-than-average per capita income may be the large number of retirees who have chosen to take up residence in this county. Even with the large percentage of residents older than 65 years of age, almost 20% of Collier County's residents are 18 years old or younger.

The Collier County school district is home to 44 public schools including 2 charter schools. The policy-making body for the school district is a five-member school board.

Getting Started

Teryl Brzeski is a skin cancer survivor. In 1986, at the age of 37, Ms. Brzeski was diagnosed with melanoma, the most deadly form of skin cancer. Her diagnosis motivated her to research the causes of skin cancer and inspired her to do all that she could to help prevent others from developing the disease. "Having a deadly disease and being lucky enough to have a full recovery is a wonderful thing. In my case, it has instilled a passion for being alive and a desire to share cancer prevention information with others."

Ms. Brzeski became especially concerned about her daughter and the other students at Seagate Elementary School. Other Collier County parents were equally concerned about their children's exposure to ultraviolet (UV) radiation. In fact, during the late 1980s, Seagate's PTO raised the $30,000 necessary to erect a pavilion on the school grounds to provide a shaded area for physical education classes. Other than the covered pavilion, however, much of the playground was not protected from excessive solar radiation, and during recess, children played in areas where there was no shade.

Determined to do something about the situation, Ms. Brzeski began her campaign for a shaded playground by researching options for providing shade on school grounds, eventually presenting her ideas to the Collier County School Board. Along with two dermatologists and a representative from the American Cancer Society, she explained to the school board why it was important to provide children, teachers, and staff with adequate protection from solar radiation. Their presentation included an architectural drawing of their vision for a shaded playground at Seagate. Informational packets were distributed to school board members, making a clear and convincing medical case for providing sun protection on a daily basis. The presenters told the school board that they were prepared to raise funds themselves, if necessary, to have the shade structures built.

Approval and Building Costs

The school board not only approved the request for Seagate, but also approved the construction of shade structures on the playgrounds of all Collier County elementary schools at a cost of $2.1 million dollars. In June 2002, Seagate Elementary School became the first county school to be fitted with a shade structure over the playground. By August 2002, before the school year began, 21 more schools in Collier County were fitted with shade structures. Funding for the project was drawn from the school district's capital budget.

Once the school board decided to build the structures, the project was outsourced to a contractor, with specifications that 95% of the playground of each school should be covered by the shade structure. At Seagate Elementary School, the structure covers 8,100 square feet of the playground.

The shade structure comprises multiple canopies. Each canopy is made of a polyethylene mesh fabric that is supported by steel cables and held up by galvanized steel poles, which are secured to concrete pilings. The canopy over Seagate's playground covers a swing set, three slides, and other playground equipment. The polyethylene mesh fabric blocks 90% to 95% of the sun's UV rays. In addition, it allows heat to escape, promoting air circulation. As a result, the temperature beneath the canopies is about 15° lower than that of the ambient air in the middle of the day.

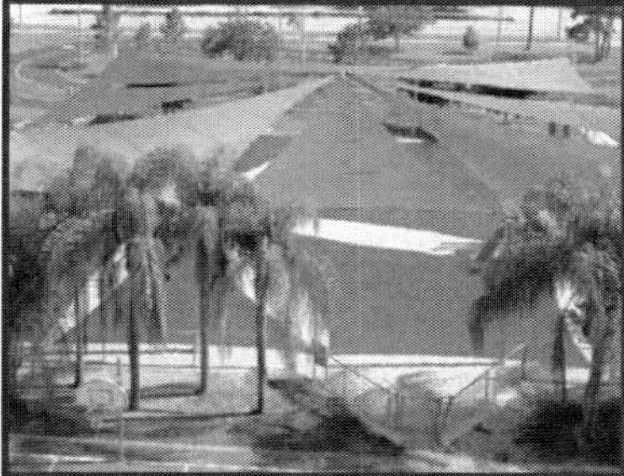

Seagate Elementary School.

Students, teachers, and staff at Seagate Elementary are now protected from ultraviolet radiation during recess.

Maintenance

After the shade structures were built, several potential modifications were identified as necessary to increase the longevity of the structures. For example, additional poles were subsequently added to guard against severe windstorms, and the sails were redesigned and restrung. In 2005 the county incurred additional expenses due to hurricane damage. Consequently, when hurricanes are forecasted, maintenance staff take down the structures. However, contractors must be hired to reassemble them. The county school board will continue their cost benefit analysis and may consider other options in the future.

Continued Efforts

To date, 25 Collier County elementary schools have been outfitted with shade structures over their playgrounds. The scope of the initial project was 22 schools, but since that time, Collier County has built three more schools and has incorporated shade structures into their design and construction.

Since the implementation of shade coverings in the Collier County school district, other neighboring school districts have seen the utility and importance of providing students, teachers, and staff with protection from UV radiation. For example, in the Lee County school district, Bonita Elementary School has begun fund-raising efforts to build a shade structure for the school. The school's parent-teacher organization has pledged to donate a portion of the funds, and solicitations of businesses and service clubs are expected to raise more. The school expects to pay $64,000 to install shade canopies over its two playgrounds.

Teryl Brzeski has won her battle with skin cancer and now fights every day to ensure that her daughter and the children of Collier County will not have to face the same battle. Her efforts to educate others on skin cancer and its prevention and to promote sun safety through the construction of shade structures at elementary schools have motivated not only her county to take action but have also influenced neighboring counties to take the same steps.

Pinellas County, Florida

Pinellas County, Florida, is located on a peninsula bordered by the Gulf of Mexico and Tampa Bay. The 280-square-mile county is home to about 921,500 year-round residents and welcomes an average of 4.5 million visitors each year. Unemployment in Pinellas County tends to be lower than the Florida state average, which tends to be lower than the national average. According to the U.S. Census Bureau, the per capita income for the year 1999 was just under $24,000, and 12.8% of the county's population lived below the U.S. Department of Health and Human Service's poverty guidelines.

With 114 elementary, middle, and secondary schools, the Pinellas County School District is the 7th largest district in Florida and the 21st largest in the United States.

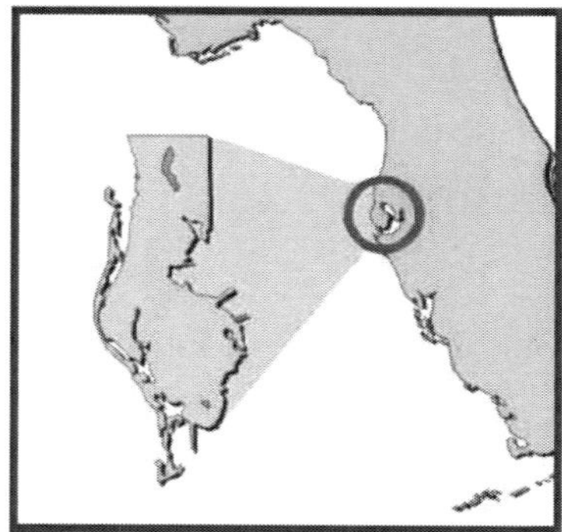

Image source: http://www.pinellascounty.org/.

Getting Started

By 1995, parents and teachers in several of Pinellas County's 82 elementary schools had become concerned about their schools' lack of indoor gymnasium facilities. Physical education classes had to be taught outdoors throughout the year and were canceled when inclement weather required it. The Parent-Teacher Associations (PTA) in those few schools took the initiative to conduct fund-raisers, such as bake sales and jog-a-thons, to collect the $35,000 that each school would need to erect a weather-protected outdoor play area. The schools tapped local expertise in determining the best design for the structures and for executing the construction.

In 2002, the local PTA efforts in Pinellas County paid off for all elementary school children in the county, prompting the Pinellas County school board to determine that all 82 elementary schools in the county should have similar structures to protect students, teachers, and staff. Walter Miller, associate superintendent of institutional services, cites health and medical concerns as the rationale for the school board's decision, "We ensure that the students, faculty, and staff have a clean and safe environment inside of the school, so it's only right that we are concerned about the environment outside of the school as well. Children and physical education teachers were exposed to extreme heat and put at risk for skin cancer, which in Florida is a major concern, so the shade structures buy students and teachers the opportunity to escape the heat and exposure to ultraviolet radiation."

Building Costs

Funding for the construction has been supported through the school district's capital budget. The school district's facilities department identified a general contractor to oversee construction of the buildings, and the contractor received bids from a number of manufacturers. A local firm was ultimately selected, because using a local builder would reduce shipping and travel costs.

To reduce costs, a single design was used for all schools, although each school determined the placement of its shade structure. The structures are 40-by-80 feet, roughly the size of a tennis court, and are constructed of metal with concrete floors. The designers had to consider the threat of strong winds associated with hurricanes or tornados, very real threats in Florida. As a result, a larger foundation was incorporated into the design to create uplift resistance in the event of a windstorm. Each structure approximately cost $60,000, which according to the director of facilities was considerably lower than it would have been if each building had been individually bid. Those schools that had begun fund-raising efforts for a shade structure were allowed to add that money to the school board's budget, and make improvements to the original design, including a larger structure, if that was what the school wanted.

Maintenance

As the oldest of the buildings begin to age, some of the maintenance requirements are becoming more obvious. Most apparent is the need to paint the steel structures regularly to prevent premature rusting. Structures that need repainting must first be sandblasted to remove old paint and rust. In some cases, as more time passes, other maintenance issues will be identified. Recently, some of the schools have experienced problems with birds nesting in the metal framing that supports the roof. Modifications to the design of future buildings and to those already constructed may solve that problem.

Continued Efforts

Currently, 66 of the 82 elementary schools in Pinellas County have shade structures. The school district expects that all schools in the county will have these structures by 2007. This tremendous accomplishment is the result of the efforts of just a few concerned parents, teachers, and principals who recognized the importance of providing sun protection to their students, teachers, and staff.

If you would like to find out more about the efforts to prevent skin cancer at Pinellas County Schools, feel free to contact:

Walter Miller, Associate Superintendent, Institutional Services in Pinellas County Phone: (727) 547-7167

Jim Ewbank, Supervisor of Pre-K Physical Education Phone: (727) 588-6078

SHADE Foundation of America and the U.S. Environmental Protection Agency's SunWise School Program

SHADE Foundation of America

In February 2001, Shonda Schilling, a 33-year old mother of four young children and wife of Boston Red Sox pitcher Curt Schilling, was diagnosed with melanoma. Having been a lifelong sunbather, Ms. Shilling felt a need to inform the public about the dangers of exposure to the sun's UV rays. She learned that although Arizona has the highest melanoma rate in the United States, the state had no organizations devoted to preventing the cancer. As a way to fill that gap, Shonda founded the SHADE Foundation.

SHADE Foundation of America is a non-profit organization dedicated to the education, prevention, and detection of skin cancer. Created in September 2002, the foundation's goal is to prevent the development of skin cancer through educational programs and free skin cancer screenings.

The U.S. Environmental Protection Agency's SunWise School Program

First piloted in May 1999, the SunWise School Program, developed by the United States Environmental Protection Agency (EPA), is an environmental and health education program designed to teach children and their caregivers how to protect themselves from overexposure to the sun. The standards-based, cross-curricular lessons in the SunWise Tool Kit were designed to foster sun-safe behaviors in children and to increase their knowledge and appreciation of the environment. In addition, the program encourages schools to create shade structures, adopt sun-safe policies, and develop additional community partnerships.

Since the year 2000, the K–8 curriculum has been available on a national basis, free of charge, to any school registering at the EPA SunWise Web site, www.epa.gov/sunwise. To participate in the SunWise program, schools must adopt a SunWise activity, which may include implementing classroom lessons, collecting and reporting UV radiation data, adopting school-wide sun-safe policies, or engaging in skin cancer prevention community outreach. Schools must also participate in a program evaluation.

Creating a Collaboration

The development of the collaboration between the SHADE Foundation and the EPA began in October 2002. Linda Rutsch, Director of the SunWise School Program at the EPA, was visiting the Web site of a melanoma foundation in Nevada when she noticed a link to the SHADE Foundation. "Usually I will check out various links in order to keep up with what's out there," Ms. Rutsch recalls. She clicked on the SHADE Foundation's link, learned about the Foundation's skin cancer prevention efforts in Arizona, and found a contact name. Ms.

Rutsch called Sue Gorham, executive director of the SHADE Foundation, and told her, "I would like to send you a SunWise Kit and tell you a little about our program."

As luck would have it, the SHADE Foundation was in the process of searching for a school curriculum on sun safety. Ms. Schilling and Ms. Gorham decided to develop a program for schools that would allow them to acquire shade structures for their campuses through the SHADE Foundation. The idea was to encourage schools to implement a sun-safe curriculum and to develop sun-safe policies within the school.

The EPA's SunWise curriculum was exactly what the SHADE Foundation was seeking, and the partnership began there. As Ms. Rutsch remembers, "That was in October of 2002 when we first started corresponding. In January of 2003, we had our first face-toface meeting where we talked about working together."

How the Program Works

The **SHADE SunWise School Program** requires schools to qualify in two steps. The first step is to request the EPA SunWise curriculum, usually via the EPA SunWise Web site. Once a school has reviewed the curriculum and made the decision to implement it, the next step is to apply to the SHADE Foundation to participate in the SHADE SunWise School Program. The written grant statement must include a description of the policy and activities the school proposes to adopt for skin cancer prevention. Upon demonstration of sustained teaching activities and the implementation of sun protection policies, the Foundation gives grants for the consideration of a shade structure.

The shade structures are an appropriate reward for the school's achievements. Besides protecting students, teachers, staff, and visitors from overexposure to UV radiation, the structures contribute to a more comfortable environment for students to enjoy outdoor physical activities. As Sue Gorham points out, "Here in Arizona, when children slide down the sliding board, it is so hot that it could take the skin off their backs. Under these shade structures, the temperatures will drop as much as 20 degrees."

Building Costs

The cost for providing a school with the 24' x 35' shade structure is between $6,000 and $10,000. The shade structures are of shade cloth, approximately 24' x 35' and hoisted on metal poles. The shade cloth provides 98% protection from UV radiation. Schools have flexibility in determining where on their grounds would be the most appropriate location for their shade structure.

The SHADE Foundation assumes all costs of the shade structures, with money raised through a number of fund-raising events, ranging from auctions to golf tournaments. The first year of implementation was used to demonstrate both the program's needs and SHADE's fiscal responsibility and ability to execute the managerial and administrative duties of the project. Hoping to supplement its fund-raising efforts with grant money, the program began applying for grants in 2004. In 2005, SHADE received its first grant of $25,000 from Teammates for Kids. SHADE, now in its 4th year of giving grants, has funded approximately 50 structures across the nation at a cost of $267,000.

Though some schools have expressed concern over the required maintenance on the structures, to date this has not been a great problem, because the structures have not required much maintenance.

Continued Efforts

To date, the SHADE Foundation has constructed 50 shade structures in U.S. schools and community areas which benefit children. In the coming year, the Foundation plans to raise funds to support 95% of grant applications.

The SHADE Foundation and EPA were recognized for their work by being awarded the "2003 Excellence in Cancer Awareness Award," presented by Congressional Families Action for Cancer Awareness. This award is presented annually to the organization that best exemplifies a total commitment and dedication to assisting others in preventing cancer. This award honors the partnership between the SHADE Foundation and the EPA SunWise program in addressing the issue of skin cancer prevention. "We are so proud of our partnership receiving the award," says Ms. Gorham. "We hope that through qualifying for grants in the future, we will be able to carry on this work in all states."

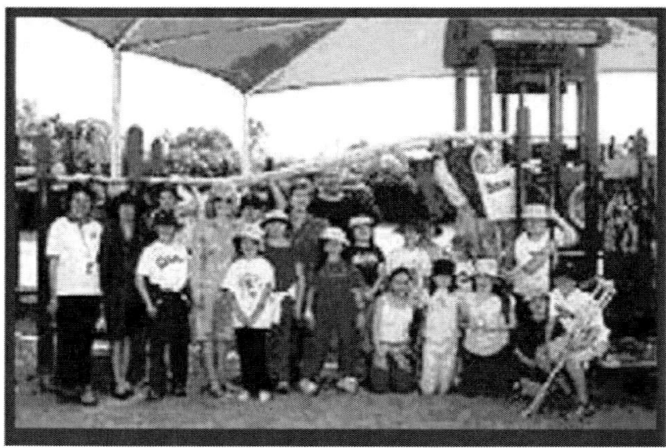

Cherokee Elementary school: the first school to graduate with the SHADE Foundation and SunWise curriculum.

If you would like to find out more about the SHADE Foundation's efforts to prevent skin cancer, feel free to contact:

Sue Gorham Executive
Director of the SHADE Foundation
www.shadefoundation.org
Phone: (480) 614-2278
Fax: (480) 614-2279
E-mail: sue@shadefoundation.org
To find out more about the EPA's SunWise School Program, contact:
Linda Rutsch
Director of the SunWise Program
www.epa.gov/sunwise
Phone: (202) 343-9924
Fax: (202) 343-2362
E-mail: rutsch. linda@epa.gov

Key Terms and Concepts

Latitude is a north-south measurement of any position on the Earth. Measured in degrees, latitude is 0° at the equator and 90° at the North and South Poles. The line that connects all locations of the same latitude is called a parallel. Shade planning teams will need to know the latitude to determine where a tree or structure will cast its shadow throughout the day.

Longitude is a west-east measurement of any position on the Earth. The line that connects all locations of the same longitude is called a meridian. Longitude, like latitude, is measured in degrees, with 0° occurring at the Greenwich Meridian or Prime Meridian. Measurements of longitude range from Prime Meridian at 0° to 180° going either west or east. The 180th meridian east is the International Date Line. Shade planning teams will need to know their longitude to determine solar noon.

Solar Noon is the time of day when the sun is aligned with true north and true south and is specific to each longitude. In the northern hemisphere, a shadow cast by a vertical pole at solar noon will point toward true north. Solar noon is also the midpoint between sunrise and sunset.

Section 5. The Earth-Sun Relationship

For any shade planning team, the primary objective is to ensure that shade falls in the right place, at the right time of day, throughout the year. A shade planning team should include members with at least a working knowledge of the Earth's relation to the sun. This section is designed to:

- Graphically illustrate the effects of daily and seasonal changes in solar angles on the length and direction of shadows.
- Provide a basic introduction, or reintroduction, to the Earth's relationship to the sun and solar geometry.
- Provide a list of resources that can assist the planning team in ensuring that shade falls in the right place, at the right time of day, throughout the year.

The Sun's Annual Path and the Creation of Shade

Shadows cast by the sun grow longer from June 21st until December 21st, and then grow shorter from December 21st until June 21st. This is a result of annual changes in the solar altitude angle. The change in shadow length is depicted graphically in the following illustration. A 36-foot tall tree with a canopy spread of 48 feet planted at the geographic center of the contiguous United States (Longitude=98°3'West; Latitude=39°0'North) tree would cast shadows at **solar noon** throughout the year as follows:

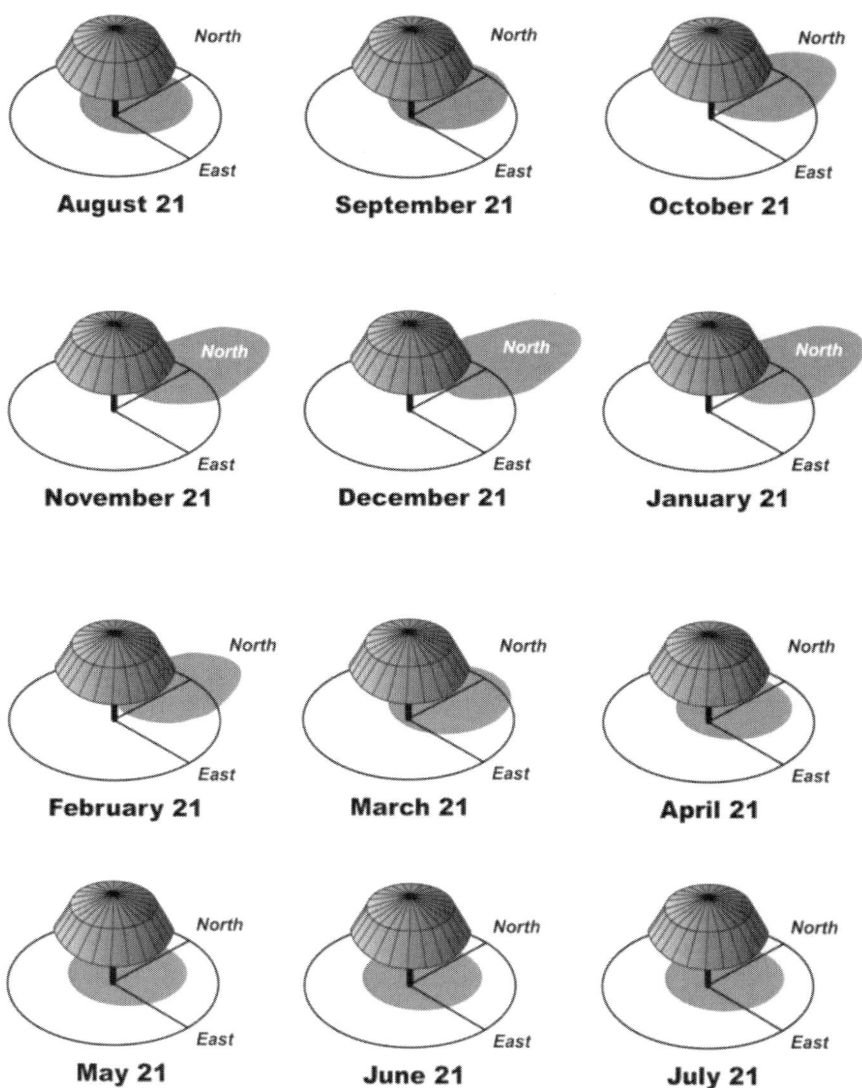

The Sun's Daily Path and the Creation of Shade

Observing that same 36-foot tall tree, the shadows that are cast move from west to east throughout the day in response to the sun's east-to-west movement. On March 21st, the shadows that would be cast throughout the school day would appear as follows:

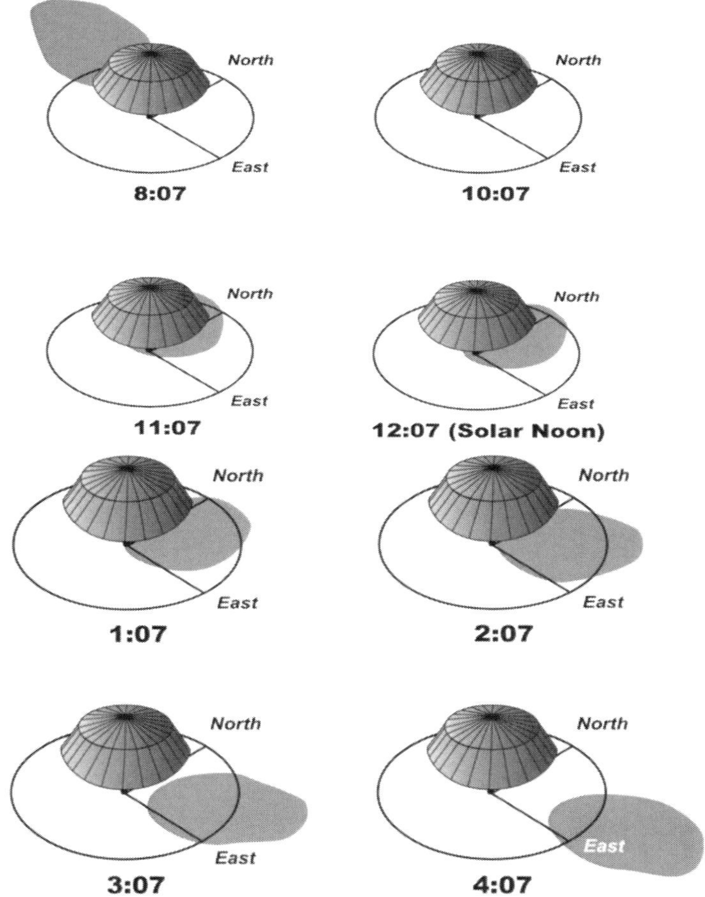

The Earth's Rotation and Revolution

Every 24 hours, the Earth makes one rotation on its axis; every 365.24 days, the Earth makes one revolution around the sun. If one were to view the Earth spinning on its axis, one would note that the axis is not perpendicular to the Earth's orbit around the sun, but is tilted at an angle of 23.5°, with the North Pole always pointing directly at the North Star. Furthermore, the Earth's orbit around the sun is not circular, but elliptical, causing the Earth's distance from the sun to vary by as much as 3 million miles throughout the year. The annual variation in the Earth's distance from the sun affects the amount of solar radiation intercepted by the Earth by as much as 7%. The changing distance from the sun, however, is not responsible for the changes in seasons. The changes in season are caused instead by the constant 23.5° tilt of the Earth and the Earth's rotation around the sun.

Summer solstice, which is on or about June 21st, marks the beginning of summer in the northern hemisphere. The Earth is positioned so that the North Pole is leaning toward the sun at 23.5°. On summer solstice, the length of the day, from sunrise until sunset is greater than 12 hours for all latitudes north of the equator, and less than 12 hours for all latitudes south of the equator. On summer solstice, the center of the sun lines up with the latitude known as the Tropic of Cancer, which is at 23.5° north.

KEY TERMS AND CONCEPTS

The Earth's axis of rotation is not perpendicular to its orbit around the sun, but is tilted at an angle of approximately 23.5°. **Solar Declination** is the angle that a given hemisphere is tilted toward the sun on any given day. It is marked by the latitude on the Earth where the location of the sun is directly overhead at solar noon. Because of the 23.5° tilt, this location is always somewhere between 23.5° north and 23.5° south, depending on the time of the year. Solar declination is 0° when the sun lines up with the equator on the equinoxes.

Equinox is one of the two periods when the declination of the sun is 0°, or the sun is lined up exactly with the equator. The autumnal equinox occurs on or about September 21st, and the vernal equinox occurs on or about March 22nd. Only on these 2 days are the hours of the day and night equal, and only on these 2 days does the sun rise due east and set due west.

Solstice is either the longest or the shortest day of the year. In the northern hemisphere, summer solstice is the longest day of the year and occurs on or about June 21st. Winter solstice occurs on or about December 22nd.

True north, also known as geographic north, is the northernmost point on the Earth as determined by the Earth's rotation. This usually differs from what a compass indicates as north. When a compass points to north, it is pointing toward magnetic north, which in some locations in the United States, may be as far as 20° from true north.

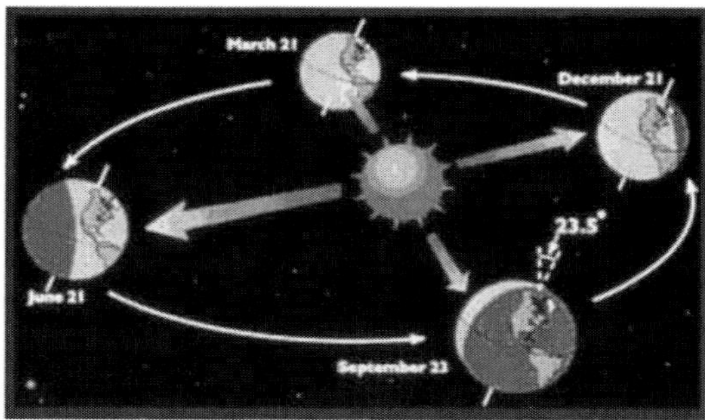

Image Source: National Geophysical Data Center.

At the winter solstice, on or about December 22nd, the Earth is positioned so that the North Pole is leaning away from the sun, and all latitudes south of the equator experience days longer than 12 hours and all latitudes north of the equator experience days shorter than 12 hours. This marks the beginning of summer in the southern hemisphere and the beginning of winter in the northern hemisphere. On winter solstice, the center of the sun lines up with the latitude known as the Tropic of Capricorn, which is at 23.5° south. On the equinoxes, those being around September 21st and March 21st, the Earth is positioned so that the North Pole points neither toward nor away from the sun. On those 2 days, the Earth's equator lines up with the center of the sun, resulting in days that are exactly 12 hours long, regardless of latitude.

KEY TERMS AND CONCEPTS

Solar azimuth angle is the angle on the horizontal plane between the point on the horizon that is directly beneath the sun and true south. The azimuth angle determines the direction of shadows.

Solar elevation angle or solar altitude angle is the angle that describes the height of the sun in relation to the nearest point on the horizon. It varies according to the time of day and the season and determines the length of shadows.

Axis Tilt and Solar Radiation

That the Earth's axis is tilted affects the amount of solar radiation reaching the Earth in three ways. First, the length of the day changes throughout the year. In the northern hemisphere, beginning on the summer solstice, the sun's daily path is increasingly lower in the sky (making shadows longer) until the winter solstice, after which the days become increasingly longer. As days grow longer, the risk of exposure to excessive ultraviolet (UV) radiation is greater.

Second, when the sun is at a lower altitude, its rays are spread over a larger area, reducing the intensity of the sun's radiation, including UV radiation.

Third, levels of solar radiation are also affected by how much of the atmosphere the sun's rays must pass through. Solar radiation levels, including UV radiation, are greatest when the sun is higher in the sky and solar radiation has a shorter path to travel through the atmosphere. When the sun is lower in the sky, solar radiation has a longer path to travel through the atmosphere, resulting in more of the sun's radiation, including UV radiation, being absorbed or scattered by the atmosphere.

Putting It All Together

In order to create shade that falls in the right place, at the right time of day, throughout the year, it is essential that the planning team model the shade that their proposed buildings and plantings will cast. To do that, the team will need to know:

- Longitude and latitude of the school's location.
- Location of true north and true south.
- Size, shape, and orientation of proposed buildings.
- Growth patterns and locations of proposed plantings.
- Time of day that solar noon occurs throughout the year at that longitude.

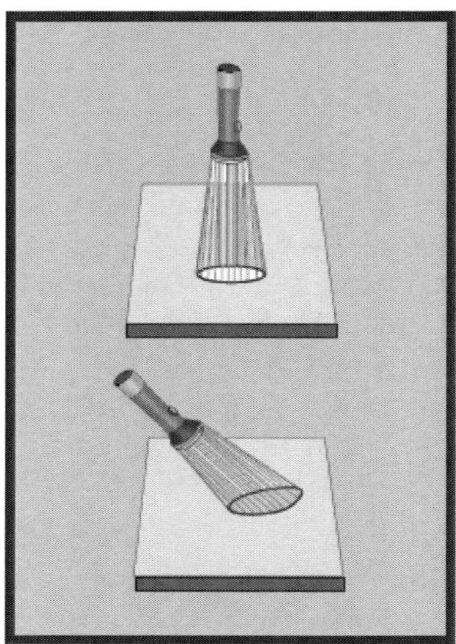

The more perpendicular a beam is to a surface, the brighter the beam will be on the surface.

Armed with that information and a working knowledge of solar geometry, it is possible to use mathematical and geometrical procedures to model the shade that will be cast by proposed structures and plantings. A number of computer software programs are available to do that work for you. Following are descriptions of two such programs, one of which has been developed for modeling sun and shade patterns for solar collectors, though it may well fit into the budgets and serve the purposes of some schools. The other is a program that has been designed specifically for shade planning.

Visual Sun Chart

www.visualsunchart.com/

Visual Sun Chart is a graphics program that was developed for visualizing solar shading to maximize the efficiency of solar collectors. It allows the user to model trees and buildings and, along with a free download, visualize the shade patterns that are cast. With Visual Sun Chart, a user can:

- Model buildings and trees.
- Export scenes to POV Ray 3.5, a free download that models shade produced by buildings and trees.
- Create reports which give information about positions of the sun, times of sunrise and sunset, horizontal and vertical shadow angles, and angles of incidence.
- View and print 3D models of sun movements.

webShade

www.shadeaudit.com.au
www.webshade.com.au

webShade is an interactive software package that allows users to prepare shade audits without the need for technical skills or expertise. Users can either scan their site plan into the computer or use a simple drawing program to create a 3D model of their site. On completion of the shade audit with webShade, the program produces a printed site plan, complete with shade solutions and simulated outcomes. Available as an internet download, a webShade user can:

- Project existing summer and winter shade patterns.
- Model alternative shade strategies.
- Project the summer and winter shade patterns for those alternatives.
- Prepare presentation-ready materials, including site-specific UV radiation information and design strategies.

Where Can I Find More Information?

To determine a location's latitude and longitude:

- www.pbs.org/wgbh/nova/longitude/find.html
- http://zipinfo.com/search/zipcode.htm
- http://geonames.usgs.gov/pls/gnis/web_query.gnis_web_query_form
- http://tiger.census.gov/cgi-bin/mapbrowse-tbl

To determine the time of day that solar noon occurs:

- http://www.srrb.noaa.gov/highlights/sunrise/sunrise.html
- http://users.vei.net/pelican/sunrise.html
- http://www.spot-on-sundials.co.uk/calculator.html

For more information on solar geometry:

- http://www.geog.ouc.bc.ca/physgeog
- http://education.gsfc.nasa.gov/experimental/July61999siteupdate/inv99Project.Site/Pages/solar.insolation.html

Section 6. How to Conduct a Shade Audit

The purpose of the shade audit is to document the usage patterns of the school grounds and determine the amount and quality of existing shade. All of the information collected through the shade audit will be used by the planning group to develop recommendations for making the best use of existing shade and, if required, for creating additional shade. The final product of a shade audit is a written report or presentation of the shade team's findings and recommendations to the school community.

The process includes a series of interviews, behavioral observations, and environmental observations followed by an assessment of the findings and the generation of prioritized recommendations for achieving the goals. The entire process may take as long as 1 year. The first step in the process is to conduct stakeholder interviews.

Stakeholder Interviews

Before the first interview is conducted, the shade planning team should produce a comprehensive list of stakeholder groups that may have an interest in, or be affected by, the resulting plan. The team should identify and invite representatives from each stakeholder group to be interviewed. Ideally, each of the stakeholder groups will be represented on the planning team; nonetheless, it will be necessary to interview members of all stakeholder groups even if they are also represented on the team. For many schools the list would include:

- School administrators.
- Teachers, particularly the physical education teacher.
- Coaches.
- School nurse.
- Students.
- Building maintenance staff.
- Organizers of little league programs or others who may use the school grounds on weekends.
- Residents of the neighborhood adjacent to the school.

Interview Guides

For each stakeholder group, the shade planning team should generate a list of appropriate questions to explore in the interview process. Questions should cover topics with which the interviewee is very familiar. Some may ask the interviewee to discuss outdoor activities that they observe or in which they participate. In order to get the most out of the interviews, interviewers should ask interviewees to reference the school's site plan while describing those activities. This is a scaled drawing of the school grounds and buildings. Often such plans are prepared by surveyors or architects, and may be available from the school's principal or the office of the superintendent of the school district. Referring to a site plan during the interview process allows interviewees to reference activities in relation to the zones and features of the school grounds and allows interviewers to record the information directly onto the site plan. Through the interview process, interviewees may identify school grounds users of whom the shade planning team was not previously aware. Such newly identified stakeholders should be added to the list of interviewees. Following are examples of questions that would be appropriate for school principals, teachers, students, and other stakeholders. This is not meant to be a comprehensive list, but instead gives samples of questions that might be most appropriate for each stakeholder group. The planning team will need to tailor their questions to the issues and concerns specific to their schools.

Sample Questions for School Principals

- How many students attend the school?
- What is the age range and distribution of the students?
- Does the school have sun-safe policies in effect?
  Hats?
  Sunglasses?
  Long-sleeved shirts?
  Sunscreen?
- What are the outdoor activities in which students participate?
  Recess?
  Lunch?
  Assemblies?
  Physical education?
  Educational activities?
  Informal social gatherings?
  Extended day activities?
  Intermural and intramural athletic events?
- For each: Where do they occur? (Have interviewee refer to site plan.)
  At what time of day do they occur?
  What is the duration of the activity?
- Do you believe there is adequate accessible shade on the school grounds? If not, where is additional shade most needed? (The interviewee should be asked to refer to the site plan.)
- Is there inaccessible shade on the school grounds that could be made accessible?
- Is there a need for an area on the school grounds that is protected from precipitation?
- Are there plans for making improvements to the school, such as remodeling, adding classroom space, or landscaping projects?
- Does the school currently have problems with, or has it recently experienced problems with vandalism?
- Are there groups that have permission to use the school grounds after school hours and on weekends?
- Are there groups that, without formal permission, use the school grounds after school hours and on weekends?
- Can you think of any barriers to providing additional shade at this school?
- What type of shade do you think would work best at this school (solid-roof structure, shade cloth structure, or natural shade)?

Sample Questions for School Teachers

- What age group do you teach and how many students are in your class?
- What are the outdoor activities in which your class participates?
  Recess?
  Lunch?
  Assemblies?

Physical education?
Educational activities?
Informal social gatherings?
Extended day activities?
Intermural and intramural athletic events?

- For each: Where do they occur? (Have interviewee refer to site plan.)
  At what time of day do they occur?
  What is the duration of the activity?
- Does the school have sun-safe policies in effect?
  Hats?
  Sunglasses?
  Long-sleeved shirts?
  Sunscreen?
- Do you believe there is adequate accessible shade on the school grounds? If not, where is additional shade most needed? (The interviewee should be asked to refer to the site plan.)
- Is there inaccessible shade on the school grounds that could be made accessible?
- Is there a need for an area on the school grounds that is protected from precipitation?
- Are there times that teachers are required to be outdoors, such as to monitor the activities on the school grounds? If so, how often does this happen and for how long?
- If there were outdoor classroom space, would you use it? Do you think that other teachers would?
- Can you think of any barriers to providing additional shade at this school?
- What type of shade do you think would work best at this school (solid-roof structure, shade cloth structure, or natural shade)?

Sample Questions for Students

- How old are you?
- When you are outside, do you usually play/socailize in the sun or in the shade?
  During recess?
  During and after lunch?
  During physical education class?
  During extended day activities (if applicable)?
  Intermural and intramural athletic events (if applicable)?
- For each, where do you play? (Have student refer to site plan.)
- Does the school have sun-safe policies in effect?
  Hats?
  Sunglasses?
  Long-sleeved shirts?
  Sunscreen?
- Do you believe there is adequate accessible shade on the school grounds? If not, where is additional shade most needed? (The interviewee should be asked to refer to the site plan.)
- Are there shaded areas on the playground that you would prefer not to use? Why?
- Are there areas on the school grounds where you are not allowed to play?

Sample Questions for Building Maintenance Engineers

- Do you believe there is adequate accessible shade on the school grounds? If not, where is additional shade most needed? (The interviewee should be asked to refer to the site plan.)
- Is there inaccessible shade on the school grounds that could be made accessible?
- Is there a need for an area on the school grounds that is protected from precipitation?
- Are there plans for making improvements to the school, such as remodeling, adding classroom space, or landscaping projects?
- How would a plan to plant trees or build a shade structure be affected by the school's utility services? (On the site plan, have the interviewee mark the service lines for the school's utility services.)
- Does the school currently have problems with, or has it recently experienced problems with vandalism?
- Are there groups that have permission to use the school grounds after hours and on weekends?
- Are there groups that, without formal permission, use the school grounds after school hours and on weekends?
- Can you think of any barriers to providing additional shade at this school? For example, would watering trees or removing tree litter be a problem?
- What type of shade do you think would work best at this school (solid-roof structure, shade cloth structure, or natural shade)?

Sample Questions for Neighbors

- Do you believe there is adequate accessible shade on the school grounds? If not, where do you believe that additional shade is most needed? (The interviewee should be asked to refer to the site plan.)
- Do residents of the neighborhood utilize the school grounds for activities on weekends or after school hours?
- In what types of activities have you seen neighbors participate on the school grounds?
- For each: Where do they occur? (Have interviewee refer to site plan.)
  On what days of the week and at what time of day do they occur? What is the duration of the activity?
- Is there a need for a rain-protected area on the playground?
- Do you think that the school currently has problems with, or has recently experienced problems with vandalism?
- Can you think of any barriers to providing additional shade at this school?
- If the school were to plant additional shade trees, are there areas on the school grounds where planting them might create a problem for neighbors?
- If the school were to build a shade structure, would it create a problem for neighbors?
- Are there areas of the school grounds where a shade structure might create a problem for neighbors?

- What type of shade do you think would work best at this school (solid-roof structure, shade cloth structure, or natural shade)?

Once all interviews have been conducted, the planning group should meet to discuss their findings. Information collected from different stakeholder sources should be synthesized and clarifications on, or answers to, any resulting questions should be sought by the group.

Behavioral Observations

The next step in conducting a shade audit involves observation of students, teachers, staff, and visitors on school grounds. Visits to school grounds after hours and on weekends will be necessary to confirm non-school–related activities that might be affected by the shade plan. Information collected in the interview process should guide the behavioral observations. Observers will want to document the types of activities, their locations, the number of individuals who participate in each activity, and the duration of the activity. Once again, it will be helpful for observers to make notes regarding all activities on a site plan. Participants in this process should model good sun-protective behaviors by wearing sunglasses, hats, and long-sleeved shirts. Observations should be made on several occasions to capture the many activities that occur on school grounds and, as much as possible, observations should be made unobtrusively. Observers should note whether activities are occurring in a particular location because no other area will accommodate that activity, or if there are other locations where the activity could take place, particularly a shaded area. Once again, upon completion of this step, the planning team should meet to discuss findings. If there are discrepancies between the information collected in the interview process and the behavioral observations, the team should note the discrepancies and seek clarification.

Environmental Observations

Other visits to the site will need to be planned to take measurements on school grounds without interfering with the day-to-day activities of the school. On these visits, having an accurate site plan will be essential. If none is available, the planning team will need to draw a freehand plan of the site, taking careful measurements of the buildings and recording the location and size of each. The site plan should indicate the boundaries of the school's property, which direction is north, and indicate if it is magnetic or true north, since there is an appreciable difference between the two. Determining true north will be important to ensure that shade is cast in the right place, at the right time of day, throughout the year. (See text box on page 22 of this manual.) It may also be important to mark the locations of important features outside of the school boundaries, such as the location of neighboring homes or businesses and any buildings not on school property that cast shadows or reflect solar radiation onto the school grounds. Once at the site, the planning team should number the site plan with all buildings and play equipment on the school grounds, recording the distances between features. The planning team will need to estimate the height of each of the buildings on the school grounds and record it on a separate set of notes, along with other characteristics of the building. Attachment A is an example of a building description sheet. It may be helpful to name areas or zones of the site if they do not already have a name. Zones can be named according to their use, such as "queuing area" or "passive play area." It is also important to document any significant topographical features, such as low spots, slopes, or ravines, because they will influence decisions on which shade strategies are most appropriate.

Because ultraviolet (UV) radiation can be reflected off ground and building surfaces, the planning team should make notes regarding the surfaces and finishes of each of the buildings and play areas on the school grounds.

Creating a Tree Inventory

The next task will require a degree of horticultural expertise. The planning team should inventory each tree and planted area on the school grounds, noting for each:

- Species.
- Estimated height.
- Trunk diameter.
- Condition (e.g., broken branches, dead limbs), paying particular attention to any that appear to be unhealthy.
- Estimated diameter of the tree's canopy, that is, the upper part which includes the branches and leaves.
- Density of the tree's canopy.

Trees should be numbered on the site plan and a separate set of notes should record the team's findings regarding each. Where densely planted areas of mixed species exist, notes should be made on which ones predominate. Attachment B is an example of a tree inventory data sheet.

Estimating the Height and Trunk and Canopy Diameters of a Tree

There are many ways to estimate the height and canopy diameter of a tree. Following is one method:

a. One member of the planning team first measures his or her own height in inches or feet.
b. The team member then stands next to the tree while another team member stands about 20 paces away.
c. With one eye closed, the second team member holds a pencil vertical at arm's length and covers part of the pencil so that the visible part is the same apparent length as the team member standing next to the tree.
d. Still keeping one eye closed, the second team member then moves the pencil up the tree and measures how many times taller the tree is than the team member standing next to it.
e. Multiply that number by the first team member's height and the result is a good estimate of the tree's height.
f. To estimate the canopy diameter, the second team member again closes one eye and holds the pencil at arm's length, covering part of the pencil so that the visible part is the same apparent length as the tree height.

g. The pencil is then turned horizontal and, measuring at the canopy's widest point, used to determine how many times wider the canopy is than the tree's height.

To determine the diameter of a tree, simply measure the tree's circumference, usually at about 3 feet above the ground, and divide it by 3.14.

Describing a Tree's Canopy Density

The task of describing a tree's canopy density is somewhat subjective since there is no common metric. For the purposes of shade planning one could describe the density of a tree's canopy by rating it as "open," "moderate," or "dense." Standing beneath the tree and looking through its branches, if over 90% of the sky is blocked by the tree's canopy, it can be described as "dense." If between 50% and 90% of the sky is blocked by the canopy, it can be described as "moderate," and if less than 50% of the sky is blocked by the canopy, it can be described as "open." An open canopy provides little UV radiation protection.

Measuring Existing Shade

The final task of the shade audit is to estimate the amount of existing shade on the school grounds. Measurements should be taken of all shade, regardless of whether it is off-limits. There are two methods for measuring shade, one of which is highly technical and requires a working knowledge of both solar geometry and computer-assisted design software. The second method requires only that the planning team mark the shade patterns on the ground at the times of day that the school grounds are used. The ground can be marked with chalk, rope, or baking flour, then measured and marked to scale on the site plan. Measurements at several times during the day and throughout the school year will be neccesary to ensure that adequate shade is provided at the right time of day, throughout the year.

If the sky can be seen by those under a tree or structure, they are at risk for exposure to indirect UV radiation.

Considering Potential Shade Strategies

Having collected information regarding the activity patterns of the different users of the school grounds and the shade patterns cast by trees and buildings, it is now time for the planning team to assess their findings and make recommendations to the school community. The planning team might find that the school grounds provide adequate protection from both direct and indirect UV radiation; however, if not, the team will need to make recommendations for making more shade accessible to students, teachers, staff, and visitors. The team should first consider strategies that increase the amount of accessible shade at very low or no additional cost to the school. These might include revising school policies to allow access to off-limits shaded areas or relocating playground equipment or picnic tables to areas of the school grounds where shade already exists. The planning team will also need to consider reflected UV radiation in their recommendations. These may include modifying ground and building surfaces to reduce their reflectivity. The planning team might determine that climbing vines would be the best solution for the indirect UV radiation reflected off a smooth wall or that artificial turf would be most appropriate to reduce the UV radiation reflected from a concrete playground. The team should engage in a process to help them examine the cost effectiveness of strategies that could be employed as they are evaluating whether or not a particular strategy will accomplish the intended goal. More information about this is provided below.

The Shade Planning Matrix

The Shade Planning Matrix is a tool that can assist the planning team with comparing potential strategies for achieving their goals while examining and comparing the cost effectiveness of each of the strategies. The team's stated shade goals must be specific, both at this stage of planning and when it is time to present recommendations to the school community. The planning team should also clearly state any goals that are ancillary to providing shade, such as the construction of an outdoor classroom or the creation of a natural wildlife habitat. Matrices should be developed for each area that is being considered.

Information for completing the Shade Planning Matrix may come from a variety of sources. It could be necessary to request an informal quote from a contractor if the planning team is considering a solid-roof structure. Many vendors will provide prices over the internet if the team believes that a shade cloth structure would be an effective strategy. If a natural solution is being considered, the team will want to enlist the help of their United States Department of Agriculture County Extension Service agent, who can provide information on the most appropriate trees, shrubs, and vines for each geographical area, and the rates at which the vegetation is expected to grow. The Shade Planning Matrix is Attachment C.

Making Recommendations

When the team has considered potential strategies for achieving their shade goals and has arrived at a consensus on a set of recommendations, their final task is to formalize them in a report to the school community. Across schools and shade planning teams, considerable variability is likely in the report format. However, several components are essential:

The Rationale

Besides the most important reason, that shade provides protection from the harmful effects of solar UV radiation, the rationale should include any additional benefits that could be accrued through the strategies that the shade planning team has recommended. Those benefits might include the creation of an outdoor classroom and sheltered area for active play during inclement weather, provision of shade for athletic event spectators, or the creation of a wildlife habitat.

Statement of Goals

With as much specificity as possible, the statement of goals should include a physical description of the location, the amount of shade needed, and a description of the activities that occur. One example is the following:

The planning team has determined that there is a need to increase the amount of shade over the area of the playground bounded to the north by the south wall of the main building, to the east by the chain-link fence, to the south by the edge of the playground pavement, and to the west by the basketball courts. Based on patterns of use by the students, it is estimated that there is a need for a total of 2,500 square feet of shade. This section of the playground is home to the jungle gym and is popular for passive play as well. Because it provides an unobstructed view of the entire playground, this is where the playground monitors usually stand.

Strategies for Achieving the Goals

Strategies for achieving the goals could include moving playground equipment to a shaded area of the playground, revising school policy to make off-limit areas accessible, or building structures or planting trees to provide additional shade. The planning team should present their recommendations, but should also be prepared to discuss alternative plans.

If the team is recommending the creation of new shade, it should be prepared to discuss the performance characteristics of the materials providing shade, including:

- Where the tree(s) or shade structure will be located.
- The amount of shade that will be provided.
- Whether the need is for seasonal or year-round shade.
- The costs associated with providing the shade, including both initial and annual maintenance costs.
- The estimated lifespan of the building or tree(s) providing the shade.

Approaches for Achieving the Goals

The cost of providing shade can range from an afternoon of volunteer labor to the expense of building a large outdoor classroom with electricity and plumbing. The school district's budget for the project often cannot be known until the planning team presents their recommendations. For this reason, modifiable plans and alternate funding sources should be explored. While members of the planning team are completing the shade audit, other members can be exploring potential funding sources and volunteer resources. As the planning team presents their recommendations, they should also be prepared to present the options for advancing their plan. Options could include fund-raising efforts by the parent-teacher organization, donation of building materials by a local builder's supply store, or a tree planting project by a local Boy Scout troop.

Attachment A: Building Description

School: ______________ Date: ______________

Building Number	Name of Building	Height at Eaves	Height at Ridge	Wall Material	Wall Color

Attachment B: Tree Inventory

School: ______________ Date: ______________

Tree Number	Species	Height	Trunk Diameter	Canopy Diameter	Canopy Density	Age	Condition

Attachment C: Shade Planning Matrix

Area to be Addressed: __________

Current Status: ____________

Recommended Total _______
Square Footage of Shade:
Goal: ____________

Strategy 1:	**Initial Investment**	**Immediate Amount of Additional Shade**	**Estimated Annual Cost**	**Total Five-Year Cost**	**Total Shade at Five Years**	**Total Ten-Year Cost**	**Total Shade at Ten Years**	**Life Expectancy and Average Annual Cost**
Advantages:					**Disadvantages:**			
Strategy 2:	**Initial Investment**	**Immediate Amount of Additional Shade**	**Estimated Annual Cost**	**Total Five-Year Cost**	**Total Shade at Five Years**	**Total Ten-Year Cost**	**Total Shade at Ten Years**	**Life Expectancy and Average Annual Cost**
Advantages:					**Disadvantages:**			
Strategy 3:	**Initial Investment**	**Immediate Amount of Additional Shade**	**Estimated Annual Cost**	**Total Five-Year Cost**	**Total Shade at Five Years**	**Total Ten-Year Cost**	**Total Shade at Ten Years**	**Life Expectancy and Average Annual Cost**
Advantages:					**Disadvantages:**			
Strategy 4:	**Initial Investment**	**Immediate Amount of Additional Shade**	**Estimated Annual Cost**	**Total Five-Year Cost**	**Total Shade at Five Years**	**Total Ten-Year Cost**	**Total Shade at Ten Years**	**Life Expectancy and Average Annual Cost**
Advantages:					**Disadvantages:**			

End Notes

[1] MMWR 2002; 51(RR04):1-16. Available at http://www.cdc.gov/mmwr/review/mmwrhtm/ rr5104a1.htm

[2] American Cancer Society. What Are The Key Statistics For Nonmelanoma Skin Cancer? Available at http://www.cancer.org/docroot/CRI/content/CRI_2_4_1X_What_are_the_key_statistics_for_skin_cancer_51. asp?sitearea=

[3] American Cancer Society. What Are The Key Statistics For Melanoma Skin Cancer? Available at http://www.cancer.org/docroot/CRI/content/CRI_2_4_1X_What_are_the_key_statistics_for_melanoma_50. asp?sitearea=

[4] American Academy of Dermatology. Skin Cancer. Available at http://www.aad.org/pamphlets/ skincan.html

[5] Armstrong BK, Kricker A. How much melanoma is caused by sun exposure? *Melanoma Res*, 1993; 3: 395-401.

[6] Diffey, BL. Solar ultarviolet radiation effects on biological systems. *Physiology Medica; Biology* 1991; 36(3):299-328.

[7] United Nations Development Programme, Montreal protocol on substances that deplete the ozone layer. Available at http://www.undp.org/seed/eap/montreal.htm.

[8] Williams ML, Pennella R. Melanoma, melanocytic nevi, and other melanoma risk factors in children. *J Pediatr* 1994; 124:833-45

[9] Moore LA. Ocular protection from solar ultraviolet radiation (UVR) in sport: factors to consider when prescribing. *The South African Optometrist* 2003; 62(2):72-79.

[10] Sliney, DH. Physical factors in cataractogenesis: ambient ultraviolet radiation and temperature. *Invest Ophthalmol Vis Sci* 1986; 27(5):781-790.

[11] Hall HI, Rogers JD. Sun protection behaviors among African Americans. *Ethnicity and Disease* 1999;9(1):126-31.

[12] Olson RL, Sayre RM, Everett M A. Effect of anatomic location and time on ultraviolet erythema. *Arch Dermatol* 1996; 93(2): 211-15.

[13] Diffey BL. Ultraviolet radiation and human health. *Clinics in Dermatology* 1998;16:83-9.

[14] Gartner LM, Greer FR. Prevention of rickets and vitamin D deficiency: new guidelines for vitamin D intake. *Pediatrics* 2003;111(4 Pt 1): 908-10.

[15] West SK, Duncan DD, Munoz B, Rubin GS, Fried LP, Bandeen-Roche K, et al. Sunlight exposure and risk of lens opacities in a population-based study: the Salisbury Eye Evaluation project. *JAMA* 1998;280:714-8.

[16] Rosmini F, Stazi MA, Milton RC, Sperduto RD. Pasquini P, Maraini G. A dose-response effect between a sunlight index and age-related cataracts. Italian-American Cataract Study Group.[comment]. *Annals of Epidemiology*. 4(4):266-70.

[17] Westerdahl J, Olsson H, Ingvar C. At what age do sunburn episodes play a crucial role for the development of malignant melanoma. Eur J Cancer 1994; 30A(11):1647-54.

[18] Zanetti R, Franceschi S, Rosso S, Colonna S, Bidoli, E. Cutaneous melanoma and sunburns in childhood in a southern European population. *Eur J Cancer* 1992;28A(6-7):1172-76.

[19] Elwood JM, Whitehead SM, Davison J, Stewart M, Galt M. Malignant melanoma in England: risks associated with naevi, freckles, social class, hair colour, and sunburn. *Int J Epidemiol* 1990;19(4):801-10.

[20] Gandini S, Sera F, Cattaruzza MS, et al. Meta-analysis of risk factors for cutaneous melanoma: II. Sun exposure. *Eur J Cancer* 2005;41:45-60.

In: Encyclopedia of Dermatology (6 Volume Set)
Editor: Meghan Pratt
ISBN: 978-1-63483-326-4

Chapter 75

SUN SAFETY FOR AMERICA'S YOUTH TOOLKIT*

Centers for Disease Control and Prevention

1. ABOUT THE SUN SAFETY FOR AMERICA'S YOUTH TOOLKIT

Since 1998, the National Comprehensive Cancer Control Program (NCCCP) has provided funding and technical support to develop and implement comprehensive cancer control (CCC) plans to "reduce cancer incidence, morbidity, and mortality through prevention, early detection, treatment, rehabilitation and palliation."[1,2] Currently the Centers for Disease Control and Prevention (CDC) Division of Cancer Prevention and Control (DCPC) "funds CCC programs in all 50 states, the District of Columbia, 7 tribes and tribal organization and 7 U.S. territories" [3].

The CCC program in each state/tribe/territory/jurisdiction has a mandate to develop a plan that addresses a wide variety of cancer prevention and control priorities. This often includes skin cancer prevention. The Sun Safety for America's Youth Toolkit is designed as a resource for state/tribe/territory/ jurisdiction CCC programs interested in engaging schools and other education partners in sun safety efforts to reduce their state/tribe/territory/ jurisdiction's incidence of skin cancer. Since a majority of sun exposure occurs during childhood and early adulthood[4] and key sun protective behaviors can most easily be established at this time, addressing sun safety for young people is an important cancer control objective.

There is a wide variety of sun safety programs, materials, and resources available to organizations interested in implementing sun safety efforts, many of which are described in this toolkit and the accompanying reference documents. This toolkit builds upon lessons learned from CDC's long history of sun safety and skin cancer prevention. In 2002, CDC released the *Guidelines for School Programs to Prevent Skin Cancer* [5]. The Guidelines

* This is an edited, reformatted and augmented version of a document issued by the Centers for Disease Control and Prevention, July 2009.

provide resources and suggestions for schools to improve sun safety practices in seven major areas: policy, environmental change, education, family involvement, professional development, health services, and evaluation. To foster implementation of these guidelines, DCPC, in partnership with the Division of Adolescent and School Health (DASH), made funds available to states with Coordinated School Health Programs (CSHPs) to conduct pilot skin cancer prevention activities. In 2003, through the Skin Cancer Priority Supplement to PA03004—Improving the Health, Education, and Well-Being of Young People through Coordinated School Health Programs—three states (Colorado, Michigan, and North Carolina) were awarded funds to pilot activities to address the school skin cancer guidelines. From late 2003 through early 2007, the Department of Education in each of the three funded states received funds to implement their pilot sun safety initiatives. Each state was required to develop an annual work plan that would guide their efforts to address CDC's skin cancer guidelines and develop a partnership with their state CCC program.

This toolkit draws from these efforts and is designed to provide CCC programs with resources and information that will help them to understand the burden of skin cancer within their state/tribe/territory/jurisdiction, assess current state/ tribe/territory/jurisdiction-level sun safety interest and activity, engage in implementation of sun safety efforts with schools and key education partners, and evaluate their efforts.

The toolkit consists of four key steps that will help CCC programs move through a logical process for engaging and implementing sun safety efforts for young people:

- Step I: Identify and Recruit Sun Safety Partners
- Step II: Assess and Understand Sun Safety Needs and Resources in Your State/Tribe/Territory/Jurisdiction
- Step III: Plan and Implement Sun Safety Activities
- Step IV: Evaluate Sun Safety Efforts

Step I describes the numerous organizations and individuals CCC programs may want to engage in sun safety planning and implementation. These partners represent both state/tribe/territory/jurisdiction and local organizations that can play an important role in reaching schools and young people to implement and enhance effective sun safety strategies.

Step II provides recommendations for understanding the current state skin cancer burden and how to utilize that information to inform the development and targeting of sun safety efforts. To understand the current level of sun safety activity within the state/tribe/territory/jurisdiction, recommendations and resources are provided for conducting a sun safety program and resource inventory at the state/tribe/territory/jurisdiction level. Resources are also provided to help your CCC program understand the current legal and/or policy issues related to sun safety and how sun safety may already be integrated into existing school resources and tools.

Step III outlines a process for conducting a Strengths, Weaknesses, Opportunities and Threats (SWOT) analysis related to implementation of sun safety activities. Recommendations and resources on selection of sun safety activities are provided as well as examples of activities implemented using the *CDC Guidelines for School Programs to Prevent Skin Cancer*.

Step IV highlights the importance of evaluation of state/tribe/territory/ jurisdiction sun safety efforts and offers some examples of how to evaluate sun safety efforts locally and at the state/tribe/territory/jurisdiction level. We also provide suggestions for modification of state surveillance systems.

Within each step, we provide examples from state sun safety efforts to help CCC programs understand how these recommendations, tools, and resources have been utilized by other states.

The toolkit also includes an extensive sun safety resource list, which highlights potential sun safety partners at the state/tribe/territory/jurisdiction and national levels, and other sun safety programs and materials that are currently available.

2. Why Is Sun Safety Important for Young People?

Skin cancer is the most common type of cancer and is thought to account for half of all cancers [6, 7]. About one million cases of basal cell or squamous cell cancers, the two most common types of skin cancer, are diagnosed each year. Melanoma, the third most common type of skin cancer [5], accounts for less than 5% of skin cancer cases but causes a majority of skin cancer deaths [6, 7].

Although children are not commonly diagnosed with skin cancer, it is during childhood that much of one's lifetime sun exposure occurs and when important protective behaviors can be established. Approximately 65%–90% of melanomas are caused by ultraviolet (UV) radiation [5], and because a substantial percentage of lifetime sun exposure occurs before age 20 [4], UV radiation exposure during childhood and adolescence plays an important role in the development of skin cancer [8]. Persons with a history of more than one blistering sunburn during childhood or adolescence are at a greater risk for developing basal cell carcinoma [9] and are two times more likely to develop melanoma than those without such exposures [5].

Why Is It Important to Work with Schools?

Sun exposure preventive behaviors can yield the most positive effects if they are initiated early and established as healthy and consistent patterns throughout life [5]. In 2003, the U.S. Community Preventive Services on Reducing Exposure to Ultraviolet Light recommended that primary schools implement educational and policy strategies to improve behaviors that reduce exposure to UV light by covering exposed skin and therefore preventing skin cancer [10]. Because much time during childhood and adolescence is spent at school, schools provide a favorable environment in which to teach and model healthy behaviors.

There are approximately 50 million students attending more than 98,000 schools nationwide [11]. Schools therefore provide the most far-reaching access to young people. Schools can play a critical role in educating young people about their health and ensuring that they have a healthy environment when they are at school and engaged in school activities. However, it is important to acknowledge that schools are faced with the challenge of maintaining high academic standards and addressing a wide variety of health priorities with limited time and resources. Therefore, identifying opportunities to integrate sun safety into existing resources, activities, and curricula is critical to successful implementation and sustainability and to reducing burden on school partners.

In addition to schools, there are numerous other community organizations that provide services to young people and thus have an opportunity to educate them about the importance of sun safety. These organizations include parks and recreation departments, summer camps, museums, health education centers, and others. Because of the important role these organizations and groups serve, they have been included as potential partners for any state/tribe/ territory/jurisdiction sun safety effort.

3. Step I: Identify and Recruit Sun Safety Partners

When preparing to engage in a sun safety effort, CCC programs can complement their own cancer control expertise by identifying and engaging additional partners who are knowledgeable and skilled in working with schools and young people. Such partnerships represent an opportunity for experts in cancer control and education to bring their respective areas of expertise together to identify strategies that can be implemented in a manner that reduces the burden on the educational system. These partners can facilitate sun safety activities in a number of ways, including

- building upon existing relationships to reduce potential barriers and reluctance by schools administrators and teachers to add sun safety to an already full agenda,
- serving as critical links to educate and improve school awareness and knowledge of the importance of sun safety,
- identifying opportunities to integrate sun safety into existing school programs and curriculum, and
- serving as sun safety advocates within their own organizations.

Develop Partnerships to Facilitate Sun Safety Planning and Implementation

In 2008, DCPC developed a *Partnership Tool Kit: Program Version*[12] that helps programs navigate the process of

- determining the need for a partnership,
- developing a partnership,
- evaluating a partnership, and
- sustaining a partnership.

This tool is recommended to CCC programs to help engage partners in skin cancer prevention efforts. Key aspects of this tool are included in this toolkit, but programs are encouraged to refer to the *Partnership Tool Kit: Program Version* for additional details and guidance.

When determining the need for a partnership, programs should consider the following questions:

- What specific outcomes or products does your program hope to achieve through partnerships?
- In what ways do you need partnerships to achieve the identified out- comes or products?
- How would partnerships provide additional expertise rather than duplicating expertise in your program?

Programs can then move toward developing a new partnership. Potential questions to consider at this stage include the following:

- What potential partners has your program identified?
- In what ways could nontraditional partners be helpful in a new partnership?
- What does your program aim to achieve by working with these potential partners?
- How will these potential partners complement and strengthen your program?
- What might be some potential drawbacks to working with these potential partners?
- How would these potential partners help your program better achieve your goals and objectives?
- What might your program and the potential partners gain through this partnership?
- What resources does your program have available to contribute to new partnerships?
- Is there an existing state-level school health coordinating committee?

Identify Other State/Tribe/Territory/Jurisdiction Partners to Engage in Sun Safety Planning

After assessing the need for additional partners and partnerships to promote a state/tribe/territory/ jurisdiction sun safety effort, CCC programs can identify a number of other state government agencies and programs that may serve as critical stakeholders and resources. The list below includes some examples of possible state-level partners that could be engaged in sun safety efforts. This list is not exhaustive, so each CCC program should identify other resources and partners specific to their state/tribe/territory/jurisdiction.

State Department of Education: The State Department of Education is an important stakeholder when addressing any issue that impacts young people. Twenty-two states and one tribal government are funded to build the capacity of their school systems through CDC's Coordinated School Health Program (CSHP) [13]. The CSHP model consists of eight key components for a comprehensive health program: health education, physical education, health services, nutrition services, counseling and psychological services, healthy school environment, health promotion for staff, and family/community involvement. State health and education agencies are encouraged to develop an ongoing partnership to facilitate the implementation of effective policies and practices to promote the health and well-being of students and staff.

With or without funding for a CSHP, the State Department of Education represents a key partner in sun safety for young people and can provide valuable linkages, insight, and resources for engaging schools in sun safety. While health education classes are perhaps the most traditional mechanism for providing education on a particular topic, they are not the only avenues to be explored. Department experts or leaders in physical education, physical activity/wellness, school health services, and after-school activities are natural partners as they can incorporate sun safety into physical education classes and school sports activities. Sun safety can also be incorporated into a number of other academic areas, such as science and math (see the *Guidelines for School Programs to Prevent Skin Cancer* for additional information on incorporation of sun safety into various curricula); thus, it is important to try to identify partners beyond just the health education curriculum.

State Agency that Regulates Commercial Tanning Facilities: Every state has a state agency that is responsible for oversight, certification, and regulations related to indoor tanning/commercial tanning facilities (i.e., tanning beds). While not directly related to the schools, these organizations provide oversight to ensure that tanning facility staff are trained and that any state laws to protect minors from tanning are adhered to. Representatives from these agencies can be valuable partners for enforcement of existing state tanning laws or for development of such legislation if it does not already exist. A list of all state agencies responsible for commercial tanning facilities oversight can be found at http://www.tanningtraining.com/reginfo/state.html.

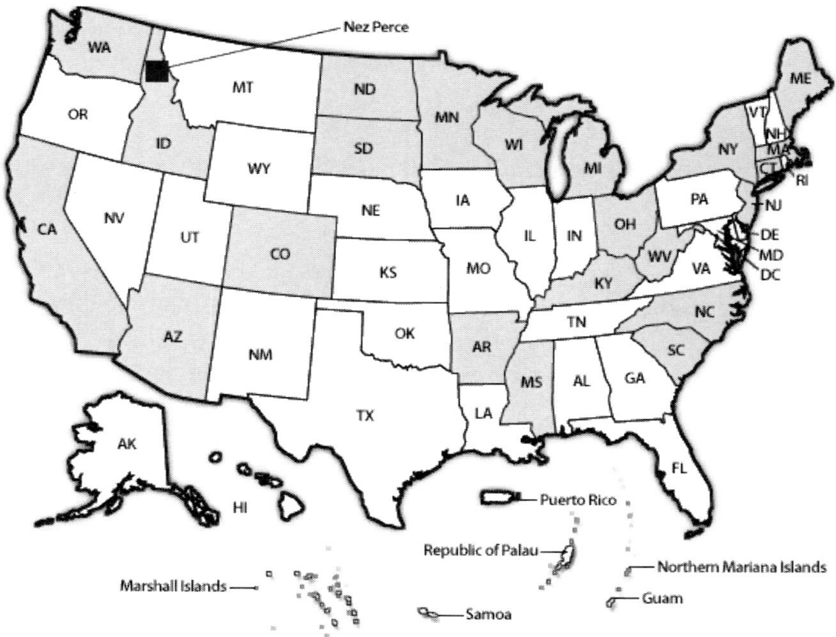

Note: State Education Agencies (SEA) that receive DASH funding are shaded. The tribal government from Nez Perce also receives CSHP funding. Source: CDC Coordinated School Health Program http://www.cdc.gov/healthyyouth/partners/ funded/cshp.htm.

Figure 1. Coordinated School Health Programs (CSHP).

State Medical Associations: Clinical partners can play an important role in advocating for sun safe behaviors with adults and young people.*

- The National Association of School Nurses has affiliate school nurse organizations in 49 states (there is no affiliate in Hawaii) and the District of Columbia. State affiliate information can be found at http://www.nasn.org/Default.aspx?tabid=60.* School nurses play an important role in training teachers and students about practicing sun safe behavior and, in some cases, may have the responsibility of administering sunscreen to students.
- The American Academy of Dermatology (AAD) has affiliate State Dermatology Society organizations that can provide resources and support to sun safety efforts. AAD offers the Seal of Recognition Program and the Skin Cancer Awareness: Intervention Plan for Tomorrow (SCRIPT) Plan. The SCRIPT Plan includes a shade structure grant program, free skin cancer screenings, advocacy for federal and state legislation to regulate indoor tanning, paid and public service advertising, and sun safety resource materials. More information on AAD and its resources can be found at http://www.aad.org/index.html.*
- The American Academy of Pediatrics (AAP) has state chapters across the United States. AAP endorses a policy statement titled *Ultraviolet Light: A Hazard to Children*. Pediatricians can provide valuable information to children and parents on sun safety and can be a valuable advocate for passing state laws addressing skin cancer and skin cancer prevention. A list of state chapters can be found at http://www.aap.org/member/ chapters/chapters.htm.*

State Athletic and Coaching Associations: Young people are exposed to the sun during a variety of outdoor activities, including participation in school or community athletic activities. Including partners who represent state athletic and coaching associations provides a valuable resource for educating adults who oversee thousands of children during outdoor sports and athletic events about the importance of sun safety while on the field.

- The National Federation of State High School Associations includes member associations in each of the 50 states and the District of Columbia. A list of member associations and their contact information can be found at http://www.nfhs.org/stateassociations.aspx.*

Colleges and Universities: State colleges and universities often have a variety of experts, resources, and programs addressing sun safety, including

* Links to non-Federal organizations found in this document are provided solely as a service to our users. These links do not constitute an endorsement of these organizations or their programs by CDC or the Federal government, and none should be inferred. CDC is not responsible for the content of the individual organization web pages found at these links.

* Links to non-Federal organizations found in this document are provided solely as a service to our users. These links do not constitute an endorsement of these organizations or their programs by CDC or the Federal government, and none should be inferred. CDC is not responsible for the content of the individual organization web pages found at these links.

- Cooperative Extension Services,
- schools of medicine,
- schools of nursing, and
- schools of public health.

American School Health Association (ASHA): ASHA has state constituent chapters in 12 states and has passed a resolution supporting sun safety school policies and education to prevent skin cancer. A list of member associations can be found at http://www.ashaweb.org/i4a/pages/ index.cfm?pageid=3317.*

Parent Teacher Association (PTA): The national PTA places an emphasis on healthy youth, and state PTA chapters can be valuable partners in implementing sun safety activities. State PTA chapters have access to local PTA chapters whose members can be educated to become suns safety advocates within their own school chapters. State PTAs can also pass resolutions and position statements in support of sun safety. State and local PTA chapters can be found at http://pta .org/jp find your pta .html.

Identify Local Partners to Engage in Sun Safety Planning

Depending on the sun safety approach and activities to be implemented, many CCC programs may also choose to engage local partners in their sun safety planning and activities. In many cases, local partners may be members or affiliates of state-level organizations that have already become engaged as sun safety partners. Local PTA chapters and individual health care providers are two examples of local organizations/members that may be closely affiliated with state-level organizations. There are a number of other local partners that can be engaged in sun safety planning and implementation.

Schools: Public, private, and alternative schools are perhaps the most obvious partners to engage in sun safety efforts, but also the most challenging. Learning how schools work is an important first step to working effectively with schools [14]. Because many policies impacting schools are implemented at the school level, it is often critical to work directly with schools and school administrators to integrate sun safety into school policies, curricula, and activities. Schools are faced with the task of addressing numerous student health issues while meeting or maintaining high academic standards. Gaining access to schools is often difficult and is most easily done by individuals and organizations that have preexisting relationships with schools and school administrators. While many schools are familiar with student health issues such as tobacco and drug use, obesity, physical activity, nutrition, and asthma, most schools are less familiar with the issue of sun safety. Engaging schools often requires time and resources to educate school decision makers on the importance of sun safety for their students and the approaches that a school can implement to protect students from the sun while in their care. Many schools have school health teams, and districts have school health councils that meet regularly to discuss school health problems and plans for improvement.

While the resources may not always be available, it is beneficial when even relatively small amounts of funding can be provided to schools interested in making improvements in sun safety policies, erecting or planting shade structures, or conducting education and awareness events and activities.

Local Education Agencies (LEAs): LEAs reside between individual schools and the Department of Education at the state level. LEAs are often considered school districts and provide administrative oversight to public schools in a particular geographic area. Like individual schools, LEAs can serve to provide leadership and guidance on school sun safety policies, shade planning, and curricula.

County or Area Parks and Recreation Organizations: While not directly related to schools, area parks and recreation organizations serve youth across the country, providing recreational sports activities, parks, and summer camps. Parks and recreation staff and the young people they oversee can benefit from educational and policy sun safety efforts. The National Recreation and Park Association was a sponsor of the Pool Cool sun safety effort aimed at improving sun safety behaviors of pool users. More information on Pool Cool can be found at http://www .poolcool .org/*

Health Education Centers: The National Association of Health Education Centers seeks to support and promote organizations that provide health education programs. Thirty-eight member organizations can be found in 22 states and the District of Columbia. A list of health education centers can be found at http://www .nahec .org/documents/2007AnnualReport .pdf .*

LESSONS FROM THE FIELD

- Recognize that cancer control and education organizations have different structures, resources, and sometimes languages. It is important to take the time to learn what they are and how they can be used most effectively to promote sun safety efforts.
- Nurture the partnership through communication, development of goals, and setting timelines.
- Include partners who are familiar with education agencies at the local level so they can share what might and might not work with local sun safety efforts. These relationships can also help engage key school personnel who may serve as advocates or potential gatekeepers.
- Work with partners to create a plan of action, rather than approaching partners once a plan has been developed.
- Many potential partners and stakeholders are not knowledgeable about the issue of sun safety. There needs to be an effort to educate and improve awareness to recruit partners before many will be willing to engage in activities.
- Plan for sustainability from the beginning. Look closely at what kinds of activities and partnerships can help ensure financial and programmatic longevity.

* Links to non-Federal organizations found in this document are provided solely as a service to our users. These links do not constitute an endorsement of these organizations or their programs by CDC or the Federal government, and none should be inferred. CDC is not responsible for the content of the individual organization web pages found at these links.

Parent Teacher Organizations (PTOs): Many schools have parent groups that are not affiliated with the national PTA; these groups are often called PTOs. There is no national or state PTO, but each PTO is independently organized and operated.

Other Community-based Organizations: Many other types of organizations that serve young people can be included in sun safety planning and program implementation, including the following:

- YMCA: http://www .ymca .net/*
- YWCA: http://www .ywca .org/
- Boys/Girls Clubs: http://www .bgca .org/*
- Boy Scouts: http://www.scouting .org/*
- Girl Scouts: http://www.girlscouts .org/*
- Museums, especially those with outdoor activities: http://www.museumca.org/usa/states.html
- Zoos, aquariums, and amusement and water parks: http://www.themeparkcity.com/USA_index.htm*
- Minor league ball parks: http://www.littleballparks .com/*
- Public or community pools

4. Step II. Understand Sun Safety Needs and Resources in Your State/Tribe/ Territory/Jurisdiction

Once major partners are identified, CCC programs should undergo a process for understanding the sun safety needs, skin cancer burden, and existing sun safety resources within their state/tribe/territory/jurisdiction. Every state/tribe/territory/jurisdiction will have different types of resources already dedicated towards sun safety; thus, prior to implementing new interventions and activities, it is valuable to work with partners to conduct an assessment of what sun safety efforts are currently in place. This assessment can then be used to identify potential gaps in resources and sun safety needs and priorities.

Within Step II, we will provide recommendations on the following:

- assessing and understanding the skin cancer burden in your state/tribe/territory/jurisdiction,
- conducting a state/tribe/territory/jurisdiction–level sun safety inventory of existing programs and resources, and
- understanding your state/tribe/territory/jurisdiction's legal and/or policy issues related to sun safety.

* Links to non-Federal organizations found in this document are provided solely as a service to our users. These links do not constitute an endorsement of these organizations or their programs by CDC or the Federal government, and none should be inferred. CDC is not responsible for the content of the individual organization web pages found at these links.

Assess and Understand the Skin Cancer Burden in Your State/ Tribe/Territory/Jurisdiction

Assessing the burden of skin cancer in your state/tribe/territory /jurisdiction will allow your CCC program to prioritize strategies and interventions, and help focus efforts on particular programmatic and geographical areas with the greatest need. As most CCC programs are aware, there are a variety of national databases that provide state/tribe/ territory/ jurisdiction–specific data on the burden of skin cancer; however, tribe, territory, and jurisdiction data is not as easily available.

National Cancer Institute and centers for Disease Control and Prevention State Cancer Profiles: The objective of the State Cancer Profiles website is to provide a system to characterize the cancer burden in a standardized manner in order to motivate action, integrate surveillance into cancer control planning, characterize areas and demographic groups, and expose health disparities. The focus is on cancer sites for which there are evidence-based control interventions. Interactive graphics and maps provide visual support for deciding where to focus cancer control efforts. The State Cancer Profiles can be found at http://statecancerprofiles.cancer.gov/.

United States Cancer Statistics: This web-based report includes the official federal statistics on cancer incidence from registries that have high-quality data and cancer mortality statistics for each year and for 2001–2005 combined. It is produced by CDC and the National Cancer Institute (NCI), in collaboration with the North American Association of Central Cancer Registries (NAACCR).[1] The United States Cancer Statistics can be found at http://apps .nccd .cdc .gov/uscs/.

Data relating to the burden of skin cancer in your area can also be found in state, territory, and jurisdiction-based resources, including your state's cancer registry. The National Program of Cancer Registries (NCPR) and NCI's Surveillance, Epidemiology, and End Results (SEER) Program together fund 50 states, the District of Columbia, Puerto Rico, the U.S. Pacific Island Jurisdictions, and six metropolitan areas to conduct surveillance and develop and maintain a cancer registry for the area. Contact information for each state/ territory/jurisdiction cancer registry can be found at http://apps.nccd.cdc.gov/ cancercontacts/npcr/contacts.asp. Information on the NCPR can be found at http://www .cdc .gov/cancer/npcr/, and information on the SEER Program can be found at http://seer.cancer .gov/about/index .html.

Other tools are also available to help demonstrate the burden of skin cancer in your area.

Cancer Mortality Maps and Graphs: This site, sponsored by NCI, provides valuable information about cancer mortality in the United States during the time period 1950–1994, based on data obtained from the National Center for Health Statistics (NCHS). Cancer Mortality Maps and Graphs provides interactive maps, graphs, text, tables, and figures showing geographic patterns and time trends of cancer death rates for more than 40 cancers for the 50 states. This is found at http://www3 .cancer .gov/atlasplus/.

Skin cancer risk factor data is more difficult to obtain.

Youth Risk Behavior Survey (YRBS): The YRBS monitors priority health-risk behaviors among young people in grades 9-12. It has included the following questions regarding routine sunscreen use and routine practice of sun safety behaviors for the previous two iterations (2005 and 2007):

- When you are outside for more than 1 hour on a sunny day, how often do you wear sunscreen with an SPF of 15 or higher?
- When you are outside for more than 1 hour on a sunny day, how often do you do one or more of the following: stay in the shade, wear long pants, wear a long-sleeved shirt, or wear a hat that shades your face, ears, and neck?

In 2007, the YRBS was conducted in 44 states (although 5 states, Alabama, Colorado, Nebraska, New Jersey, and Oregon, did not obtain weighted data), the 22 districts, including the District of Columbia, and 5 territories and jurisdictions (Territory of Guam, Territory of American Samoa, Commonwealth of the Northern Marianas Islands, Republic of the Marshall Islands, and Republic of Palau). Information on the YRBS at the state and national level can be found at http://www.cdc.gov/HealthyYouth/yrbs/index .htm.

Several states, including Colorado, Florida, and New Mexico, have included skin cancer risk factor and sun safety related question in their Behavioral Risk Factor Surveillance Survey (BRFSS) during specific years. These questions can be found in Section 6 of this toolkit (Step IV).

Another data source that can be used to help your CCC program to prioritize strategies and target efforts on particular areas with the greatest need are school-based information systems. These systems can inform CCC programs about the location and demographic make-up of the schools in their area.

School District Demographic System (SDDS): The SDDS provides access to information about demographics, social characteristics, and economics of children and school districts from the U.S. Department of Education's National Center for Education Statistics (NCES). The SDDS enables users to directly access school district geographic and demographic data. This can be found at http:// nces .ed .gov/surveys/sdds/.

LESSONS FROM THE FIELD

- Understanding the skin cancer burden in your state can help your CCC program target limited resources toward the areas with greatest need. For example, if funds are available for mini-grants to schools, recruit schools from counties or geographic areas with the greatest prevalence of melanoma.
- If your state does not currently collect data on skin cancer or sun safety behaviors, adding questions to surveillance tools can help with understanding the state skin cancer burden and with evaluation of your sun safety efforts. These data can also be used to help demonstrate need, a critical requirement when identifying funding opportunities.

Conduct a Sun Safety Inventory: What Do We Already Know about the Available Resources around Sun Safety in our State/ Tribe/Territory/Jurisdiction?

Conducting a sun safety inventory will help your CCC program understand what types of activities and resources are currently available to schools and programs that serve young people. The partners identified in Step I are extremely valuable in completing this inventory as they will be able to provide insight and information about any existing sun safety efforts currently being implemented by their organizations and partners. Once an inventory is completed, the information can be analyzed and used to identify needs and/or gaps that your CCC program's sun safety efforts can work to address, thus ensuring that sun safety resources are used wisely and do not duplicate existing efforts.

Your inventory may include a number of different resources, several examples of which are provided below. In addition, a sample sun safety inventory tracking template is included as part of this toolkit.

Existing Sun Safety Programs in your State/tribe/territory/ Jurisdiction: There are a variety of well known sun safety programs and curricula used by schools and other community partners engaged in addressing sun safety for young people. When planning CCC sun safety activities, it is helpful to know if these programs and resources are already being used. Both the SunWise program and Sunny Days Healthy Ways are examples of programs that are recommended by the *Guide to Community Preventive Services* [10].

SunWise: The U.S. Environmental Protection Agency's (EPA's) SunWise program is a free, school-based sun safety program that currently engages schools in all 50 states and the District of Columbia (http://www.epa .gov/sunwise/summary.html). The program is directed at educators in grades K-8 and includes a variety of materials and resources for the classroom, school, and community. Schools can register to be a SunWise school by completing a registration form online. As of 2008, 18,000 schools and more than one million students were engaged in SunWise (EPA, http://www.epa .gov/sunwise/evaluation.html). In spring 2009, CDC provided technical assistance to EPA as they began developing specific sun safety fact sheets for each state in the U.S.; the first fact sheets will be available soon at http://www .epa .gov/sunwise/.

As a part of your CCC program sun safety assessment, the SunWise program can provide your CCC program with a list of the schools that have registered with SunWise. While this does not ensure that a school is implementing all components of SunWise, it can serve as an indicator of school interest in sun safety and may help to target resources appropriately.

Sunny Days Healthy Ways: The Sunny Days Healthy Ways curriculum is designed for students and educators in grades K-8. The curriculum provides a wide variety of resources that can be tailored to the specific needs of schools and teachers. The curriculum also provides resources on incorporating sun safety into a variety of national and state health and science education standards (http://sdhw.info/standards/3 standards .asp).*

* Links to non-Federal organizations found in this document are provided solely as a service to our users. These links do not constitute an endorsement of these organizations or their programs by CDC or the Federal government, and none should be inferred. CDC is not responsible for the content of the individual organization web pages found at these links.

As a part of your CCC program sun safety assessment, the Sunny Days Healthy Ways program administrator, Klein Buendel, Inc., can provide you with a list of the schools that have purchased the Sunny Days Healthy Ways curriculum. As with SunWise, this does not ensure that a school is implementing all components of Sunny Days Healthy Ways it can serve as an indicator of school interest in sun safety and may help to target resources appropriately.

Another popular sun safety campaign is the ***Slip, Slop, Slap*** sun safety media campaign and materials from Australia. Having launched Slip, Slop, Slap in 1981, Australia has one of the most well-established sun safety programs. This campaign encourages people to slip on a shirt, slop on some sunscreen, and slap on a hat. Most recently, the campaign has added seek shade and slide on some sunglasses [15]. This campaign has been used in several U.S. states and has been very successful in Australia. In addition to Slip, Slop, Slap, the Cancer Council Australia has a SunSmart Schools program that has engaged 2,500 schools and 3,500 daycare centers across the country [16].

Other sun safety programs and resources that may be identified through an inventory include those presented in Table 1.

Organizations Already Engaged in Sun Safety: Step I of this toolkit provides examples of organizations that could be included as key sun safety partners. Many of the key organizations engaged in sun safety may have already been identified through this process. Additional organization may be identified by working with your state/tribe/territory/jurisdiction partners to brainstorm other potential organizational sun safety resources.

financial Resources for Sun Safety Activities: Identification of financial resources for implementation of sun safety efforts is often a critical component that determines whether schools and other organizations implement sun safety activities. A wide variety of free or inexpensive program materials are available to organizations interested in implementing sun safety activities, policies, and curricula. Many of these materials can be easily downloaded via the Internet. See the list of program resources included in this toolkit for links to many of these materials.

Table 1. Sun Safety and Skin Cancer Prevention Programs for Young People

Program	Sponsoring Agency	Website Information
Pool Cool	Rollins School of Public Health and the National Recreation and Park Association	http://www.poolcool.org/index.html*
Sun Safe for the Early Years and SunSafe in the Middle School Years	Norris Cotton Cancer Center	http://www.cancer.dartmouth.edu/melanoma/sunsafe_early.shtml* http://www.cancer.dartmouth.edu/melanoma/sunsafe_middle.shtml*
Block the Sun, Not the Fun	The Sun Safety Alliance	http://www.sunsafetyalliance.org/blockthesun.html*
Project S.A.F.E.T.Y (Sun Awareness For Educating Today's Youth)	M.D. Anderson Cancer Center	http://www.mdanderson.org/patient-and-cancer-information/cancer-information/cancer-education/prevention-programs/project-safety/*

For projects around shade planning, a few grants and funding opportunities are available from national sun safety partners. The American Academy of Dermatology offers a small number of shade structure grants directly to schools each year, but these grants are highly competitive. Similarly, the SHADE Foundation of America offers occasional funding for the construction of shade structures at schools and play areas.

Sun Safety in existing School resource materials and education Standards: In many states, the Department of Education has incorporated sun safety and skin cancer prevention into existing standard course of study materials, curriculum standards, and benchmarks. Sun safety has also been incorporated into many of the national health education standards and proficiency indicators (www.cdc.gov/healthyyouth/sher/standards/index.htm) and science education standards. An inventory should look to identify where sun safety is already included in school resources and standards and to identify potential opportunities for sun safety to be incorporated.

Human Resources: Because skin cancer affects millions of people across the United States, it is not difficult to find valuable advocates for skin cancer prevention and promotion of sun safety. These advocates can be found serving as school teachers, nurses and administrators, dermatologists, pediatricians, parents, grandparents, and skin cancer survivors. The identification and involvement of sun safety champions can be a valuable resource for implementation of sun safety activities. School health advocates often serve on district-level school health councils and school-level health teams.

Table 2. States with Laws Addressing Skin Cancer and Skin Cancer Prevention (enacted through March 2009)

State	Tanning Facilities	Prevention	School Health	Awareness	Health Education	Screening Reimbursement
Arizona	•	•	•			
Arkansas	•					
California	•	•				•
Connecticut	•					
Florida	•			•	•	
Georgia	•					
Indiana	•					
Kentucky	•	•	•			
Louisiana	•					
Maryland	•	•				
Massachusetts	•					
Michigan	•					
Minnesota	•					
Mississippi	•					

Table 2. (Continued)

State	Tanning Facilities	Prevention	School Health	Awareness	Health Education	Screening Reimbursement
New Hampshire	•					
New Jersey	•					
New York	•	•	•	•	•	
North Carolina	•					
North Dakota	•					
Ohio	•					
Rhode Island	•	•				
Tennessee	•					
Texas	•					
Utah	•					
Virginia	•					
Wisconsin	•					
Total	**25**	**6**	**3**	**2**	**2**	**1**

Source: National Cancer Institute [17].

Understand Your State/Tribe/Territory/Jurisdiction's Legal and/or Policy Issues Related to Sun Safety

There are a variety of legal and policy issues related to sun safety and skin cancer prevention that are important to understand and consider during the planning phase of any state sun safety effort.

Legislation related to Sun Safety: As of March 2009, 26 states had passed legislation regarding skin cancer or skin cancer prevention. This legislation is summarized in Table 2. Twenty-five states currently have legislation addressing access to and use of indoor tanning facilities. Between February and March 2009, three states (Montana, South Dakota, and Wyoming) failed to pass similar proposed legislation. Two states, Florida and New York, have passed laws promoting or requiring skin cancer education in schools [17]. A much smaller number of states have passed legislation regarding prevention, school health, skin cancer awareness, and skin cancer screening reimbursement.

Several resources are available to help CCC programs understand the current laws addressing skin cancer and skin cancer prevention.

- ***The National Cancer Institute's State Cancer Legislative Database Program*** provides a variety of resources on legislation related to cancer, including skin cancer and skin cancer prevention. It includes a searchable database to obtain information on skin cancer–related bills and resolutions: http://www .scld-nci.net/index.cfml.*
- ***The National Conference of State Legislatures*** provides a list of newly introduced and current legislation that addresses tanning restrictions for minors. A brief description of the restrictions is provided for each state along with links to each state statute: http://www.ncsl .org/programs/health/tanningrestrictions .htm

School Policies: In addition to legislative regulations related to sun safety, there is a variety of school policy issues that should be examined during a sun safety inventory. Many schools and/or local education agencies have established policies that impact sun safety, such as allowing hats and sunglasses to be worn at school and use of sunscreen by students. Each CCC program should have an understanding of what policies currently exist within their state/tribe/jurisdiction/territory and where school policy decisions are made (i.e., at the state, local, or school level) to inform effective implementation of sun safe policies that reduce youth exposure to UV radiation. The National Association of State Boards of Education (NASBE) maintains the State School Healthy Policy Database, which "contains brief descriptions of laws, legal codes, rules, regulations, administrative orders, mandates, standards, resolutions, and other written means of exercising authority. While authoritative binding policies are the primary focus of the database, it also includes guidance documents and other non-binding materials that provide a more detailed picture of a state's school health policies and activities"[18] The database can be searched using state, topic, or key word searches.

LESSONS FROM THE FIELD

- Policies that impact schools are not always enacted through legislation at the state/jurisdiction/territory level. In many cases school districts, and in some cases individual schools, determine their own policies. It may be helpful to partner with individuals who work with schools to understand what local school policies are common in your state/tribe/jurisdiction/territory.
- Sun safety policy may not always be directly related to schools. Many states have policies that prohibit people under the age of 18 from using indoor tanning facilities. When assessing your state/tribe/jurisdiction/territory sun safety policy, do not limit your search to just school policies; expand it to include more broad sun safety policies.

* Links to non-Federal organizations found in this document are provided solely as a service to our users. These links do not constitute an endorsement of these organizations or their programs by CDC or the Federal government, and none should be inferred. CDC is not responsible for the content of the individual organization web pages found at these links.

5. STEP III: PLAN AND IMPLEMENT SUN SAFETY ACTIVITIES

Once you have identified partners and have a thorough understanding of the current sun safety resources and issues within your state/tribe/territory/ jurisdiction, you can move toward identification of sun safety priorities and strategies.

Conduct a SWOT Analysis

A Strengths, Weaknesses, Opportunities, and Threats (SWOT) analysis is a valuable process for most public health planning activities. The process helps an organization to identify strengths and weaknesses within an organization, and opportunities and threats outside of the organization that can help with planning and decision making. A detailed description of SWOT analysis is available at the University of Kansas Community Tool Box (http://ctb. ku.edu/tools/en/sub section main 1049 .htm[*]); a brief description of the brainstorming process is provided here.

Table 3. Sample Structure for Tracking SWOT Analysis Information

internal		external	
Strengths	**Weaknesses**	**opportunities**	**threats**

A SWOT analysis can help your CCC program explore options for new sun safety efforts and can help organize the information you have gathered through your identification of partners and sun safety inventory. The process should be conducted as a group meeting with key stakeholders and partners involved in the brainstorming process. Begin by using a table to outline your strengths, weaknesses, opportunities and threats (see Table 3).

After giving participants an opportunity to introduce themselves, explain the objectives for the SWOT analysis and the process that will be used. The SWOT process can be done in a large group or by breaking stakeholders out into smaller groups, but the groups should not exceed 10 people. Because a significant amount of work has already gone into the sun safety inventory, it may be helpful to provide SWOT analysis participants with a summary of what has already been found so that this may inform the brainstorming activity.

Allow 20–30 minutes for the group or groups to brainstorm various strengths, weaknesses, opportunities and threats as they relate to the implementation of a sun safety effort. Examples of possible internal and external factors are included below.

[*] Links to non-Federal organizations found in this document are provided solely as a service to our users. These links do not constitute an endorsement of these organizations or their programs by CDC or the Federal government, and none should be inferred. CDC is not responsible for the content of the individual organization web pages found at these links.

Internal Factors: Strengths and Weaknesses

- **Human resources:** CCC staff, state Cancer Control Consortium members, other state government agencies involved in sun safety, state sun safety partners, local sun safety partners
- **Physical resources:** CCC program offices, existing sun safety equipment or materials, partner offices in the communities or geographic areas where you may want to conduct sun safety activities
- **Financial:** CDC funding for sun safety activities, other state funding or resources that can be directed towards sun safety, funding from other sun safety or skin cancer prevention organizations
- **Activities and processes:** sun safety materials or resources managed by the CCC program or sun safety partners, existing surveillance systems
- **Past experiences:** the reputation and networks of the CCC program and key sun safety program partners (e.g., Department of Education) that will help facilitate new sun safety efforts, previous sun safety efforts implemented

External Factors: Opportunities and Threats

- **Future trends:** in cancer control (Is sun safety a priority given other cancer control needs?) and in student and youth education and safety (How can sun safety "compete for attention" with more well funded student health issues such as obesity and tobacco use?)
- **The economy:** local, state, or national (How will the current economy impact school resources and priorities for incorporating sun safety into current curriculum and activities?)
- **Funding sources:** state and national budget priorities, funds available from sun safety or skin cancer prevention organizations
- **Legislation and policy:** What skin cancer and skin cancer prevention legislation is already in place? How supportive has the state legislature been in addressing skin cancer and skin cancer prevention? What current school-level policies facilitate or inhibit sun safety practices?
- **Partners/partnerships:** What resources do partners have access to in order to facilitate implementation of sun safety activities? What partners are not yet involved but would be helpful?

Once the brainstorming time is over, a group leader can begin to ask each group to report on what they identified for each box (strengths, weaknesses, opportunities, and threats). A recorder should capture the contributions from each group, allowing for discussion while groups share their input or holding off on discussion until after all groups have contributed their thoughts. Continue gathering information from all groups until the table is complete.

What Do You Do with the SWOT Results?

Once the group has completed identifying strengths, weaknesses, opportunities, and threats, the group can do several things:

- develop consensus about the most important items in each category,
- relate the findings to the group's visions, mission, and goals for implementing a sun safety initiative for schools and youth, or
- begin to translate the findings into action plans and strategies for implementing sun safety efforts.

The SWOT analysis should help your CCC program and partners to "build on your strengths, minimize your weaknesses, seize opportunities, and counteract threats ."[19]

Select and Implement Sun Safety Activities

Building on what has been learned from sun safety partners, the sun safety inventory, and the SWOT analysis, a CCC program will be ready to explore what sun safety programs and activities should be implemented. There are a wide variety of school-based sun safety efforts, curricula, and activities that CCC programs can implement to keep young people sun safe. The U.S. Preventive Services Task Force has found that educational and policy interventions within primary schools have a positive impact on sun protective "covering up" behavior to reduce UV exposure [10].

This includes wearing protective clothing, such as hats, shirts, or pants while outside. The evidence is limited as to the effectiveness of other skin cancer prevention interventions and activities, but there is still a great deal to be learned, so evaluation of sun safety efforts is of critical importance.

In 2002, CDC released the *Guidelines for School Programs to Prevent Skin Cancer*, which outlines seven guidelines schools can use to reduce the risk of skin cancer among students [5]. These guidelines, found at http://www .cdc .gov/ mmwr/PDF/rr/rr5104.pdf, provide resources and suggestions of how schools can work to improve sun safety practices in seven major areas:

1. Policy
2. Environmental change
3. Education
4. Family Involvement
5. Professional Development
6. Health Services
7. Evaluation

LESSONS FROM THE FIELD

- Determine what teachers and schools are currently doing to address sun safety and how it may already be included in the curriculum. Where possible, look for opportunities to integrate sun safety into existing activities, resources, and curricula. Asking a school or partner to look for ways to incorporate sun safety in their existing activities will reduce any sense of burden that may accompany a request to add an entirely new topic to an already full list of responsibilities.
- School-related policy decisions in are often made at the local level rather than statewide, so rather than push for all schools in a state to change, advocates need to work within each school district or even within each school. Addressing these issues with each school can take more time and effort than would be required for a statewide policy.
- The school year ends in the summer, which is the prime time for people to think about sun safety issues. Motivating schools to think about sun safety in the fall and winter can be difficult because the topic may not seem as relevant at that time.
- CCC staff and partners may need to "sell" the idea of sun safety to schools and other organizations that serve young people. One valuable way of doing this is to identify ways to link sun safety with higher priority issues, such as physical activity, playground safety, and athletic/sports activities.

These guidelines serve as a natural starting point for any CCC program focusing on sun safety efforts aimed at impacting schools and young people. For those not familiar with the *Guidelines*, it is recommended that all guidelines be reviewed, and then programs select one or two to focus their efforts. When selecting guidelines to implement, it is important to work with your partners and utilize the lessons learned from the sun safety inventory and SWOT analysis to determine the strategies that are most appropriate.

In 2003, through the Skin Cancer Priority Supplement to PA03004, Improving the Health, Education, and Well-Being of Young People through Coordinated School Health Programs, three states (Colorado, Michigan, and North Carolina) were awarded funds to pilot activities to address the seven skin cancer guidelines. As a requirement of this funding, partnerships were established between each state's Department of Education and CCC program. Each state implemented activities using the guidance provided in the *Guidelines for School Programs to Prevent Skin Cancer* [5]. Examples of the types of activities implemented by these pilot states to address each of the seven guidelines are provided below.

When selecting activities, it is important to consider the level of intervention at which your CCC program would like to intervene. Activities can be implemented at the local level (e.g., individual schools or LEAs, museums, YMCAs) or the state/tribe/territory/jurisdiction level (e.g., state PTA, legislature). Some guidelines are more easily applied at one level or another but which guidelines and activities are selected will be largely dependent on the type of activities your CCC program is interested in implementing. Each of the three pilot states funded under the Skin Cancer Priority Supplement to PA03004 utilized mini-grants to provide schools and partner organizations with funding to implement sun safety activities. The amount of funding varied but ranged from several hundred dollars to several thousand dollars. In one state, a large amount of funding was provided to the state PTA, which then distributed it in the form of smaller mini-grants to local PTA chapters interested in sun safety. Providing a small amount of funding to schools and organizational partners served as an incentive for learning more about and implementing sun safety activities. An example of a mini-grant RFP is included as part of this toolkit.

The following are provided for each of the seven guidelines:

- a brief description of the guideline and why it is important to school- based skin cancer prevention efforts
- examples of program activities that have been implemented to address each of the guidelines.

The examples are largely drawn from states who implemented activities to address the *Guidelines* through a partnership between the State Department of Education and CCC program. Please note that the evidence base of proven effective sun safety interventions is very limited. These activities are provided as examples of possible activities, but your CCC program should remain up to date on new evidence of effective sun safety interventions.

In addition to the information below, this toolkit includes a list of available resources to help your state CCC program address each of the seven guidelines.

Guideline 1: Policy – Establish Policies that Reduce Exposure to UV Radiation

Why Is Sun Safety Policy Important?

"An effectively crafted skin cancer prevention policy provides a framework for implementing the six other guidelines. The policy demonstrates institutional commitment and guides school and community groups in planning, implementing and evaluating skin cancer prevention activities… Although a comprehensive policy is preferable, more limited policies addressing certain aspects of skin cancer prevention also can be useful" (p. 7) [5].

Sample Activities

Local

- Offer mini-grants to schools and organizations to implement sun safety activities and require that each recipient include policy change in their efforts, in addition to any other activities.
- Provide sample sun safety policies to organizations and partners interested in implementing policies to remove the burden of developing new policies.
- Provide training and technical assistance to schools and other organizations on how to develop and implement sun safety policies. This can include training individuals who work with young people, such as teachers, school nurses, coaches, and PTA/PTSA groups.

- Disseminate resources such as *Fit, Healthy, and Ready to Learn* and CDC's *Guidelines for School Programs to Prevent Skin Cancer* to school boards and other decision making bodies. (Both of these documents are included as reference materials in this toolkit.)
- Help schools form school health teams and districts form school health councils to address health problems and promote health.

State/tribe/territory/jurisdiction

- Work with state PTA partners to pass a sun safety resolution.
- Incorporate development of sun safety policy into state CCC plan.
- In states where current legislation does not exist, work with state agencies that regulate indoor tanning facilities to develop legislation to restrict tanning bed use by minors.

Guideline 2: Environmental Change – Provide and Maintain Physical and Social Environments that Support Sun Safety

Why Is Environmental Change Important?

"Policies can promote the provision of supportive resources for skin cancer prevention (e.g., shade, protective clothing and hats, sunscreen at a reduced price or free, and highly visible information and prompts for sun protection) in the physical and social environment. These policies help establish routine personal behaviors and social norms that promote skin cancer prevention in the context of organized group activities" (p. 9) [5].

Sample Activities

Local

- Conduct a shade audit using CDC's Shade Planning for America's Schools tools.
- Engage students in the research and design of shade structures that are appropriate for their school.
- Provide mini-grant funding to schools to build shade structures, plant trees, or purchase portable shade structures to be used at school events.
- Provide funding so that sunscreen can be purchased and provided to students and staff during school events (e.g., field trips, sports events, and field days). If necessary, obtain informed consent from parents so that students can use the sunscreen provided.
- Encourage school staff and students to wear sunglasses, sun safe hats, and shirts with sleeves when participating in outdoor activities.
- Produce and distribute sun safety fact sheets to parents, students, coaches, and teachers.
- Work with area parks, museums, health education centers, zoos, and community pools to provide shade structures for visitors.

State/tribe/territory/jurisdiction

- Include questions on state school assessment tools to help schools identify ways to change the physical environment of their school to address sun safety. One example is the Healthy School Action Tool (HSAT) in Michigan. The SunSafe Colorado website also contains an assessment tool that can be used to assess the physical environment of schools.

Guideline 3: Education – Provide Health Education to Teach Students the Knowledge, Attitudes, and Behavioral Skills They Need to Prevent Skin Cancer

Why Is Sun Safety Education Important?

"Skin cancer prevention is likely to be most effective when it is taught as part of a comprehensive health education curriculum that focuses on understanding the relations between personal behavior and health (126) and that provides students with the knowledge and skills outlined by the National Health Education Standards (112). ... In addition to health classes, skin cancer prevention can also be integrated into other subject areas. ...This type of integrated approach requires collaborative planning and curriculum development among teachers to optimize skin cancer prevention education and to ensure consistency of messages and practices" (p. 10) [5].

Sample Activities

Local

- Host an anti-tanning pre-prom fashion show that includes educational information about the dangers of tanning.
- Develop and disseminate anti-indoor tanning press kit to student newspapers and journalists.
- Partner with summer camps and parks and recreation organizations to implement a sun safety program for youth attending day camps and to train camp staff on staying sun safe.
- Provide UV detectors to students to increase awareness of sun exposure.
- Provide schools with sun safety information and resources, such as the Sunny Days Healthy Ways curriculum or EPA's SunWise program.

State/tribe/territory/jurisdiction

- Integrate sun safety into existing teaching resources, including standard course of study guidance.
- Develop new sun safety resources or utilize some of the many that are currently available, including the SunSafe Colorado website (see Resource from the field box)

or sun safety lessons in the Michigan Model for Comprehensive School Health Education.

RESOURCE FROM THE FIELD

The SunSafe Colorado website provides a wide variety of resources and information about sun safety for schools. The website was developed by their state partner Klein Buendel, Inc., who also developed the Sunny Days Healthy Ways curriculum. Klein Buendel has offered to work with states/tribes/territories/jurisdictions interested in modifying the SunSafe Colorado website to be specific to their state. This would require a small amount of funding from your CCC program to make the necessary changes (e.g., logos, state data). If your state is interested in learning more about adapting the SunSafe Colorado website for your state/tribe/territory/ jurisdiction, please contact:

Mary Klein Buller, M.A. President, Klein Buendel, Inc.
1667 Cole Blvd., Suite 225
Golden, Colorado 80401 mbuller@kleinbuendel .com
303-565-4330 (phone)
303-565-4320 (fax)
www.kleinbuendel.com

Guideline 4: Family Involvement – Involve Family Members in Skin Cancer Prevention Efforts

Why Is Family Involvement in Sun Safety Important?

"Involving family members in skin cancer prevention efforts increases the likelihood that they will adopt and thus model healthful sun-protection behaviors of students (122). At a minimum, parents or guardians can be informed concerning school initiatives and policies and knowledgeable regarding how their cooperation is needed to ensure child health. Parents and guardians also can be encouraged to provide children with sun-protective clothing and sunglasses for outdoor activities. In addition, parents and guardians can serve as advocates for sun-protective policies and practices in schools" (p. 11) [5].

Sample Activities

Local

- Develop print or electronic resources specifically for educating parents about sun safety issues.
- Partner with state and/or local PTA groups to increase awareness of sun safety through presentations and, if possible, provide funds to PTA groups for sun safety activities.
- Include sun safety policies and information in student and parent hand-books and student planners.

- Distribute informed consent forms to parents asking permission for students to use sunscreen in school or at school activities and explaining the need for sun safety awareness.
- Distribute notes to parents about the importance of sun safety prior to field trips, field days, graduation ceremonies, and other outdoor events.
- Distribute sun safety information and sunscreen at community events, festivals, and celebrations that are held outdoors.

State/tribe/territory/jurisdiction

- Partner with newspapers, parents' magazines, and organizational news-letters to publish and distribute articles and information on sun safety.
- Work with other state children's health organizations to identify other resources, publications, and meetings that could be used to educate families about sun safety (e.g., Cooperative Extension Children's Environmental Health Program).
- Partner with state and local media outlets to issue UV alerts.

Guideline 5: Professional Development-Include Skin Cancer Prevention Knowledge and Skills in Preservice and Inservice Education for School Administrators, Teachers, Physical Education Teachers and Coaches, School Nurses, and Others Who Work with Students

Why Are Professional Development Opportunities around Sun Safety Important?

"Appropriate and effective professional development efforts should be conducted for decision makers and care givers at all levels. Professional development activities, including certification programs and inservice education, are provided routinely for teachers and other school staff (e.g., coaches and school nurses). Skin cancer prevention can be integrated into those activities. All school staff should receive basic information concerning the importance of sun safety and key strategies for skin cancer prevention" (p. 11) [5].

Sample Activities

Local

- Train school staff and administrators on sun safety policy development and skin cancer prevention.
- Train camp counselors and others who work outside with youth during the summer on how to protect themselves and the youth they work with from sun exposure.
- Identify schools in regions with the highest melanoma rates and focus trainings in those communities first.

State/tribe/territory/jurisdiction

- Collaborate with state sports/athletic associations to develop and/or provide training to coaches of outdoor sports teams.
- Provide training sessions on sun safety at other training or continuing education workshops for school staff, nurses, and teachers.

Guideline 6: Health Services – Complement and Support Skin Cancer Prevention Education and Sun Safety Environments and Policies with School Health Services

Why Is It Important to Engage Health Services in Sun Safety?

"School health services provide an opportunity for nurses, health educators, and school health resource specialists to promote and reinforce skin cancer prevention practices. Health professionals in the community, including pediatricians, primary care providers, nurses, pharmacists, and dermatologist are credible sources of information and guidance for skin cancer prevention. They can be advocates for skin cancer prevention policies, environmental changes, and programs, and support school programs through presentations, professional training, demonstrations, and classroom visits" (p.12) [5].

Sample Activities

Local

- Include school nurses in any trainings or workshops offered to teachers or other school staff.
- Provide mini-grant funding or other support to teen health centers to implement sun safety activities with teens and parents.
- Work with nurses and school administrators to discuss parental consent for sunscreen application at school.

State/tribe/territory/jurisdiction

- Provide sun safety resources to your state Association of School Nurses and offer to attend and present at their meetings and conferences.

Guideline 7: Evaluation – Periodically Evaluate Whether Schools Are Implementing the Guidelines on Policies, Environmental Change, Education, Families, Professional Development, and Health Services

Why Is Evaluation of Sun Safety Activities Important?

Evaluation questions can be used "to determine whether their programs are consistent with CDC's *Guidelines for School Programs to Prevent Skin Cancer*. These questions can be used to (1) assess whether schools in their jurisdiction care providing effective education to prevent skin cancer and (2) identify schools that would benefit from additional training, resources, or technical assistance" (p.12) [5].

Sample Activities

Local

- Collect progress reports and final reports from mini-grant recipients to track their activities and progress.
- Track and document sun safety policies implemented by schools and other community partners.
- Conduct focus groups with teachers, principals, coaches, and school nurses to identify challenges and needs regarding sun safety activities.
- Conduct pre-post training evaluations to assess training events and changes in participants' knowledge, attitudes, and skills related to sun safety.
- Train mini-grant recipients on the importance of evaluation, evaluation expectations, and how to conduct an appropriate evaluation activity.

State/tribe/territory/jurisdiction

- Add sun safety questions into state surveillance and data collection tools (e.g., BRFSS, YRBS).
- Identify state-specific surveillance tools that include sun safety items (e.g., NC Child Health Assessment and Monitoring Program, NC School Health Education Profiles, Michigan Healthy Schools Action Tools, Colo- rado Child Health Survey).

6. Step IV: Evaluate Sun Safety Efforts

Evaluation of your CCC sun safety effort is important for understanding and measuring the impact your program has on sun safety practices within your state and ultimately changes in state melanoma incidence. Evaluation is also important as a way to track progress toward meeting the goals and objectives in your state cancer plan. Evaluation results can be used to help identify and leverage additional sources of funding for your sun safety efforts and to inform program development and future sun safety program efforts.

The evaluation strategies your CCC program utilizes will need to be tailored to the unique goals and objectives of your cancer plan and to the types of sun safety strategies implemented. Evaluation planning should be conducted on an ongoing basis and should be initiated at the beginning of the program planning process to ensure that it is well integrated into your state efforts. There is a wide variety of evaluation resources available to your program. As an introduction to evaluation, please refer to CDC's *Framework for Program Evaluation in Public Health* [20]. Evaluation guidance and tools for schools are available from http://www.cdc.gov/healthyyouth/evaluation/ resources .htm. Several examples of local and state evaluation strategies are included under Guideline 7: Evaluation in the preceding section.

LESSONS FROM THE FIELD

- Schools have limited resources for evaluating local sun safety efforts, so be specific about what evaluation data are required and be prepared to offer evaluation support.
- Include evaluation planning in your program planning process. It is helpful develop your evaluation plan while planning your program activities rather than waiting until activities are being implemented or have been completed.

Inclusion of sun safety and skin cancer prevention questions in state surveillance tools and resources can yield important information regarding the current state of sun safety behaviors (as described in Step II under the heading Assess and Understand the Skin Cancer Burden in Your State/Tribe/Territory/ Jurisdiction). The BRFSS, YRBS, and other state surveillance systems can be utilized to assess both skin cancer burden and changes in behaviors. Tables 4–7 present examples of questions that have been used on various national and state-based surveys to assess skin cancer risk factors and sun safety behaviors for both adults and children. Since the field of sun safety for young people is relatively new, there are more questions to assess adult sun safety behaviors than there are for young people. The YRBS has utilized several of the adult-focused questions when assessing sun safety behaviors of high school–aged young people. Table 8 presents questions regarding school-based sun safety education programs, including both student education and staff development questions. These questions could be added to state or local surveillance systems as one way to evaluate program progress.

Table 4. Skin Cancer Prevention/Sun Safety: Child-focused Questions

Question	Response Options	Citation
On average, when your child goes outside on a sunny summer day for more than an hour, how often does he/she use sunscreen or sun block?	a. Always b. Nearly always c. Sometimes d. Seldom e. Never	Colorado[21]
On a sunny summer day, on average how much time does your child spend outside in the sun between 11am and 3pm?	a. _ _ hours/ minutes b. Don't know/ not sure	Colorado[22]
When your child is outside for more than 15 minutes between 11am and 3pm on a sunny summer day, how often does he/she use sunscreen with an SPF of 15 or higher?	a. Always b. Nearly always c. Sometimes d. Seldom e. Never	Colorado[22] North Carolina 2005[23]

Table 4. (Continued)

Question	Response Options	Citation
On a sunny summer day, when your child is outside for more than 15 minutes between 11am and 3pm, how often does he/she stay in the shade?	a. Always b. Nearly always c. Sometimes d. Seldom e. Never	Colorado[22] North Carolina 2005[23]
On a sunny summer day, when your child is outside for more than 15 minutes between 11am and 3pm, how often does he/she wear clothes covering most of his/ her arms and legs?	a. Always b. Nearly always c. Sometimes d. Seldom e. Never	Colorado[22] North Carolina[23]
Thinking back over the past 12 months, tell me as best you can whether your child has had any sunburns during that time. By sunburn, I mean any reddening or burn of the skin that lasts until the next day.	a. Yes b. No c. Don't know/not sure	Colorado[22] North Carolina[23]
Do you think a tan makes a child look healthy?	a. Yes b. No c. Don't know/ not sure	Colorado[22]

Table 5. Skin Cancer Prevention/Sun Safety: Adult-focused Questions

Question	Response Options	Citation
When you go outside on a sunny summer day for more than an hour, how often do you use sunscreen or sun block?	a. Always b. Nearly always c. Sometimes d. Seldom e. Never	Honey[24] Colorado[25, 26] Kansas[27]
What is the SPF of the sunscreen you use mostoften?	a. _ _ Number b. Don't know/not sure	Colorado[25, 26]
When you go outside on a sunny summer day for more than an hour, how often do you stay in the shade?	a. Always b. Nearly always c. Sometimes d. Seldom e. Never	Colorado[25, 26] Kansas[27]
When you go outside on a sunny day for more than an hour, how often do you wear a wide-brimmed hat or any other hat that shades your face, ears, and neck from the sun?	a. Always b. Nearly always c. Sometimes d. Seldom e. Never	Honey[24] Colorado[25, 26] Kansas[27]
When you go outside on a sunny summer day for more than an hour, how often do you wear long-sleeved shirts?	a. Always b. Nearly always c. Sometimes d. Seldom e. Never	Colorado[25, 26] Kansas[27]

Question	Response Options	Citation
When you are tanning, either outside or on an indoor tanning bed, what products do you usually apply to your skin?	a. Tan enhancer b. Sunscreen with SPF less than 15 c. Sunscreen with SPF 15 or higher d. I do not use any skin products e. I do not purposely tan in direct sunlight or use a tanning bed f. Other	Florida[28]
When you are outside in direct sunlight for the purpose of tanning, do you reapply sunscreen?	a. Yes b. No c. I do not purposely tan in direct sunlight d. Don't know/not sure	Florida[28]
Have you used a tanning bed or sun lamp in the last 12 months?	a. Yes b. No	Kansas[27]
Has a doctor, nurse, or other health professional ever spoken with you about taking protective measures against skin cancer? Protective measures include use of sunscreen, protective clothing, and avoiding exposure to sunlamps or tanning beds.	a. Yes, within the past year(any time less than 12 months ago) b. Yes, within the past 2 years(1 year but less than 2 years ago) c. Yes, within the past 3 years(2 years but less than 3 years ago) d. Yes, within the past 5 years(2 years but less than 5 years ago) e. Yes, 5 or more years ago f. No	Kansas[29]
Including any time that even a small part of your skin was red for more than 12 hours, have you had a sunburn within the past 12 months?	a. Yes b. No	Kansas[30]
Including times when even a small part of your skin was red for more than 12 hours, how many sunburns have you had within the past 12 months?	a. One b. Two c. Three d. Four e. Five f. Six or more	Kansas[30]

Table 6. Skin Cancer Risk Factors: Adult-focused Questions

Question	Response Options	Citations
Have you had a sunburn within the past 12 months?	a. Yes b. No c. Don't know/not sure	Honey[24] Colorado[25, 26] Florida[31]
Including times when even a small part of your skin was red for more than 12 hours, how many sunburns have you had within the past 12 months?	a. One b. Two c. Three d. Four e. Five f. Six or more g. Don't know/not sure	Colorado[25, 26] Florida[31]

Table 7. Sun Safety Perception: Adult-focused Question

Question	Response Options	Citation
Suppose that after several months of not being out in the sun, you went out in the sun without a hat, sunscreen, or protective clothing for an hour. Would you sunburn, darken without sunburn, or not have anything happen?	a. Sunburn b. Darken without sunburn c. Not have anything happen	Honey[24]

Table 8. School-based Education/Program Implementation

Question	Response Options	Citation
Now I am going to read a list of health topics. For each one, please tell me if you support school children receiving age-appropriate education about it in school.	a. Dental and oral health b. Nutrition and dietary behavior c. Human sexuality d. Sexually transmitted disease prevention e. Emotional and mental health f. Suicide prevention g. Tobacco use prevention h. Alcohol and other drug use prevention i. Violence prevention j. Sun safety	Colorado[22]
Does your school have a policy establishing sun safety guidelines for any of the following areas?	a. Encourage or allow students to apply lip balm and/or sunscreen b. New construction/ renovation projects include a plan for shade areas c. Promote or require the use of protective clothing outside (e.g., hats, sunglasses) d. Sun safety staff development opportunities for teachers e. Sun safety education for students f. Other areas	North Carolina[32]

Question	Response Options	Citation
During this school year, have teachers in this school tried to increase student knowledge on each of the following topics in a required health education course in any of grades 6 through 12? ***- Sun safety or skin cancer prevention***	a. Yes b. No	CDC[33]
During this school year, did teachers in this school teach each of the following physical activity topics in a required health education course for students in any of grades 6 through 12? ***- Weather-related safety (e.g., avoiding heat stroke, hypothermia, and sunburn while physically active)***	a. Yes b. No	CDC[33]
During the past 2 years, did you receive staff development (such as workshops, conferences, continuing education, or any other kind of inservice) on each of the following health education topics? ***- Sun safety or skin cancer prevention***	a. Yes b. No	CDC[33]
Would you like to receive staff development on each of these health education topics? ***-Sun safety or skin cancer prevention***	a. Yes b. No	CDC[33]

CONCLUSION

Protecting young people from UV exposure and teaching them how to practice lifelong sun safety behaviors is critical to reducing the rates of skin cancer in our country. As we have demonstrated, there is an abundance of informational material available to support programs and schools interested in engaging in sun safety activities. This toolkit brings together many of these resources into one package so that your program may develop and select sun safety strategies to address the needs of your state and program.

REFERENCES

[1] Centers for Disease Control and Prevention (CDC). (2009). *Coordinated School Health Program*. Retrieved May 4, 2009, from http://www.cdc .gov/healthyyouth/ partners/funded/cshp_map .htm.

[2] Centers for Disease Control and Prevention (CDC). (2009). *National Comprehensive Cancer Control Program (NCCCP)*. Retrieved May 4, 2009, from http://www .cdc .gov/cancer/ncccp/about .htm.

[3] Centers for Disease Control and Prevention (CDC). (2008/2009). *Comprehensive Cancer Control Program*. Retrieved May 4, 2009, from http://www .cdc .gov/cancer/ ncccp/cccpdf/0809_ncccp_fs .pdf.

[4] Godar, D. E. (2001). UV doses of American children and adolescents . *Photochemistry and Photobiology*, *74*(6), 787–793.

[5] Centers for Disease Control and Prevention (CDC). (2002). Guidelines for school programs to prevent skin cancer. *Morbidity and Mortality Weekly Report*, *51*(No.RR-4), 1-20.

[6] American Cancer Society (ACS). (2008). *Detailed guide: Skin cancer—basal and squamous cell. What are the key statistics about squamous and basal cell skin cancer?* Retrieved May 25, 2008, from http://www .cancer.org/docroot/CRI/content/ CRI_2_2_1X_How_many_people_ get_nonmelanoma_skin_cancer_51. asp?sitearea= .

[7] American Cancer Society (ACS). (2008) . *Detailed guide: Skin cancer—melanoma. What are the key statistics about melanoma?* Retrieved May 25, 2008, from http:// www .cancer .org/docroot/CRI/content/CRI 2 4 1X What are the key statistics for_melanoma_50 .asp?sitearea= .

[8] Gilchrest, B. A., Eller, M. S., Geller, A. C. & Yaar, M. (1999). The pathogenesis of melanoma induced by ultraviolet radiation. *New England Journal of Medicine*, *340*, 1341–1348.

[9] Kricker, A., Armstrong, B. K., English, D. R., et al. (1995). Does intermittent sun exposure cause basal cell carcinoma? A case-control study in Western Australia. *International Journal of Cancer*, *60*, 489–494.

[10] Centers for Disease Control and Prevention (CDC). (2003). Preventing skin cancer: Findings of the Task Force on Community Preventive Services on reducing exposure to ultraviolet light and counseling to prevent skin cancer, recommendations and rationale of the U.S. Preventive Services Task Force. *Morbidity and Mortality Weekly Report*, *52*(No. RR-15), 1–18.

[11] U.S. Department of Education. (2008). *Mapping America's Educational Progress 2008*.Retrieved June 21, 2008, from http://www.ed.gov/nclb/ accountability/results/ progress/nation .html .

[12] Soloe, C. (2007). *Developing, maintaining, and sustaining partnerships* . Final report prepared for CDC Division of Cancer Prevention and Control.

[13] Centers for Disease Control and Prevention (CDC). (2008). *Healthy youth! Coordinated school health program*. Retrieved June 21, 2008, from http://www .cdc . gov/healthyyouth/CSHP .

[14] Bogden, J. F. (2003). *How schools work and how to work with schools: A primer for professionals who serve children and youth* . Alexandria, VA: National Association of State Boards of Education .

[15] Cancer Council Australia. (2009). *Slip, slop, slap*. Retrieved June 1, 2009, from http://www.cancer.org.au/cancersmartlifestyle/SunSmart/ Campaignsandevents/ SlipSlopSlap.htm .

[16] Cancer Council Australia . (2009). *Sun smart schools* . Retrieved June 1, 2009, from http://www.cancer.org.au/cancersmartlifestyle/ SunSmart/ SunSmartschools.htm .

[17] National Cancer Institute. (2005). *State cancer legislative database program*. Bethesda, MD: National Cancer Institute.

[18] National Association of State Boards of Education (2009). *State school health policy database*. Retrieved June 5, 2009, from http://nasbe.org/ index.php/shs/health- policies-database.

[19] The Community Toolbox. (2009). *SWOT analysis: Strengths, weaknesses, opportunities and threats*. Retrieved May 28, 2009, from http://ctb.ku.edu/en/ tablecontents/sub_section_main_1049.htm.

[20] Centers for Disease Control and Prevention (CDC). (1999). Framework for program evaluation in public health. *Morbidity and Mortality Weekly Report*, *48*(No . RR-11) .

[21] Colorado Department of Public Health and Environment. (2006). *2002 Colorado behavioral risk factor surveillance system questionnaire*. Retrieved May 26, 2009, from http://www.cdphe.state.co.us/hs/brfss/ FinalCO02 .pdf .

[22] Colorado Department of Public Health and Environment. (2005). *2005 Colorado child health survey questionnaire*. Retrieved May 26, 2009, from http://www.cdphe. state.co.us/hs/mchdata/chs2005 .pdf.

[23] North Carolina State Center for Health Statistics. (2005). *2005 North Carolina CHAMP child health assessment and monitoring program survey*. Retrieved May 26, 2009, from http://www.schs.state.nc .us/SCHS/champ/pdf/CHAMPQ05 .pdf.

End Note

[1] U.S. Cancer Statistics Working Group. United States Cancer Statistics: 1999–2005 Incidence and Mortality Web-based Report. Atlanta: U.S. Department of Health and Human Services, Centers for Disease Control and Prevention and National Cancer Institute; 2009. Available at: www.cdc.gov/uscs.

In: Encyclopedia of Dermatology (6 Volume Set)
Editor: Meghan Pratt
ISBN: 978-1-63483-326-4

Chapter 76

Burn Diagnosis, Management, and Research

***Amy L. Strong*[1]*, Kavitha Ranganathan*[2]*, Eric T. Chang*[2]*, Michael Sorkin*[2]*, Shailesh Agarwal*[2] *and Benjamin Levi*[2,*]**

[1]Center for Stem Cell Research and Regenerative Medicine,
Tulane University School of Medicine, New Orleans, LA, US

[2]Department of Surgery, Section of Plastic Surgery,
University of Michigan, Ann Arbor, Michigan, US

Abstract

Burns are responsible for significant morbidity and mortality and are among the most devastating of all traumatic injuries, resulting in physical impairment, permanent disabilities, and emotional distress. It is conservatively estimated that each year 1 million persons seek medical care for burns and burn-related injuries with more than 50,000 patients being hospitalized for the treatment of burns. A burn occurs when some or all of the cells in the skin or underlying tissue is damaged due to thermal heat, radiation, electricity or contact with chemicals. The long-term consequences of burn injuries include: scars, severe muscle catabolism and wasting, joint contracture, heterotopic ossification, and other functional and aesthetic concerns. Nevertheless, major advances recently in the health care management of burn patients from the initial emergency room visit to the long-term physical therapy and reconstructive surgery have significantly improved patient outcomes. These recent advances highlight the significance of burn research to elucidate the pathophysiology of burns, as well as to improve the treatment of the acute and reconstructive sequelae of burn injuries to improve patients' overall well-being.

In this chapter, we will review the epidemiology of burns and the diagnosis and management of burn patients requiring medical care. We will further highlight the long-term consequences of burns on the skin, muscle, and joints, emphasizing the importance of early wound care and the advances in clinical care and basic science research to improve outcomes.

[*] Corresponding author.

1. EPIDEMIOLOGY

1.1. Incidence

In the United States, the incidence of burns is grossly underestimated at 1 million persons each year [1]. It is estimated that of those with burn injuries, 450,000 patients seek care in the emergency room, and an estimated 50,000 patients with burn injuries require hospitalization due to these injuries. Unfortunately, burn-related injuries continue to account for 3,400 deaths each year. The incidence of burns and deaths from burn injuries are associated with numerous factors, including age, race and ethnicity, intent of injury, treatment of injury, and socioeconomic status.

1.1A. Children

Infants and toddlers to the age of 4 years comprise almost one-third of burns. In fact, burns are the fifth leading cause of unintentional, non-fatal injury in infants and the third leading cause of fatal injury for newborns to children 9 years of age. Scald burns caused by hot liquids are the most common cause of pediatric burns and occur most often in the home [2-5]. The number of burns decreases from age 9 until adolescence and increases again after the age of 15, presumably due to greater exposure to hazards, experimentation, risk-taking, and employment [1]. Intentional burns account for roughly 10% of all cases of child abuse [6]. Pediatric burn victims are almost always under the age of 10, and the majority are less than 2 years old. Scalds from immersion into hot baths are the most frequent cause of these cases. Contact with heated objects including irons, curling irons, cigarettes, and heated kitchen utensils are also common causes of burn related injuries in child abuse cases.

1.1B. Adults

Flames and fire are the most common cause of burns in adults and the elderly. Flame burns account for 35 to 42 percent of hospital admissions in adults associated with burns, while scald burns account for 15 to 18 percent of hospital admissions related to burn injuries [3]. Cigarette ignition of upholstered furniture or bedding account for 47 percent of fires, and alcohol appears to be a significant contributor [7].

1.1C. Elderly

The elderly, defined by the age greater than 65 years, suffer a disproportionally higher percentage of hospitalizations due to burns in comparison to the general adult population. A 10 year analysis from 1995-2005 from the National Burn Repository of the American Burn Association revealed that individuals over the age of 65 comprised 11.9% of all burn unit admissions and that the average age of those admitted was 76.4 ± 6.6 years [8]. The most frequent cause of burns that led to death in elderly women was a result of clothing ignition during cooking [9]. Elderly burn patients treated for scald burns had relatively small burns (less than 13 percent of total body surface area [TBSA]) but had high mortality rates (30.2 percent) [10-12]. As a result, burns are the fourth leading cause of mortality among the elderly. Together, these results suggest that the medical, economic and social burdens of burn injuries will likely increase as the proportion of the elderly increases in future years.

1.1D. Race and Ethnicity

There is striking differences in susceptibility to burns by race and ethnicity. Burns are the leading cause of injury-related death in Black children between the ages of 1-9 and the rates are 2.7 times higher than in White, Hispanic and Asian/Pacific Islander children [13]. Likewise, in adults, the rate of non-fatal burns in Black Americans aged 35-39 years was 221 per 100,000 Blacks, which is remarkably higher than the 135 per 100,000 Whites with burns in the same age group [3]. The emergency room visit rate for burns from 1993 to 2004 in the United States was 62% greater among Black Americans (340 per 100,000 Black Americans) than White Americans (210 per 100,000 White Americans) [14]. The age-adjusted death rate from burns of all causes in the United States in 2006 was highest in Blacks (2.43 per 100,000) and lowest in Asians (0.44 per 100,000), with Native Americans (1.45 per 100,000), White non-Hispanics (1.11 per 100,000), and Hispanics (0.77 per 100,000) falling in between this range [3]. These trends can be translated to the elderly population, as the mortality rate for burn-related injuries in the elderly was 4.6 times greater in Black Americans than in White Americans [15].

There are also significant differences in the gender distribution of burns between age groups. Adult men more frequently seek care in the emergency department (69 percent), presumably due to the increased severity of their burns caused by industrial accidents, compared to women (31 percent) [1]. However, elderly women tend to be more highly represented among elderly burn victims than in younger populations [16, 17]. The greater preponderance of elderly women with burn injuries may reflect the decrease in workplace-related injuries among the geriatric population. In fact, the vast majority of burn injuries among elderly adults occur in a domestic setting involving cooking.

1.1E. Socioeconomic Status

Socioeconomic status (SES) factors have also been shown to increase the risk of burns. These factors include low household income, crowded household living conditions, and unemployment. In the metropolitan Oklahoma City, Oklahoma, the overall fire-related hospitalization and death rate was 3.6 out of 100,000 [18]. Stratification of the data based on household income, property values, and quality of housing demonstrated that the injury rate in lower SES was 15.3 out of 100,000 [19]. Children in the lowest SES groups requiring hospitalization for treatment in US burn centers was double the proportion of all children in the general population [3]. Furthermore, the incidence of house fires was 8 times greater in low income families in Dallas, Texas compared to high income families [20]. The higher incidence of house fires was attributed to the frequent absence of functional smoke detectors [20]. Together, these results highlight the increased need for educational seminars for lower SES groups to increase awareness to prevent household fires and burn injuries.

1.2. Etiology

Numerous entities, including fire or flame, scalds, contact, electrical conduction, and chemicals can produce burns. Between 2002 and 2011, 44 percent of burns were produced by fire or flame, 33 percent by scald, 9 percent by contact, 4 percent by electricity, 3 percent by chemical, and 7 percent defined as other (Figure 1) [21].

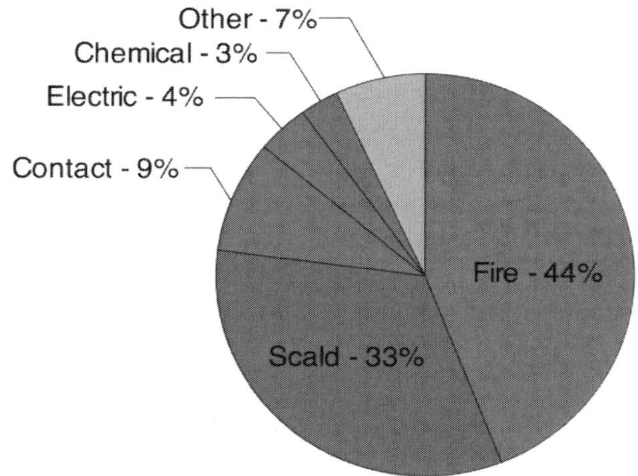

Figure 1. Causes of burn injuries.

1.2A. Thermal Burns

Thermal injuries, caused by fire or flames, are the most common burn etiology reported over the past decade [21]. Thermal injuries are associated with the highest risk of death and complications compared to all other burn etiologies. Flame burns most commonly occur at home (64 percent), while work fires and recreational fire burns account for 12 percent and 6 percent of flame burns, respectively. When considering thermal injuries, it is important to consider smoke inhalation as it significantly impacts the morbidity and mortality of patients recovering from flame burns. The majority of inhalation injuries occur while the patient was indoors or in an enclosed space and very few occur with patients who were burned while outside. Inhalation injury is present in 17 percent of patients with flame burns. The presence of smoke inhalation in burn patients is associated with an overall mortality rate of 24 percent, compared to the mortality rate of 4 percent in those patients without smoke inhalation damage.

Burns can be conceived as producing 3 concentric volumes of tissue damage: zone of coagulation, zone of stasis, and zone of hyperemia. The area most severely injured is the center of the wound or the zone of coagulation. Outside of the zone of coagulations is the zone of stasis, and beyond the zone of stasis lies the zone of hyperemia. In theory, the zone of coagulations is permanently destroyed, but with appropriate wound care, the zone of stasis can be salvageable from its ischemic state. In practice, the zone of stasis can be rescued if revascularization is achieved within a few days, preventing a superficial injury from being a full thickness injury. Extended period of ischemia in the zone of stasis, possibly from inadequate resuscitation, will result in long-term oxidative stress damage upon reperfusion, termed ischemia-reperfusion injury. This ischemia-reperfusion injury features cell death upon the return of blood to the injured areas, caused by the release of free oxygen radicals. The zone of hyperemia features inflammation due to the release of toxic metabolites caused by molecular structural alterations. The local mediators released are histamine, serotonin, bradykinin, nitric oxide, TNF-alpha, interleukins, and products of eicosanoid acid cascade [22, 23]. Histamine is an early phase mediator of increased microvascular permeability seen immediately after burns. Histamine causes large endothelial gaps to transiently form as a result of the contraction of venular endothelial cells, consequently resulting in burn edema in the skin [24]. Thus, most burn surgeons will allow at least 24 hours for the burn to progress before deciding on whether a burn has converted to a full thickness injury.

1.2B. Scald Burns

Scalds are the second leading cause of burn injuries and are the most common mechanism of burns in the pediatric population. Over 50 percent of scalds are associated with food preparation or consumption, with a smaller proportion associated with bathing [25, 26]. Common mechanisms including pulling a tablecloth or reaching up and tipping a hot container near the edge of a counter, pulling electric cords attached to heated kitchen appliances, and carrying containers with hot liquids [27, 28].

1.2C. Contact Burns

Contact burns from touching a hot object are extremely common in the pediatric population as well. Overall, contact burns make up only 9 percent of burns reported, but they are the third leading cause of burns in children.

1.2D. Electrical Burns

Electrical injuries occur more frequently in the adult than the pediatric population. As one of the most devastating and debilitating injuries cared for in burn centers, electrical injuries comprises 4 percent of all reported etiologies. Patients who have high-voltage electrical injuries, defined as greater than 1000 volts, are at elevated risk of spinal injury and require complete immobilization until spinal injury is ruled out. Bone has the highest conductance and electricity often conducts along the skeleton causing significant muscle necrosis along the bone. Whereas compartment syndrome in flame burns occurs due to a tight eschar (requiring escharotomy), compartment syndrome from electrical burns often occurs due to inflamed muscle trapped under fascia and thus requires a fasciotomy in addition to an escharotomy. Furthermore, the direct muscle damage may cause gross myoglobinuria, requiring more aggressive fluid resuscitation [29]. Patients with gross myoglobinuria caused by a severe electrical injury often require care in the intensive care unit for additional monitoring.

1.2E. Chemical Burns

While less common in the United States, chemical burns are the fifth leading cause of burn injuries. Chemical burns are a subtype of burns that are more common in developing countries. In the United States, chemical burns account for only 3 percent of burns. These burns occur most commonly as industrial accidents (34 percent) with the second most common place of occurrence being the home (32 percent). Chemical burns have also been reported in public buildings, farms, mines, and with recreational activity and sports [21]. Common agents that result in chemical burns are acidic and alkali compounds, including nitric and sulfuric acid and sodium hydroxide. Most common injured areas include the face, neck, chest, and upper limbs. Injury to the eyes is common in conjunction with facial injuries, leaving many patients partially or completely blind. In general, neutralization of chemicals should be avoided as this can cause an exothermic reaction. Removal of the chemical by immediately removing any clothing with the chemical, followed by dilution is the primary method to minimize the damage caused by chemical burns. Water irrigation is contraindicated or ineffective in several scenarios:

1. Elemental sodium, potassium, and lithium should not contact water as this will precipitate an explosion.
2. Dry lime should be brushed off, not irrigated.
3. Phenol is water insoluble and should be wiped from the skin with polyethylene glycol-soaked sponges.

Though chemicals should not be neutralized, certain chemicals require specific treatments. Hydrofluoric acid is toxic due to the fluoride ion, which binds calcium but can be neutralized with topical calcium gel (1 amp calcium gluconate in 100 g lubricating jelly). If symptoms persist, intra-arterial calcium infusion (10 mL calcium gluconate diluted in 80 mL of saline, infused over 4 hours) and/or subeschar injection of dilute (10%) calcium gluconate solution should be considered. Phenol is commonly used in disinfectants and chemical solvents with poor water solubility. Chemical burns caused by phenol results in protein disruption and denaturation, resulting in coagulation necrosis. Treatment of phenol exposure includes cleansing with 30% polyethylene glycol or ethyl alcohol followed by copious water irrigation.

1.3. Classification of Burns

To understand burn injuries, a basic understanding of the skin and underlying tissue is necessary. The outer layer of the skin, or the epidermis, arises from the stratum germinativum. As cells from the stratum germinativum layer migrate upward, they differentiate into keratinocytes and become the predominant cell type in the epidermis. The dermal layer contains epidermal appendages, including hair follicles, sweat glands, and sebaceous glands. Blood vessels, nerve endings, fibroblast, elastic, and collagen fibers reside in the dermis and provide nutrients and structural support to the skin. The subcutaneous tissue is deep to the dermis layer and contains hair follicles. Depending on the depth of the burn and the burn size, burn injuries can be classified into first degree, second degree, or third degree burns (Table 1). The depth of the injury depends on the temperature and heat capacity of the causative agent, the duration of exposure, and thickness of the skin. For instance, gasoline flame burns cause full thickness burns due to the high temperature of this flammable substance. Hot grease, which has a high heat capacity, is likely to cause deep burns as well. Mortiz and Henriques showed that irreversible damage of the basal epidermal cells in porcine skin occurring after 6 hours of contact at a temperature of 44°C, whereas increasing the temperature to 47°C required less than 30 minutes to note significant partial thickness burns [30]. At 51°C and 70°C, it required 4 minutes and 2 seconds, respectively, to cause complete destruction of the epidermis [30]. As the flash point for most cooking oils usually exceeds 200°C (and can be as high as 300°C), grease can easily cause instantaneous full thickness burns [31]. The thickness of the skin or the developmental stage of the skin also contributes to the severity of the injury. Children, who have underdeveloped skin, or the elderly, who have atrophic skin, sustain full-thickness injuries more often than young adults.

Table 1. Classification of burns injuries

Classification of Burn	Affect Skin Layers	Clinical Presentation	Management of primary burn wound
First degree	Epidermis	Red in color Dry in appearance Painful with or without stimulation Blanching occurs	Minimal care needed.
Second Degree *Superficial partial-thickness*	Epidermis and Superficial layer of the dermis	Pink or red in color Moist in appearance Painful with or without stimulation Blanching occurs	Topical antimicrobial dressings to minimize infection and inflammation
Deep partial-thickness	Deep layer of the dermis	Red or white in color Dry in appearance Diminished sensation Minimized or absent blanching	Fluid resuscitation Systemic and topical antibiotic therapy Surgical debridement of injured tissue Reconstructive surgery to increase mobility due to contractures
Third Degree	Epidermis, Entire dermis, and Subcutaneous layer	Black or charred in color Dry and leathery in appearance Painless with or without stimulation Absent blanching	Fluid resuscitation Systemic and topical antibiotic therapy Surgical debridement of injured tissue Reconstructive surgery to increase mobility due to contractures

1.3A. First Degree Burns

Burns are categorized based on the depth of burns and the burn size of the epidermis, dermis, and subcutaneous tissue that is damaged. A burn that remains confined to the epidermis is termed a first-degree burn. An example of a common first-degree burn is a non-blistering sunburn. The skin is usually red and dry in appearance and very painful with or without stimulation. These burns rarely require immediate medical attention and heal rapidly as the injured epithelium peels away from the healthy skin. Burn size estimations for the purposes of pain control and fluid resuscitation is not required for first-degree burns.

1.3B.Second Degree Burns

A burn that involves the entire epidermis and extends into the dermis is termed a second-degree burn or a partial-thickness burn. If only the superficial layer of the dermis is involved, it is often termed a superficial partial thickness burn, and these wounds are pink or red in color, wet in appearance, and painful. Wounds will blanch when pressure is applied, suggesting that the underlying blood vessels are still intact, and often heal without the need for skin grafting within 3 weeks. Blistering scald burns are a common example of such burns. Deeper involvement of the dermis is classified as a deep partial-thickness burn. These wounds are red or white in color and, unlike partial thickness burns, are dry in appearance (some describe as lobster red). Since most of the dermis is damaged in deep partial-thickness burns, sensation may be diminished and blanching is sluggish or absent. These burns heal by re-epithelization after more than 21 days and can generally benefit from skin grafting.

1.3C. Third Degree Burns

A burn involving the entire depth of the dermis and the epidermal appendages is termed a third-degree burn or a full thickness burn. All layers of the skin are destroyed and the burn extends into the subcutaneous tissue. Burn wounds appear black or white, dry, and non-blanching when pressure is applied. Texturally, these wounds can appear leathery and charred without elasticity. Patients with third-degree burns will not experience pain as the nerve endings in the dermis layer are destroyed. These burns only heal by contraction from the edges over prolonged periods of time, if at all, and require debridement and skin grafting. Deep partial thickness and full-thickness burns will often require the estimation of TBSA for proper treatment.

1.4. Incidence of Complications Related to burn

Burn complications, including joint contracture and heterotopic ossification, often present after the initial burn incident and may take several months to years to develop. The incidence of joint contracture following burn injuries is between 28 to 42 percent, depending on the severity of the burn injury. Heterotopic ossification (HO), defined as bone formation in soft tissue at abnormal anatomical sites, occurs in 0.1 to 3 percent of burn patients but rises to 60 percent in patients with severe burns. In most cases, HO occurs secondary to full-thickness burns or when more than 20 percent of TBSA is compromised.

Table 2. Imaging Techniques for Diagnosis of Burns and Secondary Complications

Imaging Technique	Description	Advantages	Disadvantages
Laser doppler imaging (LDI)	Measures cutaneous blood flow by utilizing the Doppler effect from reflected light on red blood cells	FDA registered device used to assist in assessing burn wounds	Inability to detect deeper wounds with damaged or thrombsed microvasculature
Near infrared spectroscopy (NIRS)	Utilizes infrared technology to monitor tissue oxygenation based on absorbance peaks	Aid in diagnosis of earlier than conventional tools due to high contrast Able to identify	Inability to distinguish between hemoglobin and myoglobin Skin pigmentation may skew

Imaging Technique	Description	Advantages	Disadvantages
		active areas of oxygen extraction Able to assess deeper tissue levels	measurements Expensive
Laser speckle imaging (LSI)	Captures two images of the same wound bed milliseconds apart to detect the velocity and volume of trafficking red blood cells	Faster than LDI technology with all the advantages of LDI	Limited use in clinical practices and research
Spatial frequency domain imaging (SFDI)	Utilizes imaging patterns obtained by NIRS and combines the measurements of peak absorbance of water, oxygenated hemoglobin, and deoxygenated hemoglobin at different depths of the wound	Captures a 3D image of the activity and perfusion of the tissue and different depths	Limited use in clinical practices and research
Computed tomography (CT) scans	Utilizes computer process X-ray images to acquire digital images of specific areas of the body	Provide precise volumes of bone mass in afflicted organs	Able to detect mature bone (generally 6-8 weeks after development of HO) Exposure to radiation
MRI	Utilizes the properties of nuclear magnetic resonance to image the nuclei of atoms inside the body	Detect areas of muscle edema, spasm, necrosis and hemorrhage in soft tissues to correlate the development of HO	Indirect measure and detection of HO Limited sensitivity Incompatible with patients with ferromagnetic implants
Ultrasound	Utilizes oscillating sound pressure waves to visualize muscles, tendons, and bone	Detect the presence of HO	Unable to detect deeper layers of the skin or bone Heavily operator-dependent as retrospective review of images provide limited information
Raman spectroscopy	Relies on inelastic scattering of monochromic light, usually visible, near-infrared, or near ultraviolet lasers	Able to detect early development of HO after 5 days of onset for early diagnosis Able to determine bone maturity	Require optimization of instrumentation to increase sensitivity of detection

2. Diagnostics

2.1. Diagnosing Burn Injuries

The early diagnosis of burns, in both extent and severity, allows earlier decision making on burn excision and grafting, which results in faster healing, reduced hospital length of stay, lower costs, lower infection rates, and less hypertrophic scarring [32]. Superficial burns, which do not require excision, heal well without intervention and are easy to identify by most clinicians. At the other end of the spectrum, full thickness burns, with their characteristic insensate, pale, and leathery appearance, are obvious to identify and make the decision to excise and graft clear. The burns most difficult to identify that would benefit from early surgical intervention are the partial thickness burns. Superficial partial thickness burns will heal on their own, while deep partial thickness burns require excision and grafting. A punch biopsy, with examination under light microscopy, of the burn tissue remains the gold standard to assess burn depth, but its use is limited given its invasiveness and its limited ability to assess the entire wound. Serial clinical assessment is typically used; however, studies have shown that the accuracy of even an experienced burn surgeon is 50 to 75% [33]. Recent advances in Doppler and optics have allowed for the development of novel tools to investigate the severity of the burn prior to visible clinical presentation, including laser Doppler imaging, near infrared spectroscopy, *laser speckle imaging and spatial frequency domain imaging, Raman spectroscopy* (Table 2).

2.1A. Laser Doppler Imaging

Laser Doppler imaging (LDI) is a widely recognized, noninvasive, optical burn assessment tool that is United States Food and Drug Administration registered to assist in the assessment of burn wounds. It measures cutaneous blood flow by utilizing the Doppler effect from reflected light on red blood cells. Minor burn inflammation causes increased localized blood flow from vasodilation. Deeper wounds, however, have damaged, thrombosed microvasculature and thus are more difficult to detect. Its correlation with the need for surgical excision and grafting has been shown to be accurate 95% of the time [34]. With recent advances, the image acquisition process now takes approximately 6 seconds per image while still retaining its accuracy [35]. Despite their accuracy in measuring vascularity, these tools do not always predict tissue viability.

2.1B. Near Infrared Spectroscopy

Near infrared spectroscopy (NIRS) has an advantage over devices using visible light because of its ability to assess deeper tissue levels. Deoxy-hemoglobin and oxy-hemoglobin have different absorption peaks and thus allows the NIRS device to determine areas of tissue with active blood flow as well as areas of oxygen extraction. Tissues damaged due to burn injury present with cellular metabolic changes that may occur sooner than microvascular injury and thrombosis. As a result, NIRS would allow for proper diagnosis earlier than conventional therapies, allowing for appropriate treatment sooner. The subtle edema changes that occur due to capillary leakage in burn injury can also be distinguishing by NIRS to differentiate superficial and deep partial thickness wounds. With some NIRS devices being able to detect denatured collagen, the predictive reliability improves with the each integration of data points collected with NIRS as a whole [36].

2.1C. Laser Speckle Imaging and Spatial Frequency Domain Imaging

Recent development of optical technique allows for the combined capture of two images of the same wound bed milliseconds apart. The resulting image results in speckles corresponding with the speed and volume of blood cells that reflect laser light. This laser speckle imaging (LSI) results in a two-dimensional map of the wound microvasculature in a fraction of the time it takes for LDI. Another novel optical technique recently developed is spatial frequency domain imaging (SFDI). SFDI utilizes the imaging patterns obtained by NIRS and combines the measurements of the peak absorbance of water, oxy-hemoglobin, and deoxy-hemoglobin at different depths of the wound. This captures a three dimensional image of the metabolic activity and perfusion of the tissue. Although promising, additional studies are necessary to advance the technology into clinical practice as the data is currently limited to animal studies [37, 38].

2.2. Diagnosis of Heterotopic Ossification

Historically, good clinical exams as well as plain films were the mainstays of HO diagnosis. After the injury, patients can develop HO symptoms starting as early as 2 weeks or as late as 12 months: erythematous change, range of motion limitation of the affected joint, and painful swelling. Plain films typically do not show positive finding of HO until a month after the presentation of the initial symptoms. With the development of computed tomography (CT) scan technology, a three phase bone scan has become the standard method for early detection as well as serial HO monitoring given its sensitive imaging modality [39]. MRI has also been shown to be sensitive within the first 3 weeks of symptom onset by detecting areas of muscle edema, spasm, necrosis, or hemorrhage [40]. Utilizing MRI as a diagnostic tool, a classic “zone phenomenon” describes the appearance of the centrifugal bone maturation, typical of HO [41]. Another readily available diagnostic tool for HO is ultrasound testing. While ultrasound testing for HO has not gained much popularity, its lack of radiation, point of care testing, and noninvasive nature may be an alterative in certain situations.

2.2A. Raman Spectroscopy

Raman spectroscopy offers a promising novel non-invasive method for HO diagnosis. Transcutaneous Raman spectroscopy relies on inelastic scattering of monochromatic light, usually from a visible, near infrared, or near ultraviolet laser. The laser light interacts with photons, shifting the energy of the photons. This increase in energy is picked up by the spectroscope and visualized as vibrations. Recent animal studies have been shown to detect HO formation 5 days post achilles tenotomy with concurrent burn injury, while micro-CT was unable to detect any evidence of HO until 3 weeks [42]. If validated for the clinical setting, this technology could provide clinicians with early data to help identify those patients who could benefit from prophylaxis and therapy.

Table 3. Summary of the Systems Effected by Burn Injury

System	Effect	Intervention
Neurology	Severe pain at the primary injury site	Fentanyl to limit pain, with barbituates as second line due to possible delirium Can use methadone to decrease narcotic demands
Ophthalmology/ HEENT	Increase in intraocular pressure or corneal abrasion with facial burns	Check intraocular pressure, eye lubrication
Cardiovascular	*First 24 hours:* Decrease CO, increase SVR *Second 24 hours:* Increase CO, decrease SVR General increase in vessel permeability	Cardiovascular support with fluids first and then vasoconstrictors, if necessary Levophed is often first line, while vasopressin can be added to decrease levophed doses
Respiratory	Bronchoconstriction secondary to histamine, serotonin and thromboxane A2 release	Early bronchoscopy and intubation if warrented Use best positive end-expiratory pressure (PEEP) practice to avoid high pressures
Renal	Hypoperfusion, vasoconstriction, and myoglobinuria	Support hemodynamics with fluids Increase fluid rate if myoglobinuria and avoid lasix
Gastrointestinal	Decrease absorption of fatty acids, glucose uptake amino acid Increase in gut permeability and caloric demand	Start enteral feeding with post pyloric feeding tube within 18 hours
Musculoskeletal	Muscle wasting, Increase body temperature, joint contractures, and heterotopic ossification	Early physical therapy involvement
Endocrine	Insulin resistance	Close glucose monitoring and keep <180
Hematology	Clotting factor deficiency in large burns, including vitamin K, fibrinogen	Replace factors, if clinical signs of bleeding are present
Immunology	Decrease IgG, decreased neutrophil, macrophages, B lymphocyte proliferation, helper T cells, leukocyte function and lymph activation Increase in TNF alpha, IL-7, rate of phagocytosis complement activation, and susceptibility to infection.	Remove dead tissue early to eliminate bioburden. Do not give empiric antibiotics. If clinical signs of infection, culture and treat accordingly.

3. Management

While the care of a patient suffering from burn related injuries is often divided into time frames during which clinicians should consider certain management strategies and interventions designed to prevent burn-related sequelae, the implementation of aggressive, prompt, and focused forms of multidisciplinary care cannot be compromised and should occur in a uniform fashion from start to finish (Table 3). The importance of such care is the reason burn related healthcare expenditures are as high as four billion dollars per year in the United States. Although efforts focused on the prevention of thermal injuries have the potential to exert the most change over time, the management of both acute and chronic burn injuries, if conducted properly, also has the ability to transform the lives of patients, families, and caregivers to optimize overall quality of life.

3.1. Initial Assessment

The initial care of a burn patient can be likened to that of any trauma patient. Over time, guidelines such as Advanced Trauma Life Support and Advanced Burn Life Support have standardized the care of trauma patients and have improved overall patient outcomes (Figure 2). Thus, given the extent of injuries that a burn patient may present with, it is important to follow a standard algorithm. A complete history and physical should be performed with specific focus placed on the cause and timing of the injury, concomitant injuries, and treatments received prior to arrival to the hospital. The ultimate goal is to stabilize the patient and ensure a proper assessment of the burn so that further care can be transitioned to a burn center, if necessary (Table 4).

Table 4. Burn Injuries Requiring Referring to Certified Burn Centers

According to the American Burn Association, burn injuries that should be referred to a burn center include:
1. Burn degree Partial thickness burns > 10% of TBSA Third degree burns 2. Type of burn Electrical burns Chemical burns 3. Location of burn Injuries involving the face, hands, feet, genitalia, perineum, or other major joints 4. Compounding factors Burn injuries in patients with preexisting conditions Burn injuries involving inhalation injury Burn injuries in patients with concomitant trauma (e.g., fractures) Burn injuries in patients requiring special social, emotional, or rehabilitative needs Burn injuries in children at hospitals without qualified personnel or equipment to care for children

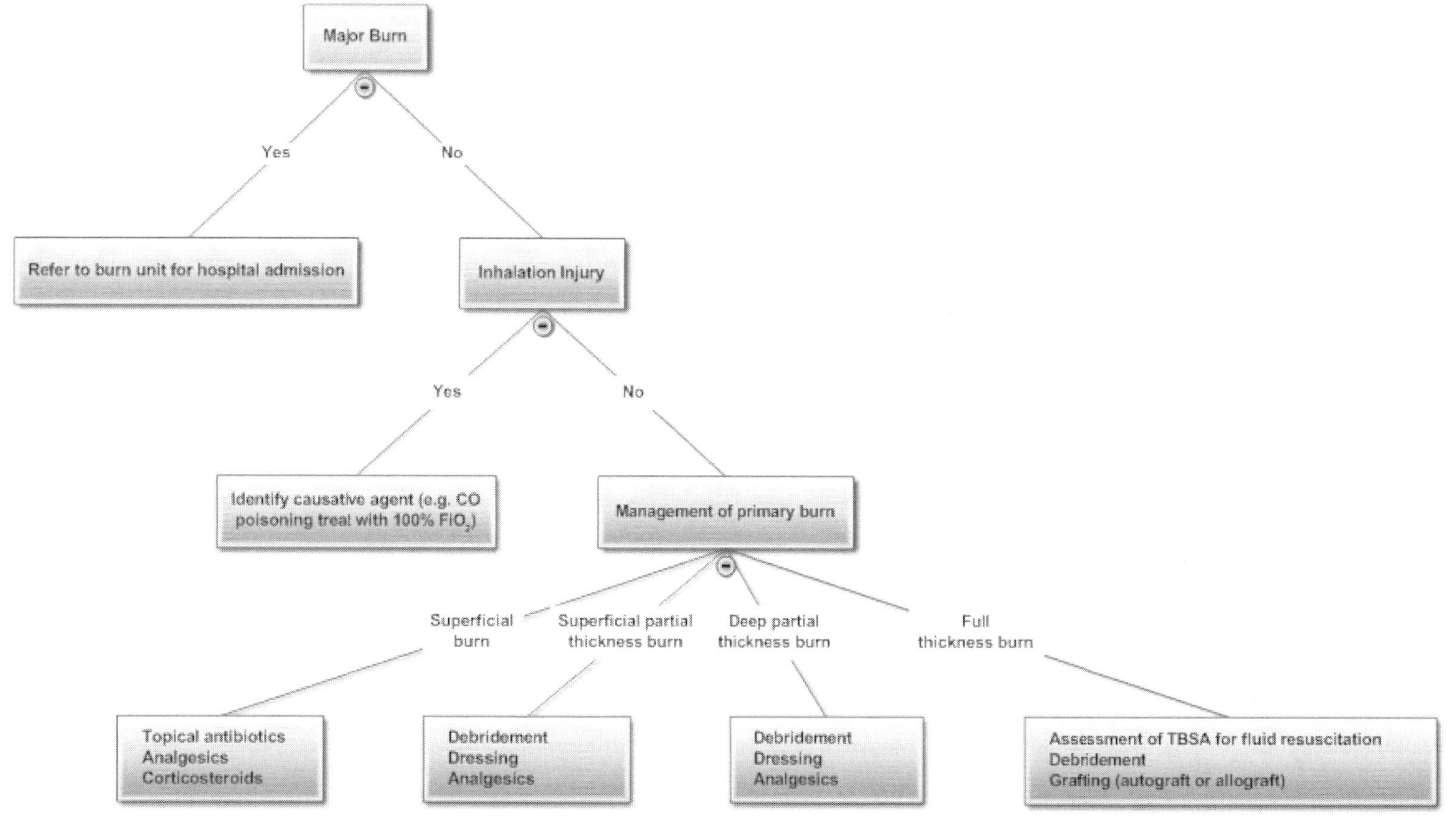

Figure 2. Algorithm for acute management of burn patients.

3.1A. Airway Assessment

Assessment should begin with evaluation of the airway, breathing, and circulation. Inhalation injuries can occur in approximately 10% of all burn patients, but are notably present in 70% of those who eventually die of their burn [43]. Thus, it is important to specifically note such findings as soon as the patient presents with nasal passage or posterior pharynx blockage, facial burns, changes in voice quality, shortness of breath, and carbonaceous sputum in the nasal or oral passages. If there is any concern that the airway is compromised, a nasopharyngeal scope or bronchoscope can be used to directly visualize the airway. Some clinicians consider the use of these tools to be mandatory in any patient who presents with facial burns, regardless of the extent of the burn itself. Although patients may not present with obvious signs of airway compromise by manifesting the symptoms as stated above, airway edema can progress very quickly causing an intubation that would have been easily performed on initial presentation to become very difficult due to progressive swelling and obliteration of anatomic landmarks. Endotracheal intubation may be required for several days until edema subsides as the mucosal slough and secretions accumulate, airway obstruction and atelectasis progresses. In severe cases, early institution of mechanical ventilation may be required to stabilize the patients.

In some instances, identifying the causative agent as well as the extent of the injury may aid in the recovery process. In particular, the possibility of carbon monoxide (CO) poisoning must also be assessed. Given the increased affinity of CO for hemoglobin molecules, oxygen becomes displaced which creates a hypoxic environment in the body. Formal diagnosis of CO poisoning is based on CO levels in the blood. Symptoms of CO poisoning typically begin with headaches at levels around 10%, while CO in the blood becomes toxic at around 50-70%. While the half-life of CO is normally 4 hours at room air, its half-life is shorten with treatment. Oftentimes, carbon monoxide poisoning is treated empirically especially in those patients presenting with agitation, reddish appearance of mucous membranes, and altered consciousness given that deliver 100% oxygen (FiO2 100%), as this therapy reduces the half-life of CO to 30-90 minutes. In patients with toxic levels of CO in the blood, more extreme measures are necessary and include the use of hyperbaric oxygen at 2.5 atm with 100% oxygen. Hyperberic oxygen will reduce the half-life of CO to 15-23 minutes. Therefore, prompt and aggressive evaluation and maintenance of the airway is the most important initial step in management of a burn patient.

3.1B. Fluid Resuscitation

After initial stabilization of the patient has been performed, the next step is to determine the extent of the burn injury for fluid resuscitation. Patients with severe burns often require significant fluid resuscitation due to both sensible fluid loss allowed by the lack of skin barriers and steady intravascular fluid loss. Extensive burns often result in the loss of external skin barriers, which allows for the physical loss of fluids. In major burn injuries, the release of inflammatory mediators, such as histamine, prostaglandins, and nitric oxide, increase capillary permeability and leads to localized burn wound edema. This reaction generally occurs within minutes to hours following the initial insult and is followed by the production of highly reactive oxygen species (ROS) during reperfusion of ischemia tissue. These ROS are toxic cell metabolites that include free radicals and cause local cellular membrane dysfunction. Cellular membrane dysfunction leads to the disruption of sodium-ATPase activity, presumably causing an intracellular sodium shift, which contributes to the hypovolemia and cellular edema. This compounded by with the release of inflammatory and vasoactive mediators, which causes local vasoconstruction, systemic vasodilation, and increased transcapillary permability, exacerbates the intravascular hypovolemia. As such, the sensible loss of fluid and steady intravascular fluid loss requires fluid resuscitation to prevent end-organ hypoperfusion and ischemia. Careful assessment of the burn will help determine the extent of the fluid resuscitation.

For superficial burns, treatment of the burn wound oftentimes requires topical antimicrobial agents to limit infection and corticosteroids to minimize inflammation, but does not require fluid resuscitation [44]. Microorganisms proliferate rapidly in burn wounds, particularly in patients with impaired immune function due to the burn. Topical antimicrobial agents delay the interval between injury and colonization and maintain low levels of wound flora. Oral antibiotics, however, should not be given unless signs of infection exist. The specific antibiotics and antiseptics for topical therapy in minor burns will be discussed in this chapter.

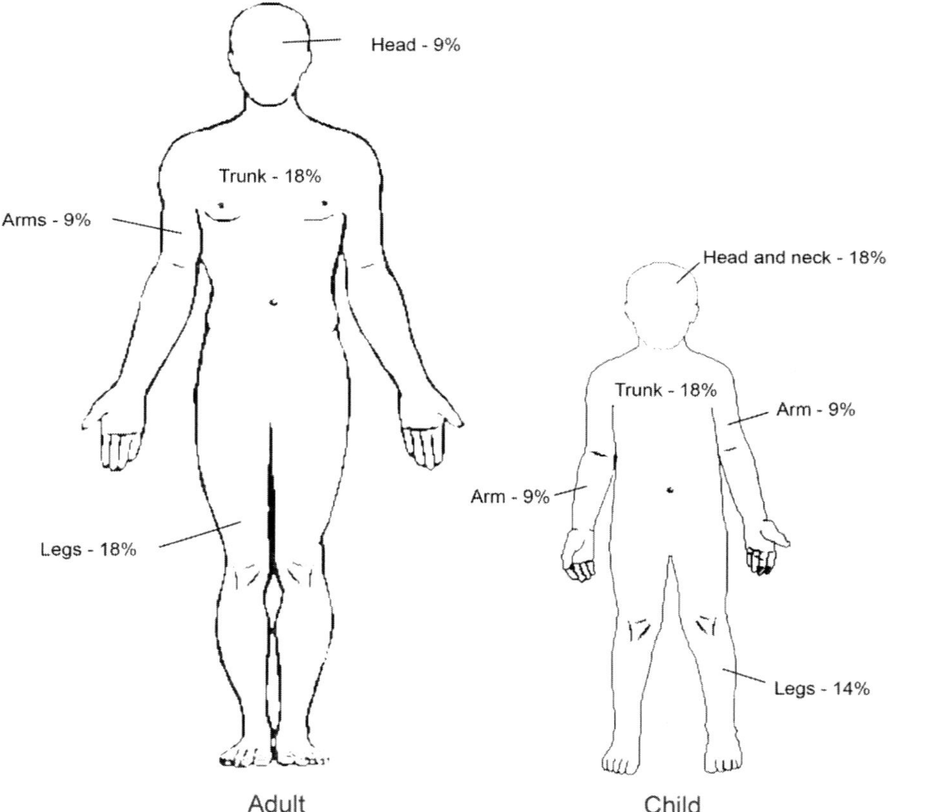

Figure 3. Rule of Nine for Total Body Surface Area.

For full-thickness burns and some deep partial-thickness burns, identifying the extent of the burn injury is crucial. TBSA is used to design fluid administration regimens and defines overall prognosis of patients. Criteria for transfer to a burn center are also based on this concept [45]. Only partial and full thickness burns are totaled to calculate TBSA. If small areas in various distributions are affected, it may be easier to use the patient as a ruler with one palm size representing 1% TBSA. Most emergency departments and burn units also have body surface charts available for use, but also follow the rule of 9s, where the body is partitioned into areas and each region constitutes 9% of the TBSA (Figure 3). Regions on the adult that constitutes 9% of the TBSA include the head and arms, while the legs, anterior trunk, and posterior trunk account for 18% of TBSA each. In children, the arms each account for 9% of the TBSA, while the legs account for 14%. The head and neck region, the anterior trunk, and the posterior trunk each account for 18% in children. Careful estimation of TBSA is essential for proper early management of burn patients, as patients who have burns of more than 20% TBSA commonly require intravenous fluid resuscitation.

The Parkland Formula is most commonly used to calculate fluid requirements within the first 24 hours [46]. It is extremely important to note that the original timing of the injury is what is used in the calculation, not the time of initial presentation.

Parkland Formula: First 24 hour requirement = 4cc X %TBSA X weight (kg)

Half of this volume is administered in the first 8 hours after the injury and the second half is administered over the next 16 hours. For example, if a 70-kg patient with 10% TBSA burns sustained at 10 a.m. presents at 12 p.m., the fluid to be administered in the first 8 hours is calculated using the following formula: [(4cc x 10% x 70kg)/2]/6. Lactated ringers is recommended to avoid complications associated with metabolic acidosis with normal saline or abnormal fluid shifts with colloid fluids [46]. Then, D5/LR is commonly used for maintenance fluids. Although such formulas exist, it is important to note that proper resuscitation is based on overall fluid status as represented by urine output, with the goal of 0.5 mL/kg/hr in adults and 1 mL/kg/hr in children, and fluids should be adjusted accordingly. Given the immobility associated with severe burn injuries and the abnormal fluid shifts that occur, aggressive hydration also accounts for potential rhabdomyolysis, leading to acute kidney injury that can occur in this setting. Pulmonary status is also an indicator of fluid status but in more of a delayed fashion. Complications such as pulmonary edema result from fluid overload and necessitate daily evaluation of oxygen requirements and ventilator settings.

Once the Parkland Formula is begun, the patient's vital signs and urine output should be closely monitored and laboratory studies should be drawn frequently. Fluids should be increased or decreased based on the response of the patient. Though the urine output is considered a "gold standard," it often lags behind and thus it may be necessary to increase fluids to compensate for increased urine output. In addition, close monitoring of the patient's laboratories are necessary to determine the trend in organ perfusion. Laboratory values that might help assess organ perfusion include lactate, base deficit, central venous O2, and/or pH. Although any one of these values alone does not provide a sensitive marker of the patient status, trending these values during resuscitation can help direct if the current fluid rate is causing a positive trend. If the organs are perfused, decreases in lactate and base deficit as well as increases in central venous O_2 and normalization of pH should be observed.

In large burns that involve the face, an ophthalmologic consultation should be obtained. As the patient becomes edematous from the resuscitation, it is imperative that the globe is kept moisturized with a lubricant. Ophthalmologic consultants can help assess globe pressure, injury to the cornea and glaucoma, which often occur in electrical injury.

Thus, while burn injuries may initially appear to be a focal area of trauma, the assessment of all systematic manifestations is paramount and must be stabilized before the burn itself is addressed.

3.2. Wound Care Assessment and Treatment

As previously discussed, the depth, location, size, and duration of the burn injury are the most important factors to consider in the assessment of a burn. Burns can present for reconstruction in the acute or chronic phase, and reconstructive options are very different depending upon when a patient presents.

Acute burn injuries require prompt intervention and serial examinations. On initial evaluation, it is important to rule out and prevent the development of circumferential burns that can lead to tissue ischemia and subsequent necrosis by limiting perfusion to the distal tissues [43]. The overarching concept, however, in acute burn reconstruction is early debridement and grafting. All blisters and nonviable tissue must be debrided upon presentation. After the initial debridement, dressing changes are initiated while the patient is stabilized from a systemic standpoint.

There are a variety of options for dressing materials, and the appearance of the burn is mainly what dictates this choice (Table 5) [46]. Although the indications for systemic antibiotic therapy have not been clearly defined within the literature, use of antimicrobial dressings is recommended. Silvadene is a silver-containing cream that has broad-spectrum coverage against both gram negative and positive bacteria. Although its use is contraindicated in patients with sulfa allergies and over wounds near the eyes, silvadene is commonly used over both partial and full thickness injuries [47]. Laboratory values including complete blood counts must be followed while patients are using this medication in the acute phase due to possible leukopenia, which is a known side effect of this medication. If leukopenia develops, silvadene should be stopped, however, patients rarely develop any serious complications. Sulfamylon is an analogous agent that is used over cartilaginous areas such as the nose or ear due to increased penetration of this dressing over these areas as compared to other dressing types. Since topical sulfamylon cream can be used without dressings, it can be used for open burn wound therapy and regular examination of the burn wound surface. However, both the cream and a 5% solution of sulfamylon are equally effective [48]. Sulfamylon has better penetration but may also cause increased pain. Patients should be monitored for complications such as hyperchloremic metabolic acidosis that can occur with utilization of this dressing due to its mechanism of action.

Other dressings include 0.5-1.0% silver nitrate and applied 3-4 times a day. However, the use of silver nitrate in burn patients remains slightly controversial as nitrates are toxic to tissues and wounds healing may be delayed by its use. The nitrates impair re-epithelization and this effect is partially offset the benefits of silver in these compounds [49]. Furthermore, it can cause leaching of cations causing hyponatremia. Additionally, it stains the skin as well as the floor and any equipment it comes in contact with.

Bacitracin and xeroform are additional examples of antimicrobial type dressing regimens. While both can be used anywhere on the body, bacitracin is commonly used for facial burns. Xeroform is often used at the donor site following the isolation of partial thickness skin for grafting. Regardless of the type of dressing used, wounds should be examined daily given the predisposition of this wound niche to become infected.

Table 5. Dressings for Burn Wounds

Type of Dressing	Mechanism of Action	Uses	Side Effects
Silvadene	Silver-containing cream with broad-spectrum coverage against both Gram-positive and Gram-negative bacteria, especially *Pseudomonas*	Used for both partial thickness and full thickness injuries Able to penetrate into various tissue types	Contrainducated in patients with sulfa allergies and over wounds near the eye Leukopenia may develop while patients are using this medication during the acute phase
Sulfamylon	Topical antimicrobial against many Gram-positive and Gram-negative organisms that reduces the bacterial flora in the avascular tissue of burn patients, specifically *clostridium*	Used for partial thickness and full thickness injuries, particularly in cartilaginous areas (e.g., nose, ear) due to increased penetration Good for treatment and prophylaxis	Contraindicated in patients with sulfa allergies or renal impairment Adverse reactions include pain, burning, rash, puritis, tachypena, hyperventilation, and metabolic acidosis
Silver nitrate	Antiseptic properties of silver limit expansion of Gram-positive and Gram-negative flora within the burn site	Useful for partial thickness and full thickness burns Excellent prophylaxis	Hyponatremia caused by the leaching of cations Transient discoloration of the skin
Bacitracin	Topical antimicrobial that disrupts the cell wall and peptidoglycan synthesis of Gram-positive bacteria	Used for facial burns (an alterative to Silvadene for burn patients with a sulfa allergy)	No major side effects
Xeroform	Fine mesh gauze impregnated with 3% bismuth tribromophenate in a petrolatum blend	Used for partial and full thickness burns Maintains a moist wound environment Deodorizes wound site	Eye and nasal passage irritation and stomatitis
Acticoat	Silver nanoparticle impregnated sheets that have antimicrobial properties	Used for partial thickness burns that may be changed every 3-5 days	Contraindicated in patients with sulfa allergies Transient discoloration of the skin Non-adhesive and dislocated from wound

For patients who are at lower risk of infection based on the appearance of wounds, dressings may be changed with less frequency to achieve a balance between pain control and the need for wound coverage. Acticoat is one such option that is mainly used in partial thickness injuries. This dressing consists of silver-impregnated sheets that have antimicrobial properties and can be changed less frequently, reducing pain and cutting costs [48]. The nanocrystalline particles in Acticoat are able to reduce wound infection and promote wound healing compared to older silver products, including silver nitrate [49]. When using Acticoat, it is important to remember to activate it with water and not normal saline as the sodium can leech out the silver.

While dressing changes are sometimes used to nourish and optimize a wound before and after operative interventions, dressings also have the potential to completely heal a wound without the need for surgical intervention depending on the overall appearance of the burn and patient as a whole. Thus, a proper wound care team must not only include a critical care physician and surgeon, but it must also include a specialized wound care nurse to appropriately address this central modality of care for any burn patient.

3.3. Operative Interventions

After initial stabilization, surgical intervention should occur as soon as possible as there are no benefits to delaying surgery [50, 51]. Early excision of devitalized tissue appears to reduce the local and system effects of mediators released from burned tissue, thus reducing the progressive pathophysiologic derangements. Tangential excision removes necrotic tissue while preserving as much of the underlying viable tissue as possible. Tissue is debrided until healthy, bleeding tissue is reached. Hemodynamic stability and correction of hematologic and metabolic derangements is helpful for such cases given that large amounts of blood may be lost during debridement. In addition to achieving a healthy and well-vascularized wound bed after debridement, it is also essential to classify and examine the wounds further during this process. At this time, the distinction between superficial and deep partial thickness burns must be made. While superficial partial thickness injuries can heal on their own with dressing changes and without grafting, deeper burns must be treated with skin grafting.

Given the association between early debridement and grafting with improved functional and scar related outcomes, the earlier this distinction is made the faster a treatment plan can be formulated. For large burns, debridement must occur within 2 to 4 days of the initial injury. Blisters and necrotic tissue may be debrided at the bedside, if the area to be treated is small, but may also need to be taken to the operating room for definitive visualization and management. Alternatively, the burn can be completely excised within the first several days after injury, and a temporary skin substitute can be used to close the wound remaining after available autologous skin has been harvested and grafted.

Using autograft, it is possible to perform a single-stage reconstruction that transforms into a vascularized environment at the site of the previous wound bed within 1-2 weeks [52]. Disadvantages, however, stem from the limited availability of tissue as well as the creation of an additional wound that must also heal over time. In contrast, allograft is available in unlimited supplies [52]. Although allograft provides temporary coverage to the traumatized wound bed, its use is limited by cost and the possible risk of disease transmission as allografts are obtained from cadavers. Nevertheless, allografts will eventually be rejected as the body recognizes the newly engrafted skin as foreign material after 10-13 days. The process is initiated by the placement of the allografts, which is associated with an inflammatory process, leading to the activation of the innate immune response. Donor dendritic cells migrate from the graft to the recipient's secondary lymphoid organs where they present donor antigens and elicit an adaptive immune response. This response results in activated effector T cells from the donor leaving the secondary lymphoid organs and infiltrating the graft where they mediate the rejection of the allograft [53].

Since allografts will ultimately result in rejection, these regions covered by allografts will need to be replaced with autograft. Oftentimes, how well the autograft takes is a sign of how well your initial debridement was. If all of the autograft does not take when placed back into the patient, this is often a sign of inadequate debridement. Additionally, if insufficient autograft exists even after temporary allograft, the surgeon should consider cultured epidermal autografts. Cultured epidermal autografts utilizes the ability to grow keratinocytes in vitro to generate cohesive sheets of stratified epithelium, which maintains the characteristics of authentic epidermis developed by Rheinwald and Green in 1975 [54]. A 3-4 cm^2 sample is taken usually from the axilla or pubic area at the same time as initial debridement, and epidermal cells are isolated form the small skin biopsy and plated onto a layer of feeder cells that act as a supporting "feeder layer" [55]. The feeder layer supports optimal clonal expansion of proliferative epithelial cells and promotes keratinocyte growth. Under optimal growth conditions, kertainocytes initiate growing colonies and after 3-4 weeks, and the CEA sheets are 8-10 cells thick [56, 57]. These constructs require advanced planning as it takes at least 2 weeks to develop. Additionally, risks and benefits should be discussed with the family and patient, as there is a high percentage of graft loss. Furthermore, case reports of squamous cell cancer developing form grafts sites do exist.

After the decision regarding the use of allograft versus autograft has been made, attention is turned to the size and thickness of the graft. Commonly, split thickness skin grafts composed of the epidermis and a thin layer of dermis are utilized to minimize donor site morbidity and optimize graft takes, since thin grafts are more likely to succeed than thick grafts. There are certain areas, however, where split thickness grafts should not be used since they cause greater secondary contracture and less color match over time as compared to full thickness grafts. Areas of function, such as the hands and feet, lose a remarkable amount of utility if afflicted by scar contracture and should not be treated with split thickness grafts, if enough tissue is available to perform a full thickness graft [58]. If split thickness is used on the feet and hands, the grafts should be harvested on the thick side and meshing should be avoided if possible. Similarly, aesthetically important areas, such as the face, are also more amenable to full thickness skin grafting to optimize color match and minimize contracture over such areas [59]. Full thickness grafts, nonetheless, are limited by increased donor site morbidity due to the need to obtain both the epidermis and dermis from a region and also require closing the tissues primarily to avoid additional wounds. There is also more difficulty with successful and complete healing of the graft given that a more robust blood supply within the wound bed is necessary to optimize take of this thicker piece of tissue. Both full and split thickness grafts can be meshed to increase the surface area that may be covered. Commonly performed in a 1:1.5 ratio, meshing also allows for fluid egress, which minimizes the risk of fluid accumulation beneath the graft, a common cause of skin graft failure. Meshing should not be performed, however, over cosmetically sensitive areas given that the meshed pattern will be quite apparent even after complete healing has been achieved. Both grafts should be bolstered once placed to minimize shear, improve contact and allow for imbibition and inosculation. The wound bed must be free of infection, defined as less than 10^5 bacteria on quantitative analysis prior to grafting, as infection is a common cause of graft failure. More specifically, wounds must be debrided properly prior to grafting to minimize this risk.

3.4. Alternatives

Integra is a newer alternative for temporary coverage of a wound after debridement. Composed of bovine collagen and silicone film, this construct is designed to mimic the epidermis and dermis of the missing tissue [45, 54]. Its structure allows for the growth of healthy granulation tissue into a wound bed to optimize the wound niche to promote greater and healthier take of the skin graft that will eventually be placed over the site of injury. This is especially important over areas of function, such as the hand, which has the potential for significant debilitation if scar or graft contracture occurs over the traumatized site. Integra is also important for areas that do not have enough viable or vascularized tissue to support a skin graft. Integra, however, often fails in burn patients due to infection and requires constant soaks with silver nitrate or sulfamylon. Additionally, clinicians should examine the Integra frequently and remove any areas of silicone under which there is concern for infection.

4. Impact

4.1. Hypertrophic Scarring

Thermal burn injures can cause tremendous morbidity, leaving the patient with not only cosmetic but also functional impairments. Hypertrophic scarring is a major complication after burn injury with a prevalence of 32 to 72%. Several risk factors have been identified that contribute to its development including the localization of the burn injury, burn depth, time to heal and skin color [62, 63]. While the precise mechanism by which hypertrophic scarring occurs by remain unclear, strong and persistent expression of TGFβ and its receptors have been associated with post-burn hypertrophic scarring. Furthermore, a critical step in the healing process that is altered is the transition from granulation tissue into normal scarring. During this remodeling process, wound epithelization and scar collagen is formed but accompany gradual decrease in cellularity due to apoptosis. However, early immature hypertrophic scars caused by burns are hypercellular and during the process of remodeling and maturing, fibroblast density do not resemble that of normal healing [64]. More specifically, apoptosis of myofibroblast occur 12 days after injury in normal wound healing, but in hypertrophic scar tissue, the maximum apoptosis occurs much later at 19-30 months [65]. These events result in a significantly higher percentage of myofibroblast and the hypertrophy of the scar tissue following severe burn injuries.

Current treatment strategies for hypertrophic scars include surgical manipulation, intralesional corticosteroid injections, cryotherapy, and laser therapy. Surgical manipulation to remove the excess skin is the traditional treatment for hypertrophic scar; however, newer approaches have shown improved outcomes. A new concept of "scar rejuvenation" has emerged with the key idea being to improve the environment of the scar without actually excision the scar. One of the key pathologic factors contributing to hypertrophic scar formation is tension. The most important step in rejuvenating the scar is releasing the tension. Rather than excising, the scar, this involves just releasing the area of greatest tension. Despite not removing any tissue, a large defect is often created once the tension is released. Adding new tissue, such as a full thickness skin grafts or a thick split thickness skin graft, can then treat this defect. Additional ways to relieve tension involves the use of tissue rearrangements, such as a Z-plasty. A Z-plasty lengthens the scar at the expense of width alleviating tension along the central access of the hypertrophic scar. In general Z-plasty rearrangements are made with 60 degree angles to maximize tissue gain, without causing excess tension on the donor site closure. Alternative V-Y advancements are useful if there is healthy tissue surrounding the scar and can be advanced into the area of the contracture.

Furthermore, recent studies investigating the role of fat grafting into scars have shown promise to further improve function and appearance [67]. Patients who have undergone fat transfer reported satisfactory results 6 months after the procedure, indicating considerable improvement in the features of the skin, skin texture, and thickness. Histological examination demonstrated new collagen deposition, neovascularization, and dermal hyperplasia in regions treated with fat grafting, which mimicked surrounding undamaged skin.

Additionally, intralesional corticosteroid suppress the inflammatory process in wounds, diminish collagen synthesis, and enhance collagen degradation [68]. Cryotherapy has been proven efficacious in the management of small scar; however, its use has also shown to increase vascular damage, tissue necrosis, and ultimately more severe hypertrophic scars [69]. Therefore the use of cryotherapy is not advised in most situations. Lastly, since the introduction of laser treatment in the mid-1980s, the therapeutic use of additional lasers with different wavelengths has been employed. The most encouraging results have been obtained with the 585 nm wavelength pulsed dye laser (PDL), which has been recognized as an excellent therapeutic option for the treatment of younger hypertrophic scars [70]. PDL induces the dissociation of disulfide bonds in collagen fibers and lead to collagen fiber realignment, decreased fibroblast proliferation, and neocollagenesis. However, repeated treatments are necessary for the desired outcome, generally between 2-6 treatments.

Recently, exciting research has demonstrated the benefits of fractional photothermolysis in the treatment of hypertrophic scarring. Though the exact mechanism is unknown, this concept uses a CO_2 laser, which is an ablative laser that targets water in the underlying tissues (10,600 nm). The laser creates columns of tissue destruction, which stimulates collagen production in adjacent uninjured columns of tissue. The adjacent uninjured tissue allows for more rapid tissue regeneration from their follicles and sweat glands. Overall, this creates a more smooth appearance and allows meshed grafts to appear less obvious. Patients have described less tightness as well as decreased pruritis [71].

4.2. Psychological Challenges

Burn victims oftentimes experience stigmatization due to disfiguring scars, leading to psychological problems of low self-esteem and depression [70]. These can significantly impact social comfort and integration in both children and adults. Early intervention has the potential to mitigate the severity of burn injury related sequelae such as depression, post-traumatic stress disorder, anxiety, and chronic pain related issues. Low body image, depression, and social discomfort have been correlated with scar severity [71]. Furthermore, emotional distress often depends on scar location and visibility, such that patients with face, head, and visible burns often report low body image and depression. For those patients who indicate that physical appearance is particularly important to them, scar severity is highly related to low body image [72]. For those who did not place high value on their physical appearance, scar severity is unrelated to body image. Burn injury victims often experience a wide range of emotions from persistent post-traumatic stress to extreme fear, anxiety, and depression. While their external wounds may heal and they may return to their daily activities, the psychological distress may last many more months to years. In order to minimize the emotional distress and improve psychological well-being, it is important to receive personal counseling and/or become a member of a burn injury survivors group at any stage in the healing process. The latter groups offer a sense of camaraderie and allow burn injury victims to talk about their emotional issues in a supportive, understanding environment. By sharing their emotional distress and discussing tips to manage pain daily, burn injury victims can help each other live fuller, more satisfying lives.

4.3. Muscle Catabolism and Wasting

Burn injury involving large areas of the human body is associated with significant pathophysiologic sequelae, which can persist even up to several years after the acute injury. Several groups observed significant changes in essential metabolic processes, which seem to shift the physiologic homeostasis to a catabolic state, specifically resulting in the loss of lean body mass. The total body surface area affected by the burn injury plays an important role, since reestablishing a functional skin barrier initially takes priority and requires a protein substrate, which is provided by skeletal muscle [73].

Muscle catabolism after burn injury is mediated by several factors, including increased energy requirement [74] and heightened inflammatory state involving the systemic release of stress hormones, catecholamines and glucocorticoids, which mediate the underlying metabolic derangements. Other factors include prolonged immobilization and the loss of a functional skin barrier, which leads to a disturbed thermoregulation requiring increased energy expenditure to maintain body temperature. The consequences can have devastating effects on the convalescence of the adult and especially the pediatric burn patients, where an increased catabolic state can lead to delayed linear growth for up to 2 years after the injury [75]. The physiologic response of skeletal muscle to anabolic stimuli is altered in pediatric patients with amino acid infusion therapy failing to stimulate a protein net deposition in skeletal muscle even after 6 to 12 months post injury, most likely due to excessive protein breakdown [76, 77].

Studies investigating the effect of burn injury on physiologic changes in skeletal muscle have uncovered a critical role for mitochondrial function showing that processes involving carbohydrate metabolism, lipid metabolism and oxidative phosphorylation are significantly altered [78]. Righi et al. elegantly demonstrated that treatment with a mitochondria targeted antioxidant in a murine burn model significantly increases mitochondrial ATP secretion and ameliorates oxidative stress, suggesting that ROS play a significant role in burn pathogenesis [79]. Improvements in skeletal muscle mitochondrial function have also been attributed to the effect of fenofibrate, a PPARa agonist used to treat impaired glucose metabolism after burn injuries to elevated stress hormone secretion. In pediatric burn patients, fenofibrate treatment improved glucose levels and insulin sensitivity [80]. Other therapeutic approaches have shown significant benefit in clinical trials, including the blockage of beta adrenergic receptors to attenuated the catecholamine effect and improved net muscle protein balance [81]. Furthermore, anabolic steroids, such as Oxandrolene, and physical exercise have been shown to increased lean body mass in children who suffered from >40% TBSA burn injury [82].

When the body is in a prolonged catabolic state due to the increase in caloric requirements, the patients must consume at least 2.5-3 g/kg/day of protein [52]. Nutritional shakes and high calorie foods are a necessity to optimize the conditions for wound healing. It is important to start feeds as soon as possible using enteric means if possible. Nasogastric and Dobhoff tubes should be inserted early in the care of burn patients if they are unable to eat. Dieticians are crucial members of the burn care team in creating individualized feeding plans and ensuring that nutrition is at the forefront of daily care. Albumin and prealbumin levels can be trended over time to ensure that adequate nourishment is achieved.

Patients should also be referred to a therapeutic exercise program should be implemented to maintain normal range of motion, strength and endurance. In order to counteract the catabolic effects of burn injuries, a program of active and active-assisted exercise is necessary. Depending the severity of the burn and the patient's willingness to tolerate the associated pain with exercise, passive range of motion exercises should be prescribed. In the event that full range of motion is not achievable, a program of stretching can be prescribed in its place. Furthermore, anesthesia can be used to assist these exercises, but should only be used in pediatric cases of patients who cannot tolerate the pain.

Range of motion exercises can also minimize skin contractures, as skin is a tissue that requires sustained mechanical stretch to facilitate lengthening of the underlying collagen and extracellular matrix compartments. Initial skin exercises should attempt to elongate the skin with repetitive low loads with differences in length. Following this initial precondition, a prolonged stretch is applied to maximize the skin laxity. Blanching is a clinical sign that capillary blood flow is impeded and is a good sign that the tissue has reached is maximum yield point. Strength exercise should follow as soon as the patient can tolerate it. Strength programs best suited for burn patients should include progressive resistive exercises. Fatigue and loss of endurance are major issues as a patient recovers. It is important to include endurance training and monitor cardiopulmonary response. Concurrently, patients should be encouraged to walk as ambulating patients have fewer lower extremity contractures, endurance problems, and venous thrombosis.

4.4. Heterotopic Ossification

Heterotopic ossification (HO) is the pathologic formation of bone in regions of soft tissue including muscle, joint spaces and often encasing major nerves. This complication of burn injury causes significant pain, joint restriction and contractures [82]. It may affect all areas of the body but is most frequently encountered in the elbow joint [83, 84]. While the etiology of HO remains elusive, common risk factors that have been identified include prolonged immobilization [85] and a delay in time to wound closure [86].

Early detection and diagnosis of heterotopic bone formation is critical in the clinical management of this complication, which oftentimes involves surgical resection. However, the success rates of surgical intervention are not well established and are oftentimes associated with a high recurrence rate. Perioperative radiotherapy has been suggested as an adjunct to surgical resection and has been shown to reduce the recurrence rate to some extent [87]. While the pathophysiologic processes underlying the development of heterotopic bone formation are poorly understood, several studies have implicated increased inflammatory signaling and the involvement of progenitor cells as crucial contributing elements, as discussed in the following section.

Pharmacological interventions have been shown to have some efficacy in limiting the severity of HO. Bisphosphonates and NSAIDs have been used for prophylaxis and treatment of HO with some success [88, 89]. However, there is no consensus on which drug should be prescribed and when treatment should begin. It has been proposed that bisphosphonates should be prescribed as soon as elevated alkaline phosphatase is noted or imaging studies establish the presence of HO. On the other hand, others have shown that NSAIDS limit the severity of HO when delivered as a preventative therapy. Additional clinical studies will need to be conducted in order to confirm whether pharmacological intervention can limit the amount of HO that develops in burn patients. It should be noted that early diagnosis of HO ensures proper and possible treatment as it is often diagnosed beyond the time at which it can be treated.

5. Clinical, Basic Science, and Translational Science Research

5.1. Clinical Research

Clinical research determines the safety and efficacy of medications, devices, diagnostic tools, and treatment regimens and has provided new insights to effectively care for burn patients. Within the last decade, critical care, wound care treatment, and burn reconstruction research has advanced in both diagnosis and identification of effective therapies to improve the overall recovery process for burn victims.

Critical care research has focused on the delivery of adequate care during the initial phase following the traumatic burn injury. Immediately following the trauma, burn patients experience severe shock due to concomitant inflammation leading to severe edema. While rigorous fluid resuscitation has shown to increase overall survival for patients with high TBSA involvement, novel resuscitation methods have recently been investigated. In a prospective randomized study, clinicians investigated the use of colloids within the first 24 hours of resuscitation [90]. Patients with a TBSA burn injury greater than 15% were either provided with crystalloid resuscitation or a mixture of crystalloid and hydroxyethyl starch. Patients given colloids required less fluids, experienced less edema, and had a lower C-reactive protein indicative of less inflammation. Additional studies have investigated the use of therapeutic plasma exchange for refractory burn resuscitation and discovered that patients had reduced lactate levels, increased mean arterial pressure, and improved urine output after treatment [91]. Our recommendation corresponds with common practice uses, which is the delivery of crystalloid rather than colloid at this time, as outcomes in burn patients have not been shown to be consistent. These studies highlight the complexity of burn shock resuscitation and the need for ongoing research in the field to identify the optimal method of fluid resuscitation.

Recent studies have also investigated the role of regulating glucose levels in burn patients during the critical phase. Stress hyperglycemia after severe burn injury has long been established as a physiological response to trauma. Additional studies have demonstrated the need for early glycemic control, as burn patients who did not have optimal glucose levels were associated with increased mortality. Delivery of intensive insulin therapy to critically ill burn patients limited the number of infections and sepsis and improved overall organ function [92]. In general, we recommend moderate glycemic control as demonstrated by the NICE-SUGAR trial [93]. Delivery of insulin also decreased inflammatory responses, as noted by decrease levels of systemic IL-6 and c-reactive protein, and improved body density, body fat, and lean body mass. Insulin therapy also reduced resting energy expenditure in the first week following the burn injury, enhanced mitochondrial function, and improved hepatic glucose metabolism [94]. Furthermore, the glucose variability experienced by a burn patient during the critical period is also associated with increased mortality rates, suggesting that consistent and tight glucose control may provide a significant survival benefit [95]. Taken together, these articles build an argument that in burn patients, intensive glucose control with insulin therapy may reduce inflammation, improve energy utilization, and improve overall prognosis.

Another important area of research is the development of new technology to aid in wound assessment and treatment. As discussed in previous sections, punch biopsy, LDI, and NIRS have been employed to diagnosis the burn depth and severity of the primary wound site. Additional studies advocate for the use of confocal laser scanning microscopy (CLSM) due to its greater contrast and sensitivity. Animal models testing this technology imaged wounds *in vivo* without any physical dissection. Using a laser source, CLSM was able to determine wound depth by assessing the number of perfused dermal papillae and was able to accurate classify burns based on the amount of perfusion [96]. Additional technology has been developed to accelerate healing. For instance, extracorporeal shock wave treatment (ESWT) has shown promise as it promotes angiogenesis, increases perfusion, and accelerates wound healing. In a pilot study, patients treated with ESWT demonstrated increase blood flow to the burn wound recorded by LDI within 3 weeks [97]. This therapy shows great promise, as it is a noninvasive measure to improve wound healing.

Advances in burn reconstruction have also been noted in the last decade. While tissue expanders have been a mainstay of burn reconstruction, several studies have surveyed the use of endoscopic assisted placement of expanders and the use of osmotic tissue expanders [98, 99]. Both endoscope assisted placement of expanders and osmotic tissue expanders offer advantages over the traditional methods, as they were more cosmetically acceptable and require fewer injections, respectively. As tissue expander technology continues to improve with new expansion techniques and devices, discovering the best technique and devices to use will be an important component of burn reconstruction. Cultured epithelial autografts, as discussed in previous sections, has gained increased interest as an alternative for cutaneous coverage for patients with large burn wounds and small potential donor sites. With final engraftment%ages as high as 73% and 90% patient survival rate, it is an attractive alterative for patients with severe and extensive burns.

5.2. Basic Science and Translational Science Research

Basic science research focuses on understanding the underlying mechanisms of disease, while translational science research focuses on the translation of bench science conducted in the lab to bedside clinical practice. Basic science and translational science research in burn injuries have significantly advanced in the last 50 years and have focused on both understanding and treating the primary wound site as well as secondary complications that arise from these traumatic burn injuries.

Within the primary wound site, hypertrophic scarring is a major focus of basic science and translational science research. Wound healing can be described in three different stages: inflammation, proliferation, and remodeling phase. Hypertrophic scarring is an aberrant form of the normal wound healing process that does not extend beyond the original wound margins. Hypertrophic scar formation involves the constitutively active proliferative phase of wound healing, resulting in high vascularity and dense extracellular matrix deposition [100]. Studies suggest that the secretion of TGF-beta1, platelet-derived growth factors, and epidermal growth factor results in a robust inflammatory response, involving mast cells, macrophages, and lymphocytes, which may underlie the excessive fibrosis seen in hypertrophic scar formation [101][102]. As translational science research from the bench to the bedside, new therapies targeted at quenching the inflammatory response, limiting fibrosis, and inhibiting angiogenesis to target the mediators of this scaring process are being developed [103, 104]. Additional basic science research aimed at understanding the wound healing process and translational science research investigating new treatment options will continue to advance our understanding and treatment of burn related injuries.

Additional studies into the precise cause of secondary complications such has HO has gained significant interest due to the increase in presence of HO in veterans who have sustained traumatic burn injuries overseas. While the precise pathophysiology behind HO is still unclear, it is thought to be related to local and systemic factors, causing osteoblastic differentiation of local cells. Previous studies have attempted to elucidate the local and systemic wound inflammatory response leading to HO, through the identification of cytokine and chemokines secreted from the wound site [105]. Serum analysis demonstrated a profound systemic inflammatory response in burn patients, as burn patients maintained increased levels of IL-6 and MCP-1 over time. Both IL-6 and MCP-1 are inflammatory agents that function in recruiting monocytes and macrophages to the site of injury, indicating sustained inflammation throughout the wound healing process. Furthermore, MCP-1 has also been implicated in bone remodeling and may be an earlier indicator of HO development. Locally, pro-inflammatory cytokine MIP-1alpha has been shown to be upregulated, indicating robust inflammation locally. This inflammatory response is believed to enhance bone regeneration; however, the precise cells and cytokines involved for this enhanced osteogenesis remains unclear. RUNX2 has also been shown to increase in the presence of macrophages and inflammatory cytokines, and this increased expression results in an increase in bone mineralization [106]. Other studies have demonstrated an increase in the tumor necrosis factor family and interleukins, including IL-1, IL6, IL-8, IL-10, IL12, and IL-18 to be contributory [107].

The most recent work in this field has focused on BMP signaling as a central mechanism that the leads to ectopic bone formation. Much of the early studies demonstrated that inhibition of transcriptional activity of BMP type I receptors with antagonists, such as noggin and chordin, has been shown to disrupt the osteoblast differentiation signaling pathways [108,

109]. Mice lacking noggin showed overactivity of BMP and displayed heterotopic ossification. The role of BMP signaling as an important regulator of ectopic bone formation, along with other mediators such as platelet-derived factor (PDGF), insulin-like growth factor 1 (IGF-1) and transforming growth factor beta-1 (TGF-beta1), continues to be the focus of research in this field. Identifying pharmacological therapies that inhibit the overactive inflammatory response may inhibit the development of HO [110].

Other studies have focused on the identification of progenitor cells responsible for HO. Nesti and colleagues identified and isolated a population of multilineage mesenchymal stem cells with osteogenic potential that were localized primarily in traumatized tissue [109]. Mesenchymal stem cells are multipotent, adult progenitor cells of great interest because of their unique immunologic properties and regenerative potential [111]. These progenitor cells have been shown to promote wound healing and regeneration of surround tissues by migrating to the site of injury, promoting repair and regeneration of damaged tissue, modulate the immune and inflammatory response, and secrete trophic factors that are important in wound healing and tissue remodeling [111-115]. Tissue resident progenitor cells are known to be highly sensitive to the surrounding inflammatory milieu [116, 117]. Interestingly, a study by Wu et al. indicates that exposure of skeletal muscle satellite cells to the serum of burned rats is sufficient to promote their osteogenic differentiation, suggesting that both systemic and local inflammation may play a role in driving stem cell differentiation. In addition, studies have recently shown that burn injury promotes HO of adipose derived stromal cells in a murine model of scald injury. Micro-computed tomography and histological analysis demonstrated increased endochondral ossification in the burn group compared to the sham control: a process which was most likely mediated through increased vascularization [118]. While resident mesenchymal stem cells seem to be implicated in the pathogenesis of HO, there is reason to believe that the immunomodulatory properties of these cells may be activated to suppress the proinflammatory microenvironment when applied externally [119].

Moreover, some groups have shown that these mesenchymal progenitor cells can be isolated from both health muscle and traumatized muscle. Both health and traumatized muscle have osteoprogenitor cells that have the potential to form ectopic bone after injury [109]. Laboratories have suggested that cells responsible for heterotopic ossification are from the endothelium of the local vasculature [120]. These studies suggest that in a setting of chronically stimulated BMP activity, muscle injury and associated inflammation sufficiently triggers heterotopic bone formation and that cells of vascular origin are essential to the development of ectopic bone formation. This cell lineage, along with stimulating factors such as BMP that create the correct environment for bone formation, could be targets for the development of therapeutic interventions to treat HO [121]. Further understanding the signaling pathways and the involvement of MSC differentiation is essential for the development of early diagnostic and prognostic tests and the development of novel prophylactic therapies.

Conclusion

Burns are responsible for significant morbidity and mortality and are among the most complex and devastating of all injuries. Early proper diagnosis of burn depth and extent allows for the delivery of appropriate treatment to ensure the best prognosis for burn patients. New technologies have advanced the method of diagnosis from punch biopsies to less invasive imaging studies, such as the LSI, NIRS, and CLSM. Diagnosis of secondary burn complications, such as joint contracture and HO, has also advanced with new imaging tools, such as the Raman spectroscopy, that may allow for earlier detection and treatment of ectopic bone formation. Nevertheless, the management of burn patients requires a team of physicians, nurses, critical care specialist, physical therapist, and counselor to provide optimal care to patients and lessen the burden of the initial burn injury. Furthermore, novel clinical, basic science, and translational science research continues to improve our understanding of the pathophysiology of burn injuries. By elucidating the pathophysiology of both the primary wound and secondary complications associated burns will assist in the treatment during the critical period and following the initial trauma and prevent secondary burn complications.

REFERENCES

[1] CDC. *Web-based injury and statistics query and reporting sytem (WISQARS).* 2009 [cited 2013 June 13]; Available from: webappa.cdc.gov/sasweb/ncipc/mortrate9.html.

[2] Association, A.B. *National Burn Repository.* 2009 [cited 2013 June 16]; Available from: www.ameriburn.org/2009NBRannualreport.pdf.

[3] Repository, N.B. *Report of data from 1999-2008.* 2009 [cited 2013 June 17]; Available from: www.ameriburn.org/2009NBRAnnualreport.pdf.

[4] Shields, B., et al., Healthcare resoure utilization and epidemiology of pediatric burn-associated hospitalizations, United States. *J Burn Care Res,* 2000. 28: p. 811-826.

[5] Conner, K., et al., Pediatric pedestrian injuries associated hospital resource utilization in the United States, 2003. *J Trauma,* 2010. 68(6): p. 1406-1412.

[6] Pressel, D., Evaluation of physical abuse in children. *Am Fam Physician,* 2000. 61: p. 3057-64.

[7] Birky, M., et al., Fire fatality study. *FIre and Materials,* 2004. 3(4): p. 211-217.

[8] Davidge, K. and J. FIsh, Older Adults and Burns. *Geriatrics and Aging,* 2008. 11(5): p. 270-275.

[9] Ryan, C., et al., A persistent fire hazard for older adults: cooking-related clothing ignition. *J Am Geriatr SOc,* 1997. 45: p. 1283-1285.

[10] Ryan, C., et al., Objective estimates for the probility of death from burn injuries. *N Engl J Med,* 1998. 338(362-366).

[11] Muller, M., S. Pegg, and M. Rule, Determinants of death following burn injury. *Br J Surg,* 2001. 88: p. 583-587.

[12] Webbenmeyer, L., et al., Predicting survival in an elderly burn patient population. *Burns,* 2001. 27(6).

[13] Bernard, S., et al., Fatal injuries among children by race and ethnicity -- United States, 1999-2002. *MMWR Surveillance Summary,* 2007. 56(SS-5): p. 1-20.

[14] Fagenholz, P., et al., National study of emergency department visits for burn injuries. *J Burn Care Res,* 2007. 28: p. 681-690.

[15] Gulaid, J., J. Sacks, and R. Sattin, Deaths from residential fires among older people, United States, 1984. *J Am Geriatr Soc,* 1989. 37(331-334).

[16] Hunt, J. and G. Purdue, The elderly burn patient. *Am J Surg,* 1992. 164: p. 472-476.

[17] McGill, V., A. Kowal-Vern, and R. Gamelli, Outcome for older burn patients. *Arch Surg,* 2000. 135: p. 320-325.

[18] Barillo, D. and R. Goode, Fire fatality study: demographics of fire vitims. *Burns,* 1996. 22: p. 85-88.

[19] Mallonee, S., et al., Surveillane and prevention of residential-fire injuries. *N Engl J Med,* 1996. 335: p. 27-31.

[20] Istre, G., et al., Residential fire related deaths and injuries among children: fireplay, smoke alarms, and prevention. *Inj Prev,* 2002. 8: p. 128-132.

[21] Repository, A.B.A.-N.B. 2012 Report. 2013 [cited 2013 June 10]; Available from: http://www.ameriburn.org/resources_factsheet.php.

[22] Ward, P. and G. Till, Pathophysiologic events related to thermal injury of skin. *Journal of Trauma,* 1990. 12 Suppl: p. S75-79.

[23] Friedl, H., et al., Roles of histamine, complement, and xanthine oxidase in thermal injury of skin. *Am J Pathol,* 1989. 135(1): p. 203-217.

[24] Till, G., et al., Role of xanthine oxidase in thermal injury of skin. *Am J Pathol,* 1989. 135(1): p. 195-202.

[25] Lowell, G., K. Quinlan, and L. Gottlieb, Preventing unintentional scald burns: moving beyond tap water. *Pediatrics,* 2008. 122(4): p. 799-804.

[26] Rimmer, R., et al., Scald burns in young children-a reveiw of Arizona burn center pediatric patients and a proposal for prevention in the Hispanic community. *J Burn Care Res,* 2008. 29(4): p. 595-605.

[27] Dissanaike, S., et al., Cooking-related pediatric burns: risk factors and the role of differential cooling rates among commonly implicated substances. *J Burn Care Res,* 2009. 30(4): p. 593-598.

[28] Drago, D., Kitchen scalds and thermal burns in children five years and younger. *Pediatrics,* 2005. 114(1): p. 10-16.

[29] DiVincenti, F., J. Moncrief, and B.J. Pruitt, Electrical Injuries: a review of 65 cases. *J Trauma,* 1969. 9: p. 497-507.

[30] Mortiz, A.R. and H. F C, Studies of thermal injury: pathology and pathogenesis of cutaneous burns: an experimental study. *Am J Pathol,* 1947. 23: p. 915-941.

[31] Bill, T.J., et al., Grease Burns of the Hand: Preventable Injuries. *Journal of Emergency Medicine,* 1996. 14(3): p. 351-355.

[32] Park, Y., Y. Choi, and H. Lee, The impact of laser Doppler imaging on the early decision-making process for surgical intervention in adults with indeterminate burns. *Burns,* 2013. 39(4): p. 655-661.

[33] Heimbach, D., et al., Burn depth: a review. *World Journal of Surgery,* 2013. 16(1): p. 10-15.

[34] Jeng, J., et al., Laser Doppler imaging determines need for excision and grafting in advance of clinical judgment: a prospective blinded trial. *Burns: Journal of the International Society for Burn Injuries,* 2003. 29(7): p. 665-670.

[35] Erba, P., et al., FluxEXPLORER: a new high-speed laser Doppler imaging system for the assessment of burn injuries. *Skin research and technology,* 2012. 18(4): p. 456-461.

[36] Kaiser, M., et al., Noninvasive assessment of burn wound severity using optical technology: a review of current and future modalities. *Burns,* 2011. 37(3): p. 377-386.

[37] Nguyen, T., et al., Novel application of a spatial frequency domain imaging system to determine signature spectral differences between infected and noninfected burn wounds. *Journal of Burn Care and Research,* 2013. 34(1): p. 44-50.

[38] Nguyen, J., et al., Spatial frequency domain imaging of burn wounds in a preclinical model of graded burn severity. *Journal of Biomedical Optics,* 2013. 18(6): p. 66010. doi:10.1117/1.JBO.18.6.066010.

[39] Mavrogenis, A., P. Soucacos, and P. Papagelopoulos, Heterotopic ossification revisited. *Orthopedics,* 2011. 34(4): p. 177.

[40] Shehab, D., A. Elgazzar, and B. Collier, Heterotopic ossification. *Journal of Nuclear Medicine,* 2002. 43(3): p. 346-353.

[41] Thomas, E., V. Cassar-Pullicino, and I. McCall, The role of ultrasound in the early diagnosis and management of heterotopic bone formation. *Clinical Radiology,* 1991. 43(3): p. 190-196.

[42] Peterson, J., et al., Early detection of burn induced heterotopic ossification using transcutaneous Raman spectroscopy. *Bone,* 2013. 54(1): p. 28-34.

[43] Bezuhly, M. and J.S. Fish, Acute burn care. *Plastic and Reconstructive Surgery,* 2012. 130(2): p. 349e-358e.

[44] Posluszny, J., et al., Surgical burn wound infections and their clinical implications. *J Burn Care Res,* 2011. 32(2): p. 324-333.

[45] Brown, D. and G.H. Borschel, *Michigan manual of plastic surgery.* Vol. Lippincott Williams & Wilkins. 2004, Philadelphia, PA.

[46] Thorne, C., *Grabb and Smith's plastic surgery2007,* Philadelphia, PA: Lippincott Williams & Wilkins.

[47] Atiyeh, B.S., et al., Review Effect of silver on burn wound infection control and healing: review of the literature. *Burns,* 2007. 33(2): p. 139-148.

[48] Falcone, P.A., et al., Mafenide acetate concentrations and bacteriostasis in experimental burn wounds treated with a three-layered laminated mafenide-saline dressing. *Ann Plast Surg,* 1980. 5(4): p. 226-229.

[49] Klasen, H.J., A historical review of the use of silver in the treatment of burns. II. Renewed interest for silver. *Burns*, 2000. 26(2): p. 131-138.

[50] Fong, J. and F. Wood, Nanocrystalline silver dressings in wound management: a review. *Nanomedicine,* 2006. 1(4): p. 441-449.

[51] Gravante, G., et al., Nanocrystalline silver: A systematic review of randomized trials conducted on burned patients and an evidence-based assessment of potential advantages over older silver formulations. *Ann Plast Surg,* 2009. 63(2): p. 201-205.

[52] Engav, L., et al., Early excision and grafting vs. nonoperative treatment of burns of indeterminant depth: a randomized prospective study. *J Trauma,* 1983. 23: p. 510-517.

[53] Gray, D., et al., Early surgical excision versus conventional therapy in patients with 20 to 40% burns: a comparative study. *Am J Surg,* 1982. 23(1001-1004).

[54] Mulholland, M.W., *Greenfield's Surgery2010,* Philadelphia, PA: Lippincott Williams & Wilkins.

[55] Benichou, G., et al., Immune recognition and rejection of allogeneic skin grafts. *Immunotherapy,* 2011. 3(6): p. 757-770.

[56] Ronfard, V., et al., Long-term regeneration of human epidermis on third degree burns transplanted with autologous cultured epithelium grown on a fibrin matrix. *Transplantation,* 2000. 70: p. 1588-1598.

[57] Atiyeh, B.S., Cultured epithelial autograft (CEA) in burn treatment: three decades later. *Burns,* 2007. 33: p. 405-413.

[58] Elliott, M. and J. Vandervord, Initial experience with cultured epithelial autografts in massively burnt patients. *ANZ J Surg,* 2002. 72: p. 893-895.

[59] Paddle-Ledinek, J.E., D.G. Cruickshank, and J.P. Masterton, Skin replacement by cultured keratinocyte grafts: an Australia experience. *Burns,* 1997. 23: p. 204-211.

[60] Sterling, J., N.S. Gibran, and M.B. Klein, Acute management of hand burns. *Hand Clinics,* 2009. 25(4): p. 453.

[61] Klein, M.B. and e. al, Primer on the management of face burns at the University of Washington. *Journal of Burn Care and Research,* 2005. 26(1): p. 2-6.

[62] Lawrence, J.W., et al., Epidemiology and impact of scarring after burn injury: a systematic review of the literature. *Journal of burn care & research : official publication of the American Burn Association,* 2012. 33(1): p. 136-46.

[63] Gangemi, E.N., et al., Epidemiology and risk factors for pathologic scarring after burn wounds. *Archives of facial plastic surgery,* 2008. 10(2): p. 93-102.

[64] Nedelec, B., et al., Myofibroblasts and apoptosis in human hypertrophic scars: the effect of interferon-alpha2b. *Surgery,* 2001. 130(5): p. 798-808.

[65] Armour, A., P.G. Scott, and E.E. Tredget, Cellular and molecular pathology of HTS: basis for treatment. *Wound Repair Regen,* 2007. 15(Suppl 1): p. S6-S17.

[66] Parnell, L.K., et al., Assessment of pruritus characteristics and impact on burn survivors. *Journal of burn care & research : official publication of the American Burn Association,* 2012. 33(3): p. 407-18.

[67] Klinger, M., M. Marazzi, and D. Vigo, Fat injection for cases of severe burn outcomes: a new perspective of scar remodeling and reduction. *Aesthetic Plast Surg,* 2008. 32: p. 465-469.

[68] Reish, R.G. and E. Eriksson, Scar treatments: preclinical and clinical studies. *J Am Coll Surg,* 2008. 206: p. 719-730.

[69] Zouboulis, C.C., et al., Outcomes of cryosurgery in keloids and hypertrophic scars: a prospective consecutive trial of case series. *Arch Dermatol,* 1993. 129: p. 1146-1151.

[70] Alster, T.S. and C. Handrick, Laser treatment of hypertrophic scars, keloids, and striae. *Semin Cutan Med Surg,* 2000. 19: p. 287-292.

[71] Manstein, D., et al., Fractional photothermolysis: a new concept for cutaneous remodeling using microscopic patterns of thermal injury. *Laser Surg Med,* 2004. 34(5): p. 426-438.

[72] Thompson, A. and G. Kent, Adjusting to disfigurement: processes involved in dealing with being visibly different. *Clinical psychology review,* 2001. 21(5): p. 663-82.

[73] Lawrence, J., et al., Epidemiology and impact of scarring after burn injury: A systematic review of the literature. *J Burn Care Res,* 2012. 33: p. 136-146.

[74] Lawrence, J., et al., Visible vs hidden scars and their relation to body esteem. *J Burn Care Rehabil,* 2004. 25: p. 25-32.

[75] Gore, D.C., et al., Quantification of protein metabolism in vivo for skin, wound, and muscle in severe burn patients. *JPEN. Journal of parenteral and enteral nutrition,* 2006. 30(4): p. 331-8.

[76] Jeschke, M.G., et al., Long-term persistance of the pathophysiologic response to severe burn injury. *PloS one,* 2011. 6(7): p. e21245.

[77] Rutan, R.L. and D.N. Herndon, Growth delay in postburn pediatric patients. *Archives of surgery,* 1990. 125(3): p. 392-5.

[78] Tuvdendorj, D., et al., Skeletal muscle is anabolically unresponsive to an amino acid infusion in pediatric burn patients 6 months postinjury. *Annals of surgery,* 2011. 253(3): p. 592-7.

[79] Porter, C., et al., Amino acid infusion fails to stimulate skeletal muscle protein synthesis up to 1 year after injury in children with severe burns. *The journal of trauma and acute care surgery,* 2013. 74(6): p. 1480-5.

[80] Padfield, K.E., et al., Burn injury causes mitochondrial dysfunction in skeletal muscle. *Proceedings of the National Academy of Sciences of the United States of America,* 2005. 102(15): p. 5368-73.

[81] Righi, V., et al., Mitochondria-targeted antioxidant promotes recovery of skeletal muscle mitochondrial function after burn trauma assessed by in vivo 31P nuclear magnetic resonance and electron paramagnetic resonance spectroscopy. *FASEB journal : official publication of the Federation of American Societies for Experimental Biology,* 2013. 27(6): p. 2521-30.

[82] Cree, M.G., et al., Insulin sensitivity and mitochondrial function are improved in children with burn injury during a randomized controlled trial of fenofibrate. *Annals of surgery,* 2007. 245(2): p. 214-21.

[83] Herndon, D.N., et al., Reversal of catabolism by beta-blockade after severe burns. The New England journal of medicine, 2001. 345(17): p. 1223-9.

[84] Przkora, R., D.N. Herndon, and O.E. Suman, The effects of oxandrolone and exercise on muscle mass and function in children with severe burns. *Pediatrics,* 2007. 119(1): p. e109-16.

[85] Elledge, E.S., et al., Heterotopic bone formation in burned patients. *The Journal of trauma,* 1988. 28(5): p. 684-7.

[86] Esselman, P.C., et al., Burn rehabilitation: state of the science. *American journal of physical medicine & rehabilitation / Association of Academic Physiatrists,* 2006. 85(4): p. 383-413.

[87] Evans, E.B., Orthopaedic measures in the treatment of severe burns. *The Journal of bone and joint surgery. American volume,* 1966. 48(4): p. 643-69.

[88] Klein, M.B., et al., Extended time to wound closure is associated with increased risk of heterotopic ossification of the elbow. *Journal of burn care & research : official publication of the American Burn Association,* 2007. 28(3): p. 447-50.

[89] Maender, C., D. Sahajpal, and T.W. Wright, Treatment of heterotopic ossification of the elbow following burn injury: recommendations for surgical excision and perioperative prophylaxis using radiation therapy. *Journal of shoulder and elbow surgery / American Shoulder and Elbow Surgeons ...* [et al.], 2010. 19(8): p. 1269-75.

[90] Orzel, J. and T. Rudd, Heterotopic bone formation: clinical, laboratory, and imaging correlation. *J Nucl Med,* 1985. 26: p. 125-132.

[91] Neal, B., et al., A systematic survey of 13 randomized trials of non-steroidal anti-inflammatory drugs for the prevention of heterotopic bone formation after major hip surgery. *Acta Orthop Scand,* 2000. 71: p. 122-128.

[92] Fearonce, G., et al., Peripherally inserted central venous catheters and central venous cathers in burn patients: a comparative review. *J Burn Care Res,* 2010. 31: p. 31-35.

[93] Neff, L., J. Allman, and H. Holmes, The use of therapeutic plasma exchange (TPE) in the setting of refractory burn shock. *Burns,* 2010. 36: p. 372-378.

[94] Cartotto, R. and A. Zhou, Fluid creep: the pendulum hasn't swung back yet! *J Burn Care Res*, 2010. 31: p. 551-558.

[95] Webbenmeyer, L., et al., The impact of opioid administration on resuscitation volumes in theramlly injuried patients. *J Burn Care Res,* 2010. 31: p. 40-47.

[96] Pidcoke, H., et al., Glucose variability is associated with high mortality after severe burn. *J Trauma,* 2009. 67.

[97] Altintas, A., et al., Differentiation of superficial-partial vs. deep partial thickness burn injuries in vivo by confocal laser scanning microscopy. *Burns,* 2009. 35: p. 80-86.

[98] Arno, A., et al., Extracorporeal shock waves, a new non-surgical method to treat severe burns. *Burns,* 2010. 36: p. 477-482.

[99] Sood, R., et al., Cultured epithelial autografts for coverage of large burn wounds in eighty-eight patients: the Indiana University experience. *J Burn Care Res,* 2010. 31: p. 559-568.

[100] Sood, R., et al., Coverage of large pediatric wounds with cultured epithelial autografts in congenital nevi and burns: results and technique. *J Burn Care Res,* 2009. 30: p. 576-86.

[101] Ehrlich, H., et al., Morphological and immunochemical differences between keloid and hypertrophic scar. *Am J Pathol,* 1994. 145: p. 105-113.

[102] Wulff, B., et al., Mast cells contribute to scar formation during fetal wound healing. *J Invest Dermatol,* 2012. 132(2): p. 458-465.

[103] Wilgus, T., et al., The impact of cyclooxygenase-2 mediated inflammation on scarless fetal wound healing. *Am J Pathol,* 2004. 165(3): p. 753-761.

[104] Peranteau, W., et al., IL-10 overexpression decreases inflammatory mediators and promotes regenerative healing in an adult model of scar formation. *J Invest Dermatol,* 2008. 128(7): p. 1852-1860.

[105] Gordon, A., et al., Permissive environment in postnatal wounds induced by adenoviral-mediated overexpression of the anti-inflammatory cytokine interleukin-10 prevents scar formation. *Wound Repair Regen,* 2008. 16(1): p. 70-79.

[106] Potter, B., et al., Heterotopic ossification following combat-related trauma. *J Bone Joint Surg Am,* 2010. 92(Suppl 2): p. 74-89.

[107] Guihard, P., et al., Induction of osteogenesis in mesenchymal stem cells by activated monocytes/macrophages depends on oncostatin M signaling. *Stem Cells,* 2012. 30(4): p. 762-772.

[108] Pignolo, R., et al., Heterozygous inactivation of Gnas in adipose-derived mesenchymal progenitor cells enhances osteoblast differentiation and promotes heterotopic ossification. *J Bone Miner Res,* 2011. 26(11): p. 2647-2655.

[109] Hannallah, D., et al., Retroviral delivery of Naoggin inhibits the formation of heterotopic ossification induced by BMP-4, demineralized bone matrix, and trauma in an animal model. *J Bone Joint Surg Am,* 2004. 86-A: p. 80-91.

[110] Nesti, L., et al., Differentiation potential of multipotent progenitor cells derived from war-traumatized muscle tissue. *J Bone Joint Surg Am,* 2008. 90(11): p. 2390-2398.

[111] Zhang, K., et al., Celecoxib inhibits the heterotopic ossification in the rat model with Achilles tenotomy. *Eur J Orthop SUrg Traumatol,* 2013. 23: p. 145-148.

[112] Uccelli, A., L. Moretta, and V. Pistoia, Mesenchymal stem cells in health and disease. *Nat Rev Immunol,* 2008. 8: p. 726-736.
[113] Caplan, A., Adult mesenchymal stem cells for tissue engineering versus regenerative medicine. *J Cell Physiol,* 2007. 213: p. 341-347.
[114] Chamberlain, G., et al., Concise review: mesenchymal stem cells: their phenotype, differentiation capacity, immunological features, and potential for homing. *Stem Cells,* 2007. 25: p. 2739-2749.
[115] Phinney, D. and D. Prockop, Concise review: mesenchymal stem cell/multipotent stromal cells: the state of transdifferentiation and modes of tissue repair. *Stem Cells,* 2007. 25: p. 2896-2902.
[116] Gimble, J., A. Katz, and B. Bunnell, Adipose-derived stem cells for regenerative medicine. *Circulation Res,* 2007. 100: p. 1249-1260.
[117] Mountziaris, P.M., et al., Harnessing and modulating inflammation in strategies for bone regeneration. Tissue engineering. *Part B, Reviews,* 2011. 17(6): p. 393-402.
[118] Nelson, E.R., et al., Heterotopic ossification following burn injury: the role of stem cells. *Journal of burn care & research : official publication of the American Burn Association,* 2012. 33(4): p. 463-70.
[119] Peterson, J.R., et al., Burn Injury Enhances Bone Formation in Heterotopic Ossification Model. *Annals of surgery,* 2013.
[120] Djouad, F., et al., Mesenchymal stem cells: innovative therapeutic tools for rheumatic diseases. *Nature reviews. Rheumatology,* 2009. 5(7): p. 392-9.
[121] Lounev, V., et al., Identification of progenitor cells that contribute to heterotopic skeletogenesis. *J Bone Joint surg Am,* 2009. 91(3): p. 652-663.
[122] Hsu, J. and M. Keenan, Current review of heterotopic ossification. *J Orthopaedics,* 2010. 20: p. 126-130.

In: Encyclopedia of Dermatology (6 Volume Set)
Editor: Meghan Pratt
ISBN: 978-1-63483-326-4

Chapter 77

PEDIATRIC BURN IN BANGLADESH: A TERTIARY LEVEL HOSPITAL EXPERIENCE

***Kishore Kumar Das*[1*], *M Quamruzzaman*[2] *and Syed Shamsuddin Ahmed*[1]**
[1]Burn Unit DMCH
[2]National Institute of Cancer and research, Dhaka, Bangladesh

ABSTRACT

Pediatric burn constitutes approximate 48 percent of the total burn patients in the burn and plastic surgery unit of Dhaka Medical College Hospital (DMCH). In Bangladesh under 12 is regarded as pediatric age group. Domestic low voltage as well as high voltage electric burns are next to scald and flame burn. Incidence of chemical burn is lower than adult but still does occur in significant number. Non accidental contact burns (torture), traditional remedy related burn; friction burns are also frequently reported. Kitchen is commonest place of accidents but burn also occur in bedrooms, yards and occasionally at neighbors house. Lot of children are employed in small industries, as domestic servants, works in hotels, restaurants and tea stalls and sustain burn injuries which is related to their jobs. Non accidental burns occur particularly in female child and maid servants.

The pattern of burn differs in the out and in patients. In outdoor cases of pediatric burn scald (63%) is highest while flame 33%, electric burn 4% and chemical burn less than 0.5%. In case of admitted patient flame 65%, scald 20%, electric 10% and chemical 1.02%.

Overall (adult and pediatric) incidence is flame burn 44%, scald 30% electric burn 18% and chemical burn 4%. Overall mortality of pediatric burn is 3%. The actual figure is much higher as many patients leave the hospital just before death to avoid post mortem.

* Corresponding author: E-mail: kishorek50@hotmail.com.

INTRODUCTION

Burn is among the first five leading cause in Bangladesh. A community survey in Bangladesh found that the rate of fatal and nonfatal burn is 0.6 per 100,000 children with permanent disability of 5.7 per 100,000 burn children [1]. However the burn unit experience contradicts the data with over 70 percent disability or deformity as the unit cannot provide total care because of huge number of patients, lack of resources and manpower. Follow up and therapy service is merely mentionable. The Dhaka Medical College Hospital burn unit is the only burn unit in Bangladesh. Since its inception in April 2004 the unit meets up 79,000 burn patient visits and admitted over 13000 burn patients till December 2012.

MATERIALS AND METHODS

The study was conducted on 2175 pediatric burn patient admitted in the burn unit as well as attending in the outpatient Department. Hospital admission records, out patient records and operation theater records were being used for data. Patients and their parents are interviewed to know the detail of the accident and condition of the child and family.

RESULTS AND OBSERVATIONS

Age

Hospital admission record shows that age range of 59% was three to seven years with highest number observed in seven year age group (16.%). Children below three years remain most of the time in the lap of the mother thus protected while children from 3 to 7 move around the mother while they are cooking and had the risk of getting burn. The incidence took a peak again after age 10 as they, particularly the girls starts helping their mother or cook independently. They start wearing long frocks (cloths) and saries at this age and the high incidences continue in the adolescent age until they get experienced in cooking. 45% of female burn occurs between ages 15 to 25 years.

Sex

Female children more commonly sustain burn injuries. About 58 percent of the pediatric burn patents were female.

Female children remain at home and helps mother during cooking, which might be cause of highest incidences among girls. Long frocks and other pattern of girl's dresses are also the cause.

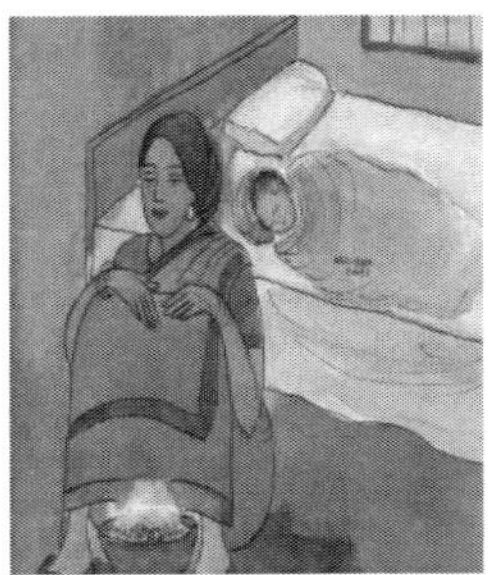
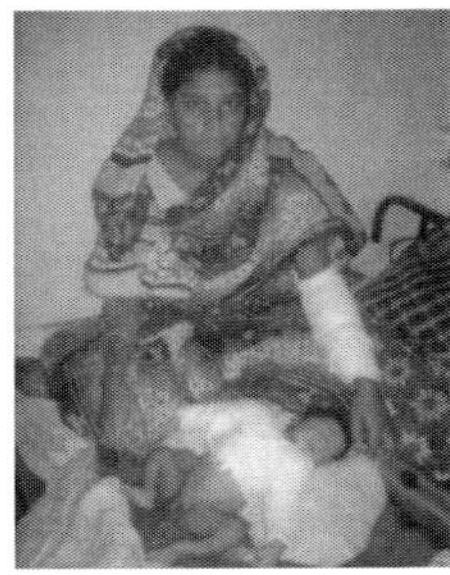

Figure 1. Both mother and newborn suffer burn injury during fumigation of birth passage after child birth.

Causes of Burn

Causes of burn differ from inpatient to out patients. Among the admitted patients flame burn is the highest while in the outpatient scald are commoner.

Outpatient

Minor burns not requiring resuscitation, ambulant patients and patients living close to the hospital are treated as outpatient. Patients themselves want to be treated as outpatient even they require admission and immediate surgery because of overcrowding in the wards and long delay in operation.

In Patient

Most severe burn occurs due to flame thus the high incidences of flame burn among admitted children. Scalds are commoner than other burns in outpatient.

Table 1. Types of pediatric burn

Causes of pediatric burn in out patients		
Cause	**Number (n-1494)**	**Percentage**
Flame	n-492	33%
Scald	n-946	63%
Electric	n-54	4%
Chemical	n-2	0.5%
Cause of pediatric burn in admitted patient		
Flame	440	65%
Scald	138	20%
Electric	70	10%
Chemical	7	1%
Contact	14	2%
Others (Ash, hot oil)	13	2%

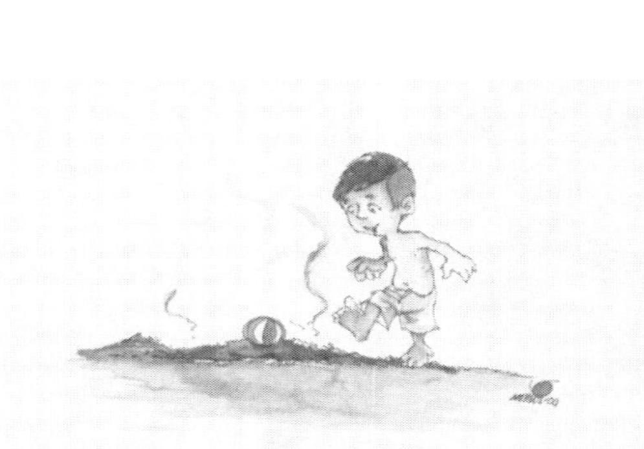
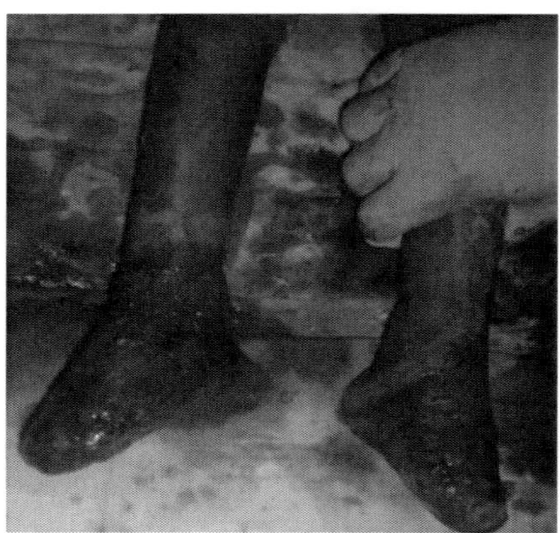

Figure 2. Burn from leftover ashes.

There is no prescribed admission criteria followed for burn patients. Admissions are often influenced by distance the patients travel from the place of occurrence in the country to the unit. Usually burs reaching the unit within 48 hours get admission as emergency patients. More delayed cases have to attend in the out patient. Acute burns needing surgery and post burn scar contractures mainly get admitted from OPD. Chemical burns and non accidental injuries are admitted.

Mechanism of Burn

Accidental Flame Burn

Table 2. source of accidental flame burn

Flame	Percentage
Accidental burn	
Open lamp, candle	29%
Chula	36.3%
Warming body	9.9%
House fire	13.2%
Drying cloths, fumigation after circumcision	4.1%
Stepping on hot ash	4.9%
Scalds	
Shower water	34.48%
Hot food (human food and animal food)	41.37%
Rice parboiling water	3.4%
Tea stall, hotel kitchen	6.8%
Road accident (engine water)	3.4%
Hot oil (residence, restaurant kitchen)	10.34%
Electric	
Roof top line	52.94%
Tree top line, Climbing up the electric pole	5.8%

Flame	Percentage
House electrification, electric fences	17.6%
Electric short-circuit, electric home appliances (TV, Freeze) putting pins or finger into sockets at home	17.6%
Biting live electric line and holding live electric wire from fallen of lines at home and at yard.	5.8%
Pediatric Chemical Burn	
Accidental chemical burn	28.57%
Attack with chemical	71.42

Note: 2.5% percent accidental burn occurred in neighbors' houses while most (97.5%) of the accidents occurred in and around their own houses.

Among the electric burn Low Voltage are 41.%, High Voltage 59%

Table 3. Types of intentional/non accidental burn

Intentional Burn (non-accidental), total 22 cases				
Flame (n-15)	**By adult (n-5)**	**22.7%**	**By children (n-10)**	**45.45%**
Scald (by adult) (n-2)	9%			
Contact (torture./maid servant, street children) (n-5)	22.72%			
Chemical	Included in the chemical burn part			

Health and safety rules and practice is virtually absent in Bangladesh.

1) Ground level chula (open hearth for cooking) is the most common source of flame burn in rural Bangladesh and in slum houses. Kerosene stoves and gas burns are also set up on the floor during cooking. These stoves and burners are made of very cheap metal sheets and materials, they often leaks gas and oil and explode.
2) Open kerosene /diesel lamps are other common sources of burn in Bangladesh. For irrigation purposes diesel engine are used all over the country. Every farmer's house there is a large can of diesel. During refueling a burning lamp from a large can explosion occur frequently resulting individual burn or often house fire. While sleeping at night people keep one lamp burning inside the room, pets or a gush of wind turn it over spreading fire. Mothers keep babies on polythene sheets as the baby's urine cannot wet the bed. These polythene sheets spread the flame rapidly when the lamps turn over.
3) People during winter make fire with sticks and straws and sits around to warm the body. Watching the adults children also make fire on the ground and gets burn from it. They go close to chula to warm body and gets burn. Warming the wounds is a common practice in Bangladesh. Mother after childbirth stands on chula or burning charcoal to fumigate or warm perineal wounds in an attempt to dry out secretions and bloods and also for rapid involution of uterus. While doing so their saries catch fire and if the newborn is close by it gets burn. Boys after circumcision also stand on fire for the purpose of rapid healing and their lungi (bottom part of a traditional Bangladeshi adult Muslim dress) catches fire. After bath sometime children dry

cloths sitting close to chula as that might the only cloth they have. While doing it they get burn.

4) House fire is common during winter when the weather is very dry. Slum houses or small factories inside house are prone to house fire. Garment factories also employ minor children and fire breaks out either they sustain burn or sometime suffer stumped. Houses and factories in Bangladesh have no fire protection and safe fire escape.
5) In the village people make fire for parboiling rice or to prepare a sweetmeat from date or palm juice. After the job is finished they do not take care of the fire and hot charcoal remains on the ground covered by a layer ash. Children frequently step in. In the city road workers leave their fire used for melting pitch after road carpeting.

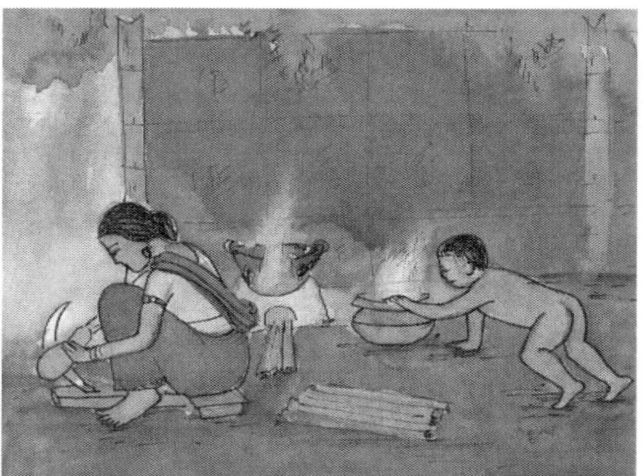
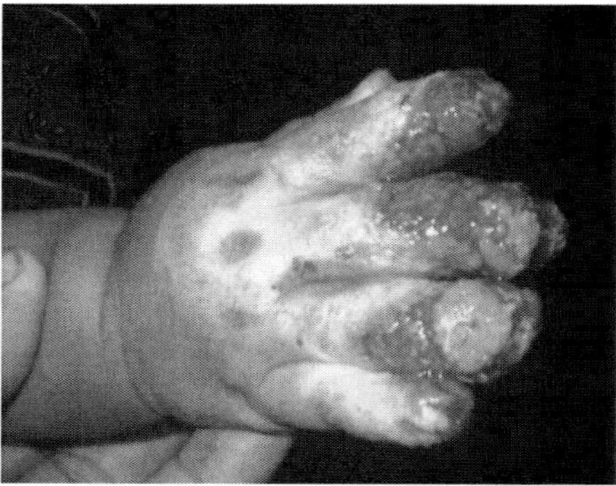

Figure 3. Cooking at ground level where toddlers can easily get accidental burn.

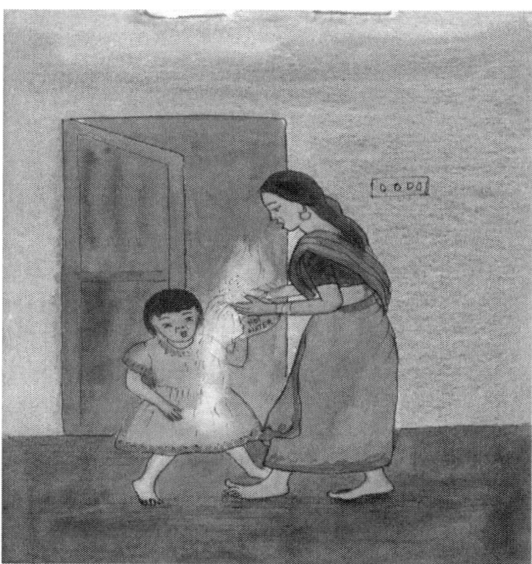

Figure 4. Collision between a child and maid servant transporting hot water is the single most common cause of scalding in Bangladesh.

Accidental Scalds

1) Scalds are commonest burn in children though more flame burn gets admitted. Hot water transportation from kitchen to bathroom for carries great risk. Maid servant or mother caring the water collide with running children while moving across the living room resulting in splashing of water on to the children and even to the transporter. A tray full of cups full of hot tea often also fall during transportation. In road side restraints children prepare and sell teas for their leavings and gets flame burn scalds and hot oil burns.
2) Hot gravy foods both made for human and animal (cows) are source of scalds. Toddlers put hands inside the bucket getting scald injury. Animal foods are produced in bulk, kept in a large bucket and children can fall on it. There are lot of rice parboiling industries across the country where rice a boiled in a large container and is a source of major scald for children as well as adults.
3) All over Bangladesh a three wheel rickshaw van has been turned into a motorized vehicle by attaching a shallow irrigation engine in it. The custom made vehicle is called VOT-VOT-E because of the sound it produce while running on the street. It contains lot of water (about ten liters) to run the engine. The water becomes very hot and when the vehicle turns over on uneven village roads frequently and is a major cause of road accident. These accident victims along with poly trauma sustain scalds. Engine water from large vehicle also causes scald.

Accidental Electrical Burn

Electric burn both high and low voltage occur in epidemic proportion in Bangladesh.

1) Roof top electric line is the commonest source of high voltage electric burn.
People build illegal houses beneath high voltage electric transmission line roof of which comes very close to the line and even a children can get hold of it. Children often playfully climb up trees or electric poles and get electrocuted. Electric poles are not protected in Bangladesh.

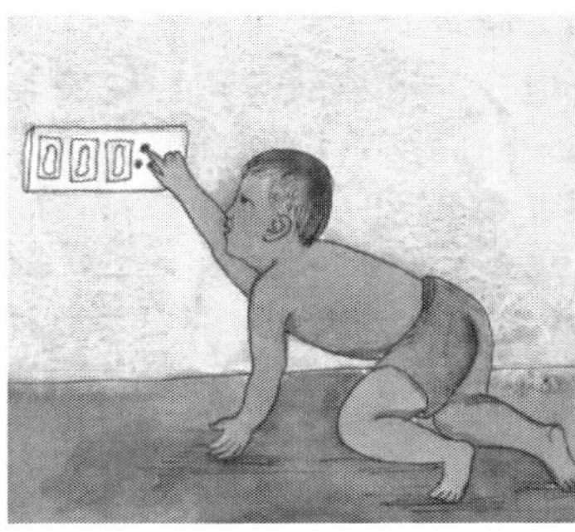
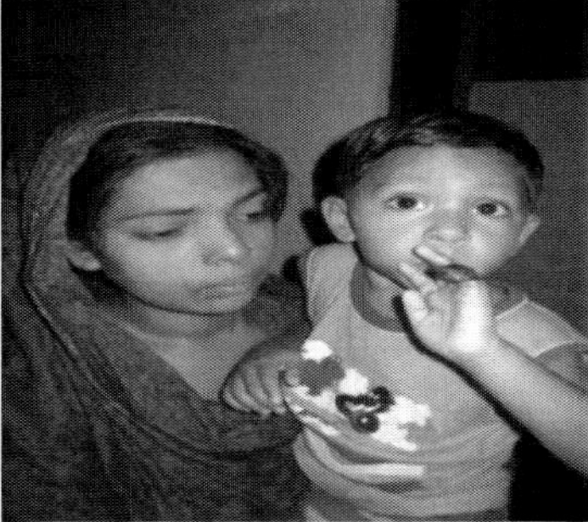

Figure 5. Electric burn from easily approachable lines.

2) Some village houses are made of corrugated iron sheets and has electric supply in it. Sometime the whole house become electrified because of faulty wiring. Children touching the walls get electric burns from it. In the city faulty electric appliances also cause electric burns in children.
3) Electric extension cords, sockets are another source. Bare electric wire fallen due to monsoon storm or being installed at children reach are another common source of electrocution. Children hold the wire sometime bites it.
4) Poultry owners fish farm owners make electric fences around the farms and keep it attached with the mainline during night to prevent stealing. They often forget to disconnect and children gets electric burn from those fences.

Chemical Burn

1) Children are not usually attacked with acids but at they remain close to their parents they gests chemical burn along with their parents. Illegitimate children, female children and in case of dispute within the family children are being targeted. Most of the time the motive behind is to kill.
2) Acid ingestion, mostly accidental but sometime intentional occur. In goldsmiths house they keep concentrated hydrochloric and Sulfuric acids in clear glass bottles and jars. Children often the adults accidentally ingest the chemicals.
3) In the rural areas people keeps carbolic acids inside houses to drive the snakes away from home. Children and women accidentally get acid burn from those as remain most of the time at home.
   No children so far reported to burn unit suffering chemical burns from industries.
4) Chemicals are transported without any safety precaution. Accidental spillage of the chemical following road accident causes chemical burn. Children are rare victim of such accident. Out of 7 chemical burn cases reported in 2008, 2 died, one was a chemical attack while the other one was following a road accident where an acid loaded truck collided with a passenger bus.

Intentional Burn

Intentional flame burn, scalds and contact burns are common in children though only 22 cases reported in 2008. Intentional flame burns are committed by adults or by older children but scald and contact burn are carried out by adults only. These victims were child labors in restaurants, maid servants or street children. Motive of the torture is punishment after breaking something or theft. Host kitchen appliances are most of the time used in case of contact burns. Hot water, oil, and cigarettes are also being used.

Fatal Case

Total 62 pediatric burn deaths were recorded which constitute approximately 3% total paediatric burn patients. Overall mortality is 9% in the unit.

Table 4. Status/provision of first aid after burn

No First Aid	94%
Water	1.9%
Egg	1.2%
Antibiotic	0.64%
Ice, Potato, mud	Less than 1%

Among the deaths 40 (64.5%) were due to acute renal failure and died within 10 days of burn while 12 (19.35%) were due to septicemia. Delay in starting fluid in pre-hospital care and inadequate fluid resuscitation in the initial periods are presumed to be the cause of deaths. While cross infection and septicemia is also common because of overcrowding, improper dressing changes and lack of early surgery facilities.

First Aid

No first aid given in 94% cases. There is a misconception in the society that if you pour water on a burn it would produce blister and blisters are considered as bad sign in case of burn. People usually give toot pest and eggs on the would but antiseptic creams, ice, meshed potato and even mud and cow dung are given on the wound.

Employment of Mother

Only 12% Mothers of the burn victims were found employed, rest of them were housewives. Employed mother do not prepare every meal. They keep maidservants and there is someone (grandparents, servants, or elder children) in the family to look after the children. Employed mothers are educated and have better knowledge on safety and are more orderly worker in the kitchen. While in case of mother who are housewife remain busy in cooking and cleaning along with keeping the children. They have to raise cattle and most of the times do not have helping hands. Most have limited or no education. They have to work as well as keep an eye on children. While keeping the children close to fire results in accidental burn on to themselves and to the children whenever concentration is being diverted.

Family Monthly Income

Burn commonly occurs in low income families who live in crowed house where there are no separate cooking areas. 62% cases the income is below 50$ US a month.

Flame burns are common among the poor while scalds are commoner among the reach. Also the reach people go to private burn hospitals.

Table 5. Family monthly income

<Tk3000	<Tk5000	<Tk10000	>Tk10000
62%	17%	10%	11%

Table 6. Complications of burn in paediatric age group

	Complications	Approximate percentage
1	Hypertrophic scaring/keloid	80%
2	Burn contracture	40%
3	Social withdrawal	30%
4	Loss of school (temporary and permanent)	90%
5	Loss of marrigability (girls only)	30%
6	Amputation and permanent disability	10%
7	Family disharmony and divorce between parents	30%
8	Psychological trauma, anxiety, fear, depression, mental retardation	30%
9	Developmental abnormality	10%
10	Fatality	3%

Outcome

A community survey in Bangladesh done by Centre for Injury Prevention an Research Bangladesh (CIPRB) found disability of 5.7 per 100,000 burn children. However the burn unit experiences differ form what has been found in the community survey. Though formal assessments of the outcome of pediatric burn are not done, here some approximate percentage are given based on clinical experiences in the unit.

Long term follow up of the patients of the burn unit is not possible because the patients lives long distant away from the hospital and cannot afford to come to the hospital for regular follow up. Patients are usually asked to come for follow up after one month but mostly do not come. There is no official set protocol for follow up.

1) Hypertrophic scaring/keloid is the most common complication. Regions are – black skin people tend to produce more hypertrophy after burn healing, grafts are done mostly on granulated wounds where hypertrophy and contracture develops long before healing process is complete or wound being grafted. Because of infection graft take is not 100% and many need second grafting of the wounds heal by secondary intension. Early splinting and post operative scar management is also absent.

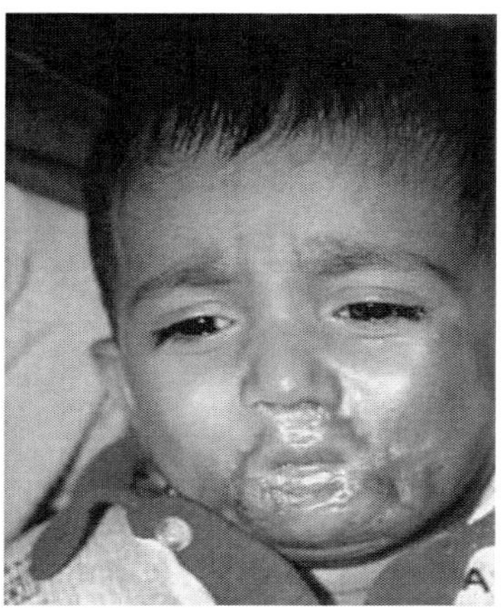

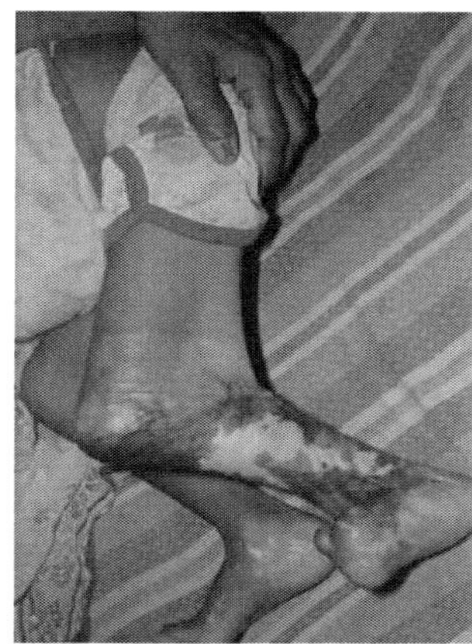

Figure 6. Severe post burn scar deformity.

They cannot afford splints and pressure garments and there is also poor compliance and ignorance. The unit has only one therapist. Early excision cannot be done because of lack of ICU facilities, unavailability of blood, and huge number of patients.

2) In a large number of cases scar contracture develops particularly in limbs. However contracture also develops in trunks hampering the curvature of the vertebral column resulting in kyphosis, chest case deformity thus hampering normal developments of the body. Permanent bone and joint changes occur in long run. Because of large bur areas and scaring of the possible donor areas make the subsequent reconstruction difficult because of scarcity of donor site.
3) Social withdrawal is another phenomenon frequently observed. Because of the change in appearance other children fear or do not want to play with a burnt child. The child usually the older ones do not want to go outside for play. They loose school either temporarily because of the long hospital stay and subsequent social adjustment delay and many never return to school because they cannot overcome the barriers.
4) Loss of marriagebility is a great issue particularly for girls [2]. Girls who got burn in their early ages cannot get married either because of the deformity or scaring. Hypo pigmentation of skin developing after burn is a get barrier for marriage here as society thinks it as a curse and might run in the family in the subsequent generation. Girls with chest wall burns loss nipple areola complex and best do not develop subsequently. This is also a barrier for getting marriage.
5) Lot of children particularly those sustaining electric injuries need amputation. With multiple limb amputation the children become dependent on others or wheel chair bound. Functional artificial limbs are not available in the country and people cannot afford to import it. Badly burnt hands and foots particularly after ash burn result in permanent physical disability.

6) Mothers are often blamed for the accident in children resulting in family disharmony and in extreme case lead to divorce between parents.
7) Long term effect of psychological development is seen commonly. Children suffer anxiety attack, the older children get depressed. Some children specially after being tortured have profound impact of the incidences in their mind needing psychiatric consultations. Some of the children were mentally handicapped before being burnt intentionally.
8) Developmental defects seen in cases of burn in early age. In case of limbs, muscle atrophy results because of disuse. Joints change permanently because of prolong abnormal position. Breast development is frequently absent in case of girls having a chest wall burn.
9) Mortality is also high. High percentage of burns, lack of first aid, inadequacy of early fluid resuscitation, lack of early surgery , lack of medical support and cross infection are the main causes of high mortality in the unit.

Discussion

Management Strategies and Recommendations

1) Prevention: Approximate 1.6 million burns a year cannot be treated properly in Bangladesh at any point of time. A few surgeons at the Dhaka city are able to manage burn. In rest of the country burn being treated by general surgeons, general practitioners and even by unqualified quacks. Prevention is a must. A campaign must be launched incorporating electronic and print media, students, fire fighters, police, community workers and most importantly the burn victims to create awareness among the people in the country. Safety legislation which is now absent should be implemented. Some preventive strategies could be incorporated in the text book for children and should be thought at school. Houses should be made safe for children. Kitchen can have barrier for children. Other methods can be devised for safe kitchen. All electric wiring and appliances should be safe and out of reach of children. Violence should be stopped through education and legislation.
2) A large epidemiological study of burn injury in the country to can be done know accurate number, causes, nature and extent of burn injury along with mortality and morbidity. The results of the study would help development of a prevention program directed at children and young adults. The long-term goal of the project would be reducing number of burns in the country and morbidity and mortality related to the accident.
3) Establishing burn centres in different districts of the country. For the initial period there should be a burn unit in each six divisional towns. At present there is not enough manpower to run those units. Even the burn unit in Dhaka is not fully equipped and there is lack of trained doctors nurses and other staffs. There should be a strategy for developing manpower along with infrastructure development. Most case burn treatment is non-rewarding. There should be incentives and encouragements for people who deals burns in those units.

4) In the present burn unit facilities for early wound coverage should be established. It needs equipments and manpower for that. Proper planning and organization of the unit is also necessary.
5) Outcome of the burn in the unit in physical, psychological and social terms should be assed. The care should be up to rehabilitation of all burn survivors in course of time. Legal support should be provided in cases of non accidental injuries.

CONCLUSION

Mortality and morbidity related with burn are declining in advanced countries where as 90 per cent of burn deaths occur in lower and middle income countries where prevention programs are uncommon and quality of care is not appropriate [3]. Bangladesh falls in lower income countries and as stated there is no prevention program and quality of care of burn patients are very poor.

Scalds are the commonest thermal injury in children [4]. Differences between accidental and intentional scalds are challenging. Our experience found that children sustain more flame burn than scalds when we consider the major burns only. Where as in cases of minor injuries scalds are common. Both accidental and non accidental burns are found. In many case non accidental nature of burn can be determined by its clinical picture but many times it is not possible as children cannot narrate the mechanism.

A framework of presentation program using low cost local resources for example a mud barrier built around the cooking area found successful in reducing accidental burn among children in rural Bangladesh [5]. It was a small scale intervention. A large scale intervention using local resources would be possible if the program is designed appropriately incorporating all level of community participation.

REFERENCES

[1] Mashreky. SR; Rahman, A; Chowdhury, SM; Giasuddin, S; SvanstrOm, L; Linnan, M; Shafinaz, S; Uha, IJ; Rahman, F. Epidemiology of childhood burns: Yield of largest community based injury survey in Bangladesh. *Burns*, 2008, 34, 856-862

[2] Bari, SM; Chowdhury, M; Mahmud, I. Acid Burn in Bangladesh, *Ann Burns Fire Diseaster*, 14, (2002) 115-118.

[3] Michael, D Peck. Epidemiology of burns throughout the world. Part I: Distribution and risk factors. *Burns*, 37, (2011), 1087-1100

[4] Maguire, S; Moynihan, S; Mann, M; Potakar, T; Kemp, AM. A systemic review of the features that Indicate intentional scalds in Children. *Burns*, 34, (2008), 1072-1081.

[5] Mashreky, SR; Rahman, A; SvansrrOm, L; Linnan, MJ; Shafinaz, S; Rahman, F. Experience from community based childhood burn prevention program in Bangladesh: Implication for low resource setting. *Burns*, xxx, (2011), xxx-xxx.

In: Encyclopedia of Dermatology (6 Volume Set)
Editor: Meghan Pratt
ISBN: 978-1-63483-326-4

Chapter 78

MULLIGAN'S MOBILISATIONS WITH MOVEMENT: A MANUAL THERAPY APPROACH TO THE REATMENT AND MANAGEMENT OF HAND BURN INJURIES

***Natalia Montes Carrasco*[1], *Maria Jesús Trancón Bergas*[1], *Carmen Oreja Sánchez*[1], *Maria Virginia Vicente Blanco*[1] and *Javier Nieto Blasco*[2]**

[1]Physiotherapist of Department of Rehabilitation
University Hospital of Salamanca, Salamanca, Spain
[2]M.D. Department of Physical Medicine and Rehabilitation.
University Hospital of Salamanca, Salamanca, Spain

ABSTRACT

Despite advances in complication management, hand burn patients suffer severe long term effects. These injuries limit performance in activities of daily living (ADLs), and have a significant impact both on the patients' psychological well-being and on their working lives, with a resulting decline in quality of life.

Burns in functional areas, as in the case of hand burns, are more difficult to treat, and more likely to present sequelae, such as hypertrophic or shrink scars and joint deformities. Pain is considered one of the most important problems arising from burn injuries. A high percentage of patients report that chronic post burn pain interferes in their daily lives and in their recovery, and physiotherapy is considered one of the factors that increase the pain.

The physiotherapy objectives are to minimize the adverse effects caused by burn injuries, mainly aimed at reducing pain, increasing the range of motion and restoring function. A range of techniques are employed to this end, such as kinesitherapy, scar massage and splinting.

From a Manual Therapy (MT) approach, Mulligan's mobilisations with movement (MWM) technique is proposed as a tool for addressing various pathologies involving pain and / or limitation of motion in peripheral joints. This technique involves the therapist sustaining pressure on the affected joint using an accessory glide, while the patient simultaneously performs the previously painful movement.

In MWM, the absence of pain during the technique application is top priority. The technique is indicated if, during application, there is a reduction in pain and improvement in function of at least 50%. This technique's active mechanism may be the activation of the descending pain inhibitory pathways or the correction of a joint positional fault.

The effectiveness of MWM in the treatment of hand burns has recently been described. The patient showed severe pain in the metacarpophalangeal and interphalangeal flexion of both hands, with limited mobility and functional deficit. Mulligan technique was performed in the affected joints and, following a low number of sessions, the patient performed full flexion with minimal pain, with subsequent functional improvement. Thus, if the treatment response is correct, the MWM technique is suggested as an alternative in the treatment of patients with burns to the hands, although we note that future studies are required to assess its effectiveness in hand burn patients with painful joint limitation.

INTRODUCTION

Despite advances in complication management, hand burn patients suffer severe long-term effects. These injuries limit performance in activities of daily living (ADLs), and have a significant impact both on the patients' psychological well-being and on their working lives, with a resulting decline in quality of life. Additionally, management in both acute phase and long term rehabilitation comes at a great cost, both economically and to the patients' health.

Approximately 1% of the world's population suffers burns each year [1], with an incidence of 60-80% in the hands [2, 3]. The dorsum of the hand and fingers is the worst affected area [4]. Though the hand constitutes only 2-3% of total body surface area (TBSA) and does not play an important role in survival, a hand burn is classified as major injury by the American Burn Association, as it leads to a loss of 57% of the individual's total independent function [5, 6]. ADLs are affected in 76% of patients [7], due to the reduced grip strength and pinch performance caused by burns and resulting deformities [8]. Most patients, after appropriate management and treatment of these burns, reach a sufficient degree of independence in self-care and mobility one year after the injury [8]. Post-burn professional activity and participation is similarly defined. These are reduced in more than half of cases [7], limiting social and work reintegration [4, 9-11]. Following a hand burn, only 54% of patients who were working at the time of the injury return to the workplace within six months, while 64% resumed their professional activity after twelve months [3].

Patients with hand burn injuries experience a 68% decline in dominant hand function and 65% in the non-dominant hand [12]. Therefore the top priority of the recovery process should always be the restoration of function, due to its high professional, economic, social and aesthetic impact [5, 6, 12].

PATHOPHYSIOLOGY

Modern advances in burn patient management and improved survival rates have created the need for an in-depth understanding of the pathophysiological changes that occur in patients following a severe burn, with the aim to palliate or prevent these injuries and restore normal physiological function [13].

A high inflammatory response is produced after a burn and a number of metabolic disorders appear in two stages. During the acute phase, spanning the first 24-48 hours, an initial reduction of metabolism occurs [14, 15]. This is followed by a second "flow phase" characterised by a hypermetabolic state, an increase in energy expenditure [13, 16, 17] and catabolic rate that can lead to physiological exhaustion [14, 15, 17, 18]. This increased metabolism affects the vast majority of the body's systems and can last up to 36 months after injury, even after wounds have completely healed [14-16, 18-20].

Among the various burn-induced pathophysiological changes, the release of catecholamines and various cytokines secondary to systemic inflammatory response [13, 15, 21, 22], combined with adrenergic stimulation, alters the kinetics of numerous metabolic substrates [13, 16, 18- 20].

One particularly important alteration in the metabolic cycles is the increase in the rate of protein breakdown in skeletal muscle, thereby increasing the intracellular availability of amino acids within the muscle [13-16, 18-20, 23]. These amino acids are used in wound healing or scarring [13-16, 18-20, 23] and in the synthesis of the proteins involved in immune function [16]. This increased catabolism causes excessive loss of protein which, coupled with high levels of cytokines, leads to rapid degradation and muscle atrophy [8, 16, 18-20].

The loss of muscle mass results in a loss of lean body mass and bone mineral density, which increases the risk of infection, impairs wound healing, affects survival outcome and limits participation in a subsequent rehabilitation program [13-18, 22].

These alterations, in burn patients, may adversely affect the function and range of motion (ROM). This can further lead to the onset of contractures or restrictions in movement [20] and interfere with the rehabilitation program [14-18], prolonging hospital stay and increasing the risk of mortality [20, 22].

In addition, burns can cause alterations of nerve structures in the burned area. The injury of peripheral nociceptors, followed by disorganised growth and healing, transforms the nervous system. This produces a state of chronic pain [24], which may be accompanied by cutaneous sensory abnormalities [25]. This alteration of the nerve fibre is of interest, not only due to the presence of pain, but also due to the rapid loss of muscle mass and strength to which skeletal muscle denervation may lead [22].

Metabolic disorders such as hypermetabolism, and inflammatory response as well as the loss of muscle mass and bone density, are considered a major cause of both short and long term morbidity and mortality in burn patients [14].

COMPLICATIONS

Burns in functional areas such as hands, face or perineum are more difficult to treat and more prone to dysfunction and sequelae [26].

Among the most common complications that may appear on the hands are the postburn scars [7]. Scar development is associated with the severity, depth and extent of the burn [27, 28], as well as with the re-epithelialisation time [27]. As the hands are a very visible part of the body during daily interaction, the aesthetic outcome influences the perception of good treatment outcome and quality of life [4, 9-11].

This cosmetic factor is associated with an increased nociceptive nerve fibre density in both scars and in normal skin, inducing chronic scar pain, which may be a generalised phenomenon among those affected [24].

Delay in wound healing is a significant risk factor for the development of hypertrophic scars (32% - 67% prevalence) and / or shrink scars [27, 29, 30], caused by the presence of myofibroblasts in the scar tissue [27]. The location of these scars in the vicinity of a joint or skin fold favours the appearance of deformities and functional limitations [31], as the replacement of flexible skin by inelastic scar tissue produces a joint range limitation [28]. The hand ranks third most common place on the body for postburn scarring [7], with especially frequent contractures in the palm, fingers and interdigital spaces [10].

Other complications that may limit the ROM are skin adhesions [32] or muscle, tendon and ligament shortening [33].

Scarring, together with the inflammatory process and the reduced ROM, can lead to severe joint deformities such as claw-hand, Boutonnière deformity, and thumb adduction [31, 33]. Flexion contracture of fingers is one of the most serious consequences of hand burns [35].

Another common complication is the apparition of burn oedema, which can cause compartment syndrome [36] and even lead to amputation, mainly of the fingers [3].

To prevent aesthetic and functional sequelae, early surgical intervention is essential [37]. Reconstruction is required, comprising skin grafting with cutaneous, fasciocutaneous, muscle or myocutaneous skin flaps [38]. Among the most common surgical techniques used for treating hand burns are sheet grafts [39] and angioplasty by transversal or cross incision to correct neosyndactyly [40].

Pain, both acute and chronic, is considered one of the most important problems arising from burn injuries. The incidence of posttraumatic stress disorder (PTSD) in burn patients is high, correlating, not with the severity of the burns, but with the pain scores shortly after injury [24]. Therefore, post burn pain control is a key part of the comprehensive approach to treatment of burn injuries [31, 41]. A high percentage of patients (45%) claim that chronic post burn pain interferes in their daily lives, while 66% report that it hinders their recovery. Physiotherapy is considered one of the factors that increase the pain [42]. The pain experienced by patients with burns during treatment sessions can be extreme and may discourage them from adhering to their therapy [41, 43, 44]. Treatment is required to prevent possible contractures or joint limitations [41]. Therefore, pain control is necessary to guarantee the patient's recovery, encouraging collaboration and tolerance to the various procedures undertaken during the treatment process [31, 41, 43]. This is done using techniques designed to modulate, inhibit or modify nociceptive signals in the spinal cord, which serves as a gate for controlling the intensity of pain signals sent to the brain [31].

Treatment Methods

Rehabilitation is an essential and integral part of burn treatment. It aims to minimise the adverse effects caused by burns in order to maintain ROM, to attenuate contracture development and the impact of scarring, and to maximise functional ability, all of which will improve the patient's psychological wellbeing and social integration [45].

Patients with burns to the hands require physiotherapy from the early stages of wound management, as finger and thumb joints are very sensitive and the ROM can be lost rapidly [46]. The hand is considered to be functional if it maintains a minimum total active range of motion (TAROM) of 220 degrees, of the normal 270; taking into account that the TAROM in the burned hand is the sum of the degree of active flexion at each finger joint, minus the sum of the extension lag at each joint [31].

Several techniques are used to achieve this functional TAROM, such as splinting which is used after skin graft on partial and complete thickness burns to prevent deformities and maintain function [7]. Following physiotherapy, splints are frequently used in static, static progressive or dynamic form, to lengthen tissue and subsequently increase ROM [7]. Splints are also used for the treatment of post-burn scars [7].

Kinesitherapy is one of the most commonly used treatment techniques. Its goals are to increase muscle strength and endurance, reduce oedema or treat and prevent deformities [7]. Passive mobilisation is mainly used in the operating room to assess potential tissue shortening and achieve full painless elongation of the various structures [7]. Active mobilisation of isolated joints is used to prevent joint stiffness. Similarly, active mobilisation of a segment as a whole is used to achieve maximum tissue elongation and to prevent scar contractures [7].

Kinesitherapy in patients with partial thickness hand burns should be active, focusing on flexion-extension movements of each digit, as this is more beneficial than passive kinesitherapy [7]. In deep burns where the extensor tendons are more brittle, full flexion is avoided due to risk of tendon damage. The technique utilises isolated metacarpophalangeal joint flexion exercises, performed actively or passively, combined with interphalangeal extension. Finger abduction and adduction, in addition to maintaining ROM, reduce swelling through dorsal and palmar interosseous muscle contraction [7]. Oedema control in the hand should be a priority in order to minimise stiffness in soft tissue, as well as loss of tendon gliding and joint mobility [7]. Due to its multiple joints, the hand is more susceptible to hypertrophic scar deformities [7]. A variety of treatment techniques, such as acupressure, are used in hypertrophic scar prevention [31]. When applied to hands and fingers in the acute phase, acupressure helps initial scar management, acting on the collagen fibres. During intermediate stages and long-term treatment, it is used to minimise scar hypertrophy [7].

Massage therapy is another technique used in the treatment of postburn scars. Its application encompasses the control of pain and sensory abnormalities, enabling a greater mobility of the scar during exercise and facilitating functional improvement [7, 31].

Pain control plays an important role in burn treatment as it can affect sleep, work and social activities as well as interfere with the therapeutic process. Pain fluctuates widely in intensity over the course of the recovery process, even in an individual patient [41, 43, 47]. Besides the actual burn nociceptive factors, various psychological factors, such as prior experience, anxiety, understanding of pain or focus of attention, influence the pain experience [41, 43]. Therefore, it is essential to avoid increasing the intensity of perceived pain during the necessary therapeutic procedures, through the use of either a pain-free approach or distraction techniques [41]. Immersion in virtual reality (VR) is used during burn rehabilitation as non-pharmacological analgesic adjuvant, resulting in a reduction in pain by more than 50%. Hoffman et al. showed that the repeated use of VR achieved an attenuation in pain, demonstrating that VR immersion technology significantly reduced pain-related activity in the brain [31]. Interactive video game use also causes a reduction in pain, and simultaneously facilitates an increase in ROM [48, 49].

Mulligan's Mobilisations with Movement (MWM): A Manual Therapy Technique

From a Manual Therapy (MT) approach, Mulligan's mobilisations with movement (MWM) technique is proposed as a tool for addressing various pathologies involving pain and / or limitation of ROM in peripheral joints. This technique involves the therapist sustaining pressure on the affected joint using an accessory glide, while the patient simultaneously performs the previously painful movement [50]. The technique is indicated if there is a reduction in pain and improvement in function of at least 50% during application [51].

In MWM, the total absence of pain during technique application is top priority. If the patient complains of pain during the performance of active movement, the treatment plane or grade of movement should be modified, until the motion is once more painless [50]. Application of this technique should be discontinued if pain persists [52].

For application at interphalangeal and metacarpophalangeal joints, the proximal end of the joint is stabilised, while the accessory glide is induced in the distal. This is carried out in translation and / or rotation, which allows the patient to perform a pain-free flexion or extension movement.

The protocol established for conducting the Mulligan technique on the peripheral joints, upon selection of the accessory movement, is at most 3 sets of 10 repetitions [50].

Regarding the application of this technique in the hand, Mulligan published the case of a patient with a fracture of the fifth metacarpal, who complained of pain on flexion of the joint. After just a few sessions, this patient experienced pain-free active mobilization [50]. Other authors have shown clinical success of this technique in the treatment of various musculoskeletal disorders of the hand [53], such as traumatic subluxation of the thumb [54].

The inicial effects of the Mulligan technique on joint ROM and pressure pain threshold (PPT) have been analysed in patients with painful limitation of shoulder movement. A randomised controlled trial has produced results which indicate an immediate positive effect on both pain and ROM [55]. In shoulder impingement syndrome, MWM, on a par with glenohumeral joint mobilisation, is the technique which produced the greatest score changes in pain scales analysed. The Mulligan technique also produced the greatest increase in joint ROM, with a high level of significance. MWM has the benefit of performance on all planes of movement, which provides an additional proprioceptive stimulus to the tissue, through the activation of the Golgi tendon organ in response to tendon stretch as well as to capsule and glenohumeral ligament stretch [56]. Similarly the effect of MWM with or without taping is being investigated in patients with shoulder pain induced by multiple causes which causes joint limitation. Both interventions improve ROM, an outcome which is maintained in the longer term with the application of tape. However, no difference in pain measures is found between groups analysed at different times [57]. Kachingwe A. F et al. suggest that the increased mobility at the glenohumeral joint is produced by a reduction in pain due to the activation of mechanoreceptors. This would cause inhibition of nociceptive stimuli through gate-control, or by facilitating synovial circulation. Other factors that allow this improved ROM may be related to capsular stretch or arthrokinetic regulation of the glenohumeral joint [56]. The effect of MWM on patients with recurrent ankle sprain injury has been studied, finding improvements in weight-bearing dorsiflexion, by analysing the differences between the performance of the technique in weight-bearing and non-weight-bearing [58].

The initial effects of the Mulligan technique on a sample of subjects with subacute ankle sprain has also been studied. This study combined a relative posteroanterior glide of the tibia on talus with an active ankle dorsiflexion, preferably in weight bearing. A significant increase in mobility is produced. However, no variation of the thermal or mechanical threshold is experienced. These results indicate that the MWM treatment for ankle dorsiflexion has a mechanical rather than hypoalgesic effect [59].

The initial effect of Mulligan's lateral glide technique in patients with epicondylalgia has also been investigated. Following application of the technique, Vicenzino et al. found an increase both in pressure pain threshold (10%) and pain-free grip strength [60]. Other studies have described similar motor effects [61].

A laboratory study was performed to evaluate the effects of lateral glide-MWM in healthy subjects with experimentally induced lateral epicondylalgia [62]. The application of the technique does not cause an increase in strength or significant analgesia in these patients, in contrast to the benefits of the application of the technique in patients with clinical epicondylalgia [60]. These unexpected results may be explained by the fact that the technique is more effective in patients with chronic manifestations than in patients with acute pain, or the effect may insufficient to modulate induced deep tissue pain. Nor was an increase in motor strength produced; this absence may be interpreted as a limited effect for the technique in musculoskeletal pain conditions associated with partial myotendinous disruption [62].

Different theories exist to account for the effects of the mobilisation with movement technique. According to Mulligan, the joint dysfunction or failure is caused by a positional fault, or a chronic situation of joint misalignment. The positional fault occurs due to changes in joint congruency, damage to cartilage or alteration of ligamentous, capsular or myotendinous fibres. This change could result in an alteration in the traction direction of these structures [63]. The technique would bring about the correct alignment of the joint or of its traction mechanisms [50].

With the aim to evaluate the positional fault theory, Hsieh et al. present the case of a patient with a seven month long pain in the right thumb, following a fall in which the finger experienced forced abduction. Joint alignment is examined using magnetic resonance imaging (MRI) prior to treatment. Both the first metacarpal and the proximal phalanx are found to have a greater degree of pronation than in the left hand. The image taken during the application of the technique shows an in-situ position of positional fault correction. Upon completion of treatment a new MR image shows no change to the initial positional fault, although the patient no longer experiences pain with movement [64]. This indicates that although the MWM technique may modify the positional fault during its application resulting in initial effects, the long-term effects should be attributed to other mechanisms.

Several laboratory studies have described the characteristics of the hypoalgesic effect of the lateral glide-MWM in epicondylalgia. Upon application of the technique, a decrease in pressure pain threshold, but not in thermal threshold, is produced [65]. This selective modulation is accompanied by signs of sympathetic nervous system activation; an increase in heart rate and blood pressure, as well as modifications in vasomotor function and sweating, with an increase in temperature of the skin, blood flow and conductance are observed [66]. These findings are consistent with outcomes of analysis of the analgesic effect produced in manipulation of animal subjects. Skyba et al. [67] have found that, following manipulation, an increase is produced in mechanical withdrawal threshold in rat ankle, which has had an experimental pain model induced by capsaicin injection into the joint.

Spinal blockade of several receptors indicates that manipulation activates pain-inhibitory serotonergic and noradrenergic mechanisms. These findings on the effects of manual therapy are consistent with those found by Sluka and Wright [68] where manipulation of the knee results in a reduction of capsaicin induced hyperalgesia.

Similarly, Paugmali et al. have analysed the effect of lateral MWM on the elbow joint in patients with epicondylalgia. Their findings show that the initial hypoalgesic effect is not antagonised by naloxone [65] and repeated application of the technique does not develop tolerance [69]. These data, together with the improvement of motor function, may indicate the relationship between the effects of MWM and the descending pain inhibitory system (DPIS) [60, 69], by activating non-opioid pain relief mechanisms and possibly noradrenergic mechanisms [70].

Regarding patients with burn injuries, Montes et al. have described the case of a patient with burns in both hands, treated using Mulligan technique. The patient had burns in 21% TBSA, affecting 2% of the surface area of each hand. Surgical treatment consisted in laminar autograft on the dorsum of both hands and fingers [71].

Upon initial examination, scars were observed on both upper limbs in relation to the grafts, as well as a shrink scar on the ventral surface of the left wrist due to compartment syndrome surgery. A pain-induced mobility limitation in active flexion of the metacarpophalangeal and interphalangeal joints, with a value of 9 in the Visual Analogue Scale (VAS) was revealed. The pain increased with passive flexion, impeding full joint ROM assessment. The overall joint ROM in the right hand was 148 degrees and left hand 108 degrees. This limitation results in a severe functional deficit, yielding a score of 80.8% in the Spanish adaptation of the Disabilities of the Arm, Shoulder and Hand Outcome Questionnaire (DASHe) [71].

The authors describe the treatment protocol followed in the application of the Mulligan technique. The accessory mobilisations sustained are medial and lateral rotation, medial and lateral glide and caudal glide. The parameters vary from session to session in the same joint. These accessory mobilisations allow the patient to achieve full pain-free flexion [71].

Pain evolution is analysed; following the third session, there is a 5-point reduction in VAS, and by the tenth session a score of 1 on the pain scale is reached. Regarding ROM limitation, the patient performs active digital palmar grip following the tenth session. With respect to function, an improvement of 40% is observed in the first assessment, reducing functional deficits to 20% after ten sessions. These effects are maintained long term, having increased functional ability, obtaining a minimum score of 9% on the DASHe Questionnaire [71]. This study demonstrates the clinical usefulness of applying MWM in a patient with burns on both hands, and how these effects are maintained over time. Furthermore, a rapid improvement in the range of flexion of all fingers is produced, as is a significant decline in pain, resulting in a reduction in the degree of functional impairment [71].

Conclusion

Biomechanical theory considers that the positional fault which originates after injury results in a restriction of movement and / or pain, and that this positional fault may be corrected through the use of Mulligan technique [50].

MWM also appears to have a neurophysiological effect, activating the descending pain inhibitory pathways, which originate in the central nervous system [69, 72].

In the hand burn case described, the variability of the parameters used in the accessory glides may indicate that the improvement is due to the reduction of a complex positional fault. Alternatively it may be due to the pain modulation induced by activation of endogenous inhibitory pain mechanisms [71]. The mechanisms by which the MWM act on pain are likely to be multifactorial, and further study of these mechanisms and their effects is required.

The benefit of Mulligan's mobilisations with movement technique is that accessory glides allow pain-free movement and limitation in joint range of motion is rapidly reduced. In addition to the absence of pain during movement, treatment response is immediate and outcomes are maintained in the long term. Mulligan suggests that failure to obtain pain-free active movement indicates that the therapist has not found the correct accessory glide plane, or grade of mobilisation, or that this technique is not indicated in this case and therefore should not be used as treatment [50].

Thus, providing the treatment response is correct, the MWM technique is suggested as an alternative in the treatment of patients with burns to the hands, although we note that future studies are required to assess its effectiveness in hand burn patients with painful joint limitation.

Acknowledgments

Thanks are due to Dr. Angel Hernandez for his selfless help and patience, and to Elizabeth Nestor for her linguistic assistance.

References

[1] González-Cavero, J., Arévalo, J. M., Lorente, J. A. Traslado secundario del paciente quemado crítico. *Emergencias*. 2000; 12:340-4.

[2] Kamolz, L. P., Kitzinger, H. B., Karle, B., Frey, M. The treatment of hand burns. *Burns*. 2009; 35 (3):327-37.

[3] Klein, M. B., Lezotte, D. L., Fauerbach, J. A., Herndon, D. N., Kowalske, K. J., Carrougher, G. J., et al. The national institute on disability and rehabilitation Research burn model system database: a tool for the Multicenter study of the outcome of burn injury. *J. Burn Care Res*. 2007; 28(1):84-96.

[4] Cartotto, R. The burned hand: optimizing long-term outcomes with a standardized approach to acute and subacute care. *Clin. Plast. Surg*. 2005; 32(4):515-27.

[5] McCauley, R. L. Reconstruction of the pediatric burned hand. *Hand Clin*. 2009; 25(4): 543-50.

[6] Siemers, F., Mailänder, P. Treatment of hand burns. *Der Unfallchirurg*. 2009; 112 (6): 558-64.

[7] Merilyn, L., Moore, M. L., Dewey, W. S., Richard, R. L. Rehabilitation of the burned hand. *Hand Clin*. 2009; 25(4): 529–541.

[8] Baker, C. P., Russell, W. J., Meyer, W. 3rd, Blakeney, P. Physical and psychologic rehabilitation outcomes for young adults burned as children. *Arch. Phys. Med. Rehabil.* 2007; 88(12 Suppl. 2):S57-64.

[9] Pallua, N., Künsebeck, H. W., Noah, E. M. Psychosocial adjustments 5 years after burn injury. *Burns*. 2003; 29(2):143-52.

[10] Ulkür, E., Uygur, F., Karagöz, H., Celiköz, B. Flap choices to treat complex severe postburn hand contracture. *Ann. Plas. Surg*. 2007; 58(5):479-83.

[11] Ulkür, E., Acikel, C., Karagoz, H., Celikoz, B. Treatment of severely contracted fingers with combined use of cross-finger and side finger transposition flaps. *Plast. Reconstr. Surg*. 2005; 116(6):1709-14.

[12] Mohammadi, A. A., Bakhshaeekia, A. R., Marzban, S., Abbasi, S., Ashraf, A. R., Mohammadi, M. K., et al. Early excision and skin grafting versus delayed skin grafting in deep hand burns (a randomized clinical controlled trial). *Burns* 2011; 37(1):36-41.

[13] Porter, C., Herndon, D. N., Sidossis, L. S., Borsheim, E. The impact of severe burns on skeletal muscle mitochondrial function. *Burns*. 2013; 39(6):1039-47.

[14] Pedroso, F. E., Spalding, P. B., Cheung, M. C., Yang, R., Gutierrez, J. C., Bonneto, A., et al. Inflammation, organomegaly, and muscle wasting despite hyperphagia in a mouse model of burn cachexia. *J. Cachexia Sarcopenia Muscle*. 2012; 3(3):199-211.

[15] Merrit, E. K., Cross, J. M., Bamman, M. M. Inflammatory and protein metabolism signaling responses in human skeletal muscle after burn injury. *J. Burn. Care Res*. 2012; 33(2):291-7.

[16] Borsheim, E., Chinkes, D. L., McEntire, S. J., Rodriguez, N. R., Herndon, D. N., Suman, O. E. Whole body protein kinetics measured with a non-invasive method in severely burned children. *Burns*. 2010; 36(7):1006-12.

[17] Gore, D. C., Chinkes, D. L., Hart, D. W., Wolf, S. E., Herndon, D. N., Sanford, A. P. Hyperglycemia exacerbates muscle protein catabolism in burn-injured patients. *Crit. Care Med.* 2002;30(11):2438-42.

[18] Hart, D. W., Wolf, S. E., Mlcak, R., Chinkes, D. L., Ramzy, P. I., Obeng, M. K., et al. Persistence of muscle catabolism after severe burn. *Surgery*. 2000; 128(2):312-9.

[19] Branski, L. K., Herndon, D. N., Pereira, C., Micak, R. P., Celis, M. M., Lee, J. O., et al. Longitudinal assessment of Integra in primary burn management: a randomized pediatric clinical trial. *Crit. Care Med*. 2007; 35(11):2615-23.

[20] Yasuhara, S., Perez, M. E., Kanakubo, E., Yasuhara, Y., Shin, Y. S., Kanki, M., et al. Skeletal muscle apoptosis after burns is associated with activation of proapoptotic signals. *Am. J. Physiol-Endoc. M*. 2000; 279(5):E1114-21.

[21] Natale, V. M., Brenner, I. K., Moldoveanu, A. I., Vasiliou, P., Shek, P., Shephard, R. J. Effects of three different types of exercise on blood leukocyte count during and following exercise. *Sao Paulo Med. J.* 2003; 121(1):9-14.

[22] Lych, G. S., Schertzer, J. D., Ryall, J. G. Therapeutic approaches for muscle wasting disorders. *Pharmacol. Therapeut*. 2007; 113(3):461-87.

[23] Martyn, J. A., Fagerlund, M. J., Eriksson, L. I. Basic principles of neuromuscular transmission. *Anaesthesia*.2009; 64(Suppl. 1):1-9.

[24] Wolf, S. E., Arnoldo, B. D. The year in burns 2011. Published by Elsevier Ltd and ISBI. *Burns*. 2012; 38:1096-1108.

[25] Holavanahalli, R. K., Helm, P. A., Kowalske, K. J. Long-term outcomes in patients surviving large burns: the skin. *J. Burn. Care Res*. 2010; 31 (4): 631-9.

[26] De los Santos, C. Abordaje sencillo de las quemaduras [monografía en internet]. Republica Dominicana: monografias. com; 2003 [consultado 10 Ago 2013]. Disponible en: http://www.monografias.com.

[27] Wang, X. Q., Kravchuck, O., Winterford, C., Kimble, R. M. The correlation of in vivo burn scar contraction with the level of α-smooth muscle actin expression. *Burns*. 2011; 37(8):1367-77.

[28] Richard, R. L., Lester, M. E., Miller, S. F., Bailey, J. K., Hedman, T. L., Dewey, W. S., et al. Identification of cutaneous functional units related to burn scar contracture development. *J. Burn Care Res*. 2009; 30(4):625-31.

[29] El-Ghalbzouri, A., Van Den Bogaerdt, A. J., Kempenaar, J., Ponec, M. Human adipose tissue-derived cells delay re-epithelialization in comparison with skin fibroblasts in organotypic skin culture. *Br. J. Dermatol*. 2004; 150 (3):444-54.

[30] Li, X., Liang, D., Liu, X. Compartment syndrome in burn patients. A report of five cases. *Burns* 2002; 28(8):787-9.

[31] Esselman, P. C., Thombs, B. D., Magyar-Russell, G., Fauerbach, J. A. Burn rehabilitation. State of the science. *Am. J. Phys. Med. Rehabil*. 2006; 85:383–413.

[32] Fergason, J. R., Blanck, R. 14 Prosthetic management of the burn amputation. *Phys. Med. Rehabil. Clin. N. Am*. 2011; 22(2):277-99.

[33] Bláha, J. Permanent sequelae after burns and tested procedures to influence them. *Acta Chir. Plast*. 2001; 43(4):119-31.

[34] Woo, S. H., Seul, J. H. Optimizing the correction of severe postburn hand deformities by using aggressive contracture releases and fasciocutaneous free-tissue transfers. *Plast. Reconstr. Surg*. 2001; 107(1):1-8.

[35] Grishkevich, V. M. Flexion contractures of fingers: contracture elimination with trapeze-flap plasty. *Burns* 2011; 37(1):126-33.

[36] Lowell, M., Pirc, P., Ward, R. S., Lundy, C., Wilhelm, D. A., Reddy, R. Effect of 3M Coban Self-Adherent Wraps on edema and function of the burned hand: a case study. *J. Burn Care Rehabil*. 2003; 24 (4):253-8.

[37] Tambuscio, A., Governa, M., Caputo, G., Barisoni, D. Deep burn of the hands: Early surgical treatment avoids the need for late revisions. *Burns*. 2006; 32(8): 1000-4.

[38] Voulliaume, D., Mojallal, A., Comparin, J. P., Foyatier, J. L. Severe hand burns and flaps: indications. *Ann. Chir. Plast. Esthet*. 2005; 50(4): 314-9.

[39] Demir, E., Rahnama, R., Gazyakan, E., Germann, G., Sauerbier, M. Burned palm reconstruction. Current concepts regarding grafting techniques, sensibility and hand function. *Chirurg*. 2006; 77(4): 367-75.

[40] Emsen, I. M. The cross incision plasty for reconstruction of the burned web space: introduction of an alternative technique for the correction of dorsal and volar neosyndactyly. *J. Burn Care Res*. 2008; 29 (2) 378-85.

[41] Hoffman, H. G., Patterson, D. R., Carrougher, G. J. Use of virtual reality for adjunctive treatment of adult burn pain during physical therapy: a controlled study. *Clin. J. Pain*. 2000; 16(3): 244-50.

[42] Dauber, A., Osgood, F. P., Breslau, A. J., Vernon, H. L., Carr, D. B. Chronic Persistent Pain After Severe Burns: A Survey of 358 Burn Survivors. *Pain Med*. 2002; 3(1):6-17.

[43] Das, D. A., Grimmer, K. A., Sparnon, A. L., McRae, S. E., Thomas, B. H. The efficacy of playing a virtual reality game in modulating pain for children with acute burn injuries: a randomized controlled trial. *BMC Pediatrics*. 2005; 5:1.

[44] Lee, G. K., Suh, K. J., Kang, I. W., Hwang, D. H., Min, S. J., Han, Y. M. MR imaging findings of high-voltage electrical burns in the upper extremities: correlation with angiographic findings. *Acta Radiol*. 2011; 52(2):198-203.

[45] Procter, F. Rehabilitation of the burn patient. *Indian J. Plast. Surg*. 2010; 43: 101-13.

[46] Okhovatian, F., Zoubine, N. A comparison between two burn rehabilitation protocols. *Burns*. 2007; 33(4): 429-34.

[47] Choiniere, M., Melzack, R., Rondeau, J., Girard, N., Paquin, M. J. The pain of burns: characteristics and correlates. *J. Trauma*. 1989; 29(11):1531-9.

[48] Haik, J., Tessone, A., Nota, A., Mendes, D., Raz, L., Goldan, O., et al. The use of video capture virtual reality in burn rehabilitation: the possibilities. *J. Burn Care Res*. 2006; 27(2): 195-7.

[49] Parry, I. S., Bagley, A., Kawada, J., Sen, S., Greenhalgh, D. G., Palmieri, T. L. Commercially available interactive video games in burn rehabilitation: therapeutic potential. *Burns*. 2012; 38(4): 493-500.

[50] Mulligan, B. *Manual Therapy NAGS, SNAGS, MWMs,* etc. 6th ed. Wellington, New Zealand: Plane View Service; 2010.

[51] Mulligan, B. R. Mobilisations with movement (MWM'S). *J. Man. Manip. Ther*. 1993; 1(4):154–6.

[52] Mulligan, B. The painful dysfunctional shoulder: a new treatment approach using mobilisation-with-movement. *New Zealand J. Physiother*. 2003; 31:140–142.

[53] Folk, B. Traumatic thumb injury management using mobilization with movement. *Man. Ther*. 2001; 6: 178-82.

[54] Hsieh, C. Y., Vicenzino, B., Yang, C. H., Hu, M. H., Yang, C. Mulligan's mobilization with movement for the thumb: a single case report using magnetic resonance imaging to evaluate the positional fault hypothesis. *Man. Ther*. 2002; 7:44-49.

[55] Teys, P., Bisset, L., Vicenzino, B. The initial effects of a Mulligan's mobilization with movement technique on range of movement and pressure pain threshold in pain-limited shoulders. *Man. Ther*. 2008; 13(1): 37-42. [Epub. 2006 Oct. 27].

[56] Kachingwe, A. F., Phillips, B., Sletten, E., Plunkett, S. W. Comparison of Manual Therapy Techniques with Therapeutic Exercise in the Treatment of Shoulder Impingement: A Randomized Controlled Pilot Clinical Trial. *J. Man. Manip. Ther*. 2008; 16(4): 238-47.

[57] Teys, P., Bisset, L., Collins, N., Coombes, B., Vicenzino, B. One-week time course of the effects of Mulligan's Mobilisation with Movement and taping in painful shoulders. *Man. Ther*. 2013 Feb. 4 [Epub. ahead of print].

[58] Vicenzino, B., Branjerdporn, M., Teys, P., Jordan, K. Initial changes in posterior talar glide and dorsiflexion of the ankle after mobilization with movement in individuals with recurrent ankle sprain. *J. Orthop. Sports Phys. Ther*. 2006; 36 (7): 464-71.

[59] Collins, N., Teys, P., Vicenzino, B. The initial effects of a Mulligan's mobilization with movement technique on dorsiflexion and pain in subacute ankle sprains. *Man. Ther*. 2004; 9: 77-82.

[60] Vicenzino, B., Paungmali, A., Buratowski, S., Wright, A. Specific manipulative therapy treatment for chronic lateral epicondylalgia produces uniquely characteristic hypoalgesia. *Man. Ther*. 2001; 6:205-12.

[61] Abbott, J. H., Patla, C. E., Jensen, R. H. The initial effects of an elbow mobilization with movement technique on grip strength in subjects with lateral epicondylalgia. *Man. Ther.* 2001; 6:163-9.

[62] Slater, H., Arendt-Nielsen, L., Wright, A., Graven-Nielsen, T. Effects of a manual therapy technique in experimental lateral epicondylalgia. *Man. Ther.* 2006; 11: 107-17.

[63] Mulligan, B. *Manual Therapy NAGS, SNAGS, MWMs*, etc. 5th ed. Wellington, New Zealand: Plane View Services ltd.; 2004.

[64] Hsieh, C. Y., Vicenzino, B., Yang, C. H., Hu, M. H., Yang, C. Mulligan's mobilization with movement for the thumb: a single case report using magnetic resonance imaging to evaluate the positional fault hypothesis. *Man. Ther.* 2002; 7(1): 44-49.

[65] Paungmali, A., O'Leary, S., Souvlis, T., Vicenzino, B. Naloxone fails to antagonize initial hypoalgesic effect of a manual therapy treatment for lateral epicondylalgia. *J. Manipulative Physiol. Ther.* 2004; 27(3): 180-85.

[66] Paungmali, A., O'Leary, S., Souvlis, T., Vicenzino, B. Hypoalgesic and sympatho-excitatory effects of mobilization with movement for lateral epicondylalgia. *Phys. Ther.* 2003a; 83: 374–83.

[67] Skyba, D. A., Radhakrishnan, R., Rohlwing, J. J., Wright, A., Sluka, K. A. Joint manipulation reduces hyperalgesia by activation of monoamine receptors but not opioid or GABA receptors in the spinal cord. *Pain.* 2003; 106:159–68.

[68] Sluka, K. A., Wright, A. Knee joint mobilization reduces secondary mechanical hyperalgesia induced by capsaicin injection into the ankle joint. *Eur. J. Pain.* 2001; 5:81–7.

[69] Paungmali, A., Vicenzino, B., Smith, M. Hypoalgesia induced by elbow manipulation in lateral epicondylalgia does not exhibit tolerance. *J. Pain.* 2003b; 4: 448-54.

[70] Kuraishi, Y., Harada, Y., Aratani, S., Satoh, M., Takagi, H. Separate involvement of the spinal noradrenergic and serotonergic systems in morphine analgesia: the difference in mechanical and thermal algesic tests. *Brain Res.* 1983; 273: 245-52.

[71] Montes, N., Trancón, M. J., Oreja, C., Vicente, M. V. Efectos de la técnica de Mulligan en un paciente quemado. A propósito de un caso. *Rev. Iberoam. Fisioter. Kinesiol.* 2011; 14(02): 90-3.

[72] Sterling, M., Jull, G., Wright, A. Cervical mobilisation: concurrent effects on pain, sympathetic nervous system activity and motor activity. *Manual Therapy.* 2001; 6: 72–81.

In: Encyclopedia of Dermatology (6 Volume Set)
Editor: Meghan Pratt
ISBN: 978-1-63483-326-4

Chapter 79

Epidemiological Characteristics of Burn Injuries

Bishara Atiyeh[1] and Michel Costagliola[2*]
[1]Euro-Mediterranean Council for Burns and Fire Disasters
Annals of Burns and Fire Disasters,
Plastic and Reconstructive Surgery,
American University of Beirut Medical Center,
Beirut, Lebanon
[2]Reconstructive and Aesthetic Surgery
Faculté de Médecine Toulouse-Rangueil, Toulouse, France

Abstract

Although natural disasters cannot be avoided, accidents and in particular accidental burns that are among the most devastating of all injuries, are mostly preventable. Unfortunately, burn injuries continue to be responsible for significant mortality and morbidity worldwide and are the fourth leading cause of death from unintentional injury. Like other injury mechanisms, the prevention of burns requires adequate knowledge of the epidemiological characteristics and associated risk factors. It is hence important to determine its magnitude and determinants and necessary to define clearly, the social, cultural and economic factors, which contribute to burn causation.

Burn epidemiology in developing countries is said to be different from that in the developed world. Moreover, burns in developing countries are much more common than in the USA and Europe or other affluent developed countries, due to poverty, overcrowding, and illiteracy, and are associated with higher mortality rates. Unfortunately, burn injuries in most low and middle-income countries (LMICs) are grossly under-reported and there is a palpable lack of comprehensive data documenting the extent of the burn injuries problem to guide policy makers and medical personnel.

* Michel Costagliola, MD; Emeritus Professor of Plastic, Reconstructive and Aesthetic Surgery; Faculté de Médecine Toulouse-Rangueil. 3 rue du Languedoc 31000 Toulouse, France. e-mail: costagliola.m@wanadoo.fr

The current review highlights the epidemiologic characteristics of burn injuries with special focus on LMICs in which burn injury remains endemic and associated with a high mortality rate.

INTRODUCTION

Burn injuries are among the most devastating of all injuries and represent a diverse and varied challenge to medical and paramedical staff. They are responsible for significant mortality and morbidity worldwide. Apart from high numbers of deaths, the pain, suffering and agony of burn survivors are immeasurable with outcomes spanning the spectrum from physical impairments and disabilities to emotional and mental consequences [1, 2, 3]. The suffering caused by burns is even more tragic as the vast majority of burns occurring in the world are accidental hence so eminently preventable [4, 5, 6, 7, 8]. In order to understand and overcome the challenges in the management and prevention of burns, and in order for the approach to burn prevention be effective in a particular area, a close look at the epidemiology and etiological patterns of burns as well as causal factors involved is required. It is also necessary to understand the local economic constraints and the available health-care infrastructure taking into account the geographical variations and socioeconomic differences in burn epidemiology [3, 9].

Like other injury mechanisms, the prevention of burns requires adequate knowledge of the epidemiological parameters and associated risk factors [1]. With proper identification of the population groups at risk and in presence of adequate material resources necessary to deal with this complex public health problem, improved management and prevention strategies have resulted in important declines in morbidity and mortality in high-income countries (HICs) [7, 9]. Successful community-based prevention programs in countries such as Norway have resulted in a 52% reduction in burn-related hospital admissions [9, 10]. In the United States a 50% decline in burn-related mortality and hospital admissions over a 20 year period could be achieved [9, 11]. While much has been accomplished in many HICs in the areas of primary and secondary prevention of fires and burns due to sustained research on the descriptive epidemiology and risk factors, the same cannot be said of developing or low- and middle-income countries (LMICs) where most of these advances and accomplishments did not occur [7, 12]. Moreover, a sharp contrast is evident when comparing burn related mortality rates in high and low-income countries [9].

WORLDWIDE BURN INCIDENCE AND FIRE INJURIES BURDEN

In 2012, 450,000 patients with burn injuries received medical treatment in the USA with a total population of more than 312 million for an incidence of about 0.15/10,000. 40,000 patients were admitted to hospitals among which 30,000 to specialized hospital burn centers. In the same year, 2,550 patients died from residential fires, 300 from vehicle crash fires, and 550 from other sources (approximately 150 deaths from flame burns or smoke inhalation in non-residential fires, 400 from contact with electricity, scalding liquids or hot objects) [13].

Epidemiologic data of burn admissions to burn centers from 2002 to 2011 demonstrated that males were affected more than twice as females (69% vs 31%). 59% were Caucasians, 19% African-Americans, 15% Hispanics, and 7% of other ethnicities. 44% were admitted due to fire/flame burns, 33% secondary to scalds, 9% contact, 4% electrical, 3% chemical, and 7% due to other causes. 69% of burn injuries occurred at home, 9% were occupational, 7% street/highway, 5% Recreational/Sport, and 10% in other locations. Overall survival rate was 96.1% [13]. Hospital admission of burned patients represent 2.4% of all admitted trauma cases and are responsible for 1.6% of the traumatic deaths. Based on hospital admissions and death registers in the US, burns due to fire and flames are fatal in 6.1%. Scalds and contact burns are fatal in 0.6% [14].

Despite the fact that exact European figures about burn injuries requiring medical attention are still unavailable, and most European countries do not yet have a national registration system of hospitalized patients with severe burn injury, a systematic literature search conducted about burns from 1985 to 2009 revealed an annual severe burns incidence of 0.2 to 2.9/10,000 inhabitants with a decreasing trend in time. Almost 50% of patients were younger than 16 years, and about 60% were male patients. Flames, scalds, and contact burns were the most prevalent causes in the total population, but in children, scalds clearly dominated. Mortality was usually between 1.4% and 18% and is decreasing in time [14].

Unfortunately, burn injuries are much more common in developing countries than in the US and Europe or other affluent developed countries. The exact incidence of burns in developing or LMICs is difficult to determine because of under reporting, inadequate records, and unreliable available data. At present, it can only be estimated. Globally, the incidence of burns severe enough to require medical attention in 2004 was nearly 11 million people and ranked fourth in all injuries [15]. However, the WHO estimates indicate that there were globally more than 7.1 million fire related unintentional burns in 2004 giving an overall incidence rate of 110 per 100,000 per year [16]. A report published in 2010 estimated the worldwide number of patients seeking medical help for burns annually to be 6 million, however, the majority are treated in outpatient clinics [14]. Another report published in 2010 estimated the incidence of burns in the Eastern Mediterranean Region to be 187 per 100,000 per year compared to the lowest estimated incidence in the Americas of 19 and the highest incidence in South East-Asia of 243 per 100,000 per year [16]. Judicious extrapolation suggests that India for example, with a population of over 1 billion, has 700,000-800,000 burn admissions annually. In view of the complexities and high cost of burn care as well as the reported high fire-related burn burden expressed as days lost particularly highest in the South-East Asia region, this high incidence makes burn injuries an endemic health hazard in LMICs [2, 17, 18].

In high-income countries (HIC), the incidence of injuries is decreasing at a slower rate than the incidence of illness. In contradistinction in LMICs, both death and disability from injuries is increasing very rapidly [15]. Globally, 5.8 million people die each year as a result of accidental injuries or intentional violence equivalent to more than nine people dying every minute. This accounts for 10% of the total world's deaths, 32% more than the number of fatalities resulting from malaria, tuberculosis and HIV/AIDS combined [19, 20]. The three leading causes of injury and violence-related deaths are road traffic accidents, falls and suicides, and homicides [19, 20]. Nonetheless, a large number of deaths occur each year from fires alone, with more deaths from scalds, electrical burns, and other forms of burns, for which global data are not available [7]. LMICs are unfortunately disproportionately affected. Across the world, 90 to 95% of the reported 322,000 global fire-related deaths in 2002 occurred in lower middle or low-income countries. Slightly more than 7% occur in high middle-income countries. Only 3% of burn deaths occur in HIC [7, 9, 12, 15]. The WHO Global Burden of disease database has reported an over 10 fold difference between mortality rates in South East Asia and Europe (11.6 vs 0.7 per 100 000 population respectively) [9, 18]. South East Asia alone accounts for just over one-half of the total number of fire-related deaths worldwide with females in this region having the highest fire-related burn mortality rates [7, 12]. Fire injuries related burden in LMICs is compounded by the resulting serious disfigurement and disabilities of survivors that cannot be supported adequately due to lack of sufficient resources and inexistent infrastructures.

Most burn injuries are however minor and do not require special in hospital care. It is reported that among patients treated for burns at emergency departments in the USA only 4% are admitted and only 4% of those are transferred to burn centers [15]. It appears that anywhere from 5 to 16 burn patients per 100,000 population require hospital admission for treatment of their injuries [15]. Similarly, a survey in Ethiopia showed that 1.2% of the population is burned each year. Even though burns were the second most common injury to children under 15 years of age and the annual incidence of burns severe enough to restrict activity for one or more days was 80 per 1000 children, over 80% of these burns occurred at home, and 90% healed without any complications. Only 1% of the burn victims died [15]. During 2003 in Bangladesh, the overall incidence of non-fatal burns was 166 per 100,000, and about 288 per100,000 children suffer moderate to severe burns each year with a mortality rate of 0.6 per 100,000 [15]. Other studies confirm the relative infrequency with which burn patients require hospitalization [16]. Fortunately, the absolute number of emergency department visits for burn has decreased over the last two decades in many high-income countries. A similar trend is being observed in India and elsewhere in LMICs [15, 21, 22].

Global Epidemiology of Burns

Knowledge of burns epidemiology is affected by the sources of data including national and regional public health registries, hospital and/or burn center registries, and community surveys as well as by differences in methodologies and classification systems used [14, 15]. It is reported that developing countries due to high population density, illiteracy, and poverty, have a high incidence of burn injuries, creating a formidable public health problem [17]. In HICs, higher burn injury incidence is associated with a lower standard of life and ethnic minorities [14]. However, published data vary considerably and sometimes are not coherent. Nevertheless, even though epidemiologic parameters vary greatly among different countries and regions depending on local economic and cultural factors, there are still common universal general trends worldwide.

Globally, children, especially those under 5 years of age whose physical abilities, reasoning, and judgment are still developing, are invariably at increased risk for burns and burn related mortality and constitute the highest risk group for burn injuries [1]. Children account for almost half of the population with severe burn injury (40% to 50%) and even more in some countries. Children younger than 5 years account for 50% to 80% of all childhood burns [21]. In LMICs, infants and toddlers from birth through 4 years of age have a disproportionately higher number of burn injuries [12]. In many settings like Brazil, Cote d'Ivoire, and India, this age group was found to account for nearly half of all childhood burns [22]. With an aging population in the Western world, an increasing proportion of elderly is being encountered with severe burns (10% to 16% of the total population with severe burn injury) resulting in an increased mean age of severely burned patients [14].

In several studies, an overall male predominance is described probably because adult burns are often work related [14]. In the pediatric populations, 60% to 65% are boys, but in the elderly population, a female predominance of up to 65% may be found [14]. Many studies, however, based on all age groups report conflicting results regarding gender distribution with considerable variation in gender ratio for differing age groups [12]. In India for example, most domestic burns are sustained by women aged 16–35 years and almost 70% of these injuries are due to the traditional practice of cooking at floor level, or over an open fire, compounded by the wearing of loose fitting clothing made from non-flame retardant fabric [1].

Flames, scalds (including steam), and contact burns are the top three causes of severe burns in most studies [14]. In some studies scalds are more prevalent than flames (up to 63%) [14]. In children presenting in the emergency department, scalds are most common (35% to 80%), followed by contact burns (13% to 47%), and flame burns (2% to 5%) [14]. Children younger than 2 years are at high risk for scalds. While scald injury is more common in early childhood accounting for 60% to 75% of hospitalized patients followed by flame and contact burns, flame injury predominates with increasing age and in some countries can be the most common cause of burn in children 6–17 years old [1, 14].

The vast majority of childhood burns is reported to occur in the home, while adult burns are reported to occur in the home, outdoors, and at work places in approximately equal proportions [12]. For all age groups, the kitchen is the most common scene of burns, followed by the backyard, house yard, or veranda for younger children, and the living room and the home vicinity for older children. Among the elderly population, the bathroom is also reported as a common scene of burns [1]. Among the various age groups, children under 5 years and the elderly (i.e., those aged over 70 years) have the highest fire-related burn mortality rates [7] moreover, fire-related deaths rank among the 15 leading causes of death among children and young adults 5-29 years [7].

Burn injuries in LMICs are said to possess a different epidemiology than that in the developed world [18]. It has been reported that the preponderance of burns seen during childhood and among the elderly in HICs is rarely seen in LMICs [1, 12]. Children and elderly people may be at relatively less risk because many households still exist as joint families, and the system safeguards these age groups to some extent. More recently, however, studies in LMICs have demonstrated a high number of burns in persons older than 60 years. Previously reported low incidence is probably due to lack of data on the elderly [1, 12].

Interestingly, studies done at US burn centers regarding recovery from severe burn injury clearly show that that the ability to adjust following injury is less dependent on the physical characteristics of the burn (such as burn size, burn depth or location), and more dependent on the status of the burn victim's pre-injury level of adjustment, coping skills, family and community support, and general psychological health [15, 23]. This means that burn survivors from struggling family backgrounds that deny them the opportunity to recover from even a small burn injury, in particular in LMICs, are likely to suffer from serious reintegration problems and have little chance of recuperation [15].

BURN EPIDEMIOLOGY CHALLENGES

The vast majority of burns are not fatal [15] and many patients with minor burns never report to an emergency health care facility for treatment. As a consequence, most surveys and studies reporting epidemiology of burns whether in HICs or LMICs fail to provide a realistic view about the true incidence of burn injuries. Population surveys carry an inherent margin of error and most retrospective or prospective reported studies are undertaken in specialized burns centers. Their study population is definitely not representative of the whole population at risk of burn injuries. These studies are about a special group of patients suffering from the most serious injuries and do not account for the minor burns that do not require specialized hospital care [1, 2, 16].

Despite the lack of a large-scale registration of burn injury in HICs, available epidemiologic data in these countries was sufficient to initiate effective burn prevention campaigns and achieve a net reduction in severe burn injury incidence. However, available epidemiologic data in most LMICs is less than adequate. In many LMICs the vast majority of studies focus on childhood burns and all but a few are hospital or clinic-based [12].

The deficiencies of hospital and burn centers based epidemiologic research in LMICs are great and their validity may be compromised by inadequate access to medical care, admission policies, financial difficulties, and still widespread traditional beliefs regarding home treatment of burns.

In most LMICs many severely burned patients may simply not have access to health care for various reasons or simply because health care facilities are inexistent particularly in rural and remote areas. Moreover, retrospective studies based on data from hospital records are prone to the usual limitations of accuracy, inconsistency, and completeness and result mainly in underestimation of the true burden of burn injuries [1, 2, 16].

It may be argued that the determination of the exact incidence of burn injuries may not be relevant. It is sufficient to account only for the burn injuries severe enough to necessitate special care whether as out or in-patient and these can be determined from available hospital emergency department or admission records. Nevertheless, these records are definitely not enough to assess adequately the magnitude of the challenges generated by burn injuries to the health care systems. Many patients are treated by private family physicians. Many more use over the counter remedies without even consulting a physician.

DISCUSSION

Epidemiology depends on valid data that may be gathered by tools including surveys, surveillance, analysis of program data, or rapid assessment [24]. However, every tool has limitations [24]. Data based on surveillance, or disease registries are used to estimate population disease burdens and to quantify the degree to which risk factors and humanitarian interventions affect population health. It may also be used to study associations between exposures and outcomes [24, 25].

Surveillance is a centuries old tool that has been an essential component of public health systems in developed countries for decades and in countries with highly developed comprehensive surveillance systems, disease reporting to healthcare authorities range from voluntary to mandatory reporting by law [25]. However, potential for various sources of biases in reporting cannot be completely prevented due to differences in disease reporting practices and inconsistencies in case definitions and diagnoses among healthcare professionals and medical institutions, along with differences in the health seeking behavior of populations [25]. However, in most LMICs where centralized, population-based comprehensive disease surveillance systems are not well developed, some attempts at small-scale, focused, disease-specific surveillance projects, have been fairly successful. Nevertheless, failure to follow one standard approach and the resulting variation, make gathered data even more vulnerable to bias [25]. Moreover, very often, particularly in LMICs or in an emergency situation, the ability to gather data is severely restricted due to insecurity preventing survey workers from carrying out data collection or lack of resources preventing health workers from submitting surveillance data. Lack of access may also be due to difficulties in communication and transport to remote areas [24]. A high degree of skepticism must be kept always assuming that many cases are not reported when analyzing surveillance data [24].

Primary data collection for estimating disease or injury burden in any given population is often restricted by limited resources. As a result, particularly in LMICs, institutional databases such as hospital records are frequently utilized for estimating population disease burdens and testing research hypotheses. However, like surveillance data, the institutional databases have their own limitations [25].

The validity of epidemiologic research findings utilizing hospital data may be uncertain due to Berkson's bias in particular when hospital-based case-control studies are performed to determine associations between risk factors and diseases [25]. Moreover, many individuals, usually with minor symptoms or injury, are not diagnosed or do not even seek treatment in an outpatient or emergency department of a healthcare facility which leads to under-reporting by accounting only for the more serious cases [25].

Under reporting may also be due to reduced health-seeking behavior which is partly determined by the low educational level and health knowledge of individuals of communities in many LMICs. Additionally, over the counter distribution of prescription medicines contributes as well to under reporting by promoting self-medication providing patients with an alternative to seeking a qualified healthcare professional [25]. On the other hand, overestimation of disease or injury burden may result from projecting on the population seriously biased data generated in a tertiary care center that attracts patients with certain conditions such as specialized burn centers [25].

Errors in determining disease population burden may result also from inaccuracies in applying the International Classification of Diseases (ICD) more likely to be encountered in LMICs [25].

Conclusion

Even though burn injuries are not a leading cause of mortality, the devastating effects of burns are long lasting at both an individual and societal level [9]. Millions are left with lifelong disabilities and disfigurements, often with resulting stigma and rejection [7]. Unfortunately, these impacts are compounded in resource-poor settings that are lacking adequate resources in first-aid as well as acute surgical management and rehabilitation facilities and where the human and material resources necessary to deal with this complex public health problem are lacking, patients that do survive their burn injuries often have poor, disfiguring and disabling long term outcomes [3, 9].

It remains painfully clear that people living in poorer economic situations suffer disproportionately from burns, as well as from many other types of injuries and diseases. Poverty, lack of parental education, large families, and substandard housing have all been associated with increased risk of burns, in particular childhood burns [1]. In addition to reducing severe burn injury incidence, developed countries have achieved ideal burn care through costly burn centers, units, and equipment certainly not available in most LMICs [26]. As M.H. Keswani [27] said in 1986, "The challenge of burns in India lies not in the successful treatment of a 100 per cent burn, but in the 100 per cent prevention of all burn injuries." This saying applies as well to all LMICs.

For planning and implementing prevention programs, the approach has to be multi-disciplinary and co-ordinated and most importantly based on valid epidemiologic data. Unfortunately, a burn prevention strategy that fits all is not at hand because the epidemiological factors of burns vary in different countries [3]. Sadly enough, valid epidemiologic data is still dramatically deficient in many LMICs. Awareness of these limitations is crucial to making the correct decisions [24]. Unfortunately there are no easy solutions to eliminating inherent biases related to surveillance or hospital-based data [25].

Implementation of national and preferably also international registration systems with consensus definitions of hospitalized patients with burn injury as well as all burn patients necessitating some form of medical care will facilitate research through more extensive databases and hence will enable detection of possible relations between risk factors. Consequently, a more accurate registration and description of the population with burn injury may allow improved targeting of prevention campaigns and cost-effectiveness of total burn care [14].

Unfortunately, major challenges still face intervention research and epidemiologic studies and surveys in many countries but particularly in LMICs. Challenges related to the population include illiteracy and poverty. However the most important hurdle that needs to be overcome in LMICs remains generalized lack of access to health care particularly in rural and remote areas. As for the potential research teams in those countries, most suffer from inadequate training; moreover, review committees lack expertise, training and above all independence.

References

[1] Atiyeh BS, Costagliola M, Hayek SN. Burn prevention mechanisms and outcomes: Pitfalls, failures and successes. *Burns* 2009; 35:181-193.

[2] Atiyeh B, Masellis A, Conte C. Optimizing Burn Treatment in Developing Low and Middle Income Countries with Limited Health.

[3] Kumar S, Ali W, Verma AK, Pandey A, Rathore S. Epidemiology and mortality of burns in the Lucknow Region, India-A 5 year study. Burns. 2013 May 7. pii: S0305-4179(13)00110-1. doi: 10.1016/j. Burns 2013.04.008. [Epub ahead of print]

[4] American Burn Association. Burn prevention. http:// www.kumed.com/bodyside.cfm?id=2027. Accessed January 1, 2008.

[5] Edelman LS. Social and economic factors associated with the risk of burn injury. *Burns* 2007; 33:958–65.

[6] Ghosh A, Bharat R. Domestic burns prevention and first aid awareness in and around Jamshedpur, India: strategies and impact. *Burns* 2000; 26:605–8.

[7] World Health Organization (WHO). Violence and Injury Prevention: Burns. http://www.who.int/violence_injury_prevention/other_injury/burns/en/index.html. Accessed May 25, 2013.

[8] Michael D. Peck Epidemiology of burns throughout the World. Part II: Intentional burns in adult. *Burns* 2012; 38:630–637.

[9] Burn Management http://ptolemy.library.utoronto.ca/sites/default/files/reviews/2008/October%20-%20Burn%20Management.pdf . Accessed May 25, 2013.

[10] Forjuoh SN, Guyer B, Strobino DM, Keyl PM, et al. Risk factors for childhood burns: a case-control study of Ghanaian children. *J. Epidemiol Community Health* 1995; 49:189-193.

[11] McGwin G Jr, Cross JM, Ford JW, Rue LW 3rd. Long-term trends in mortality accoding to age among adult burn patients. *J. Burn Care Rehabil* 2003; 24:21-25.

[12] Forjuoh SN. Burns in low- and middle-income countries: a review of available literature on descriptive epidemiology, risk factors, treatment, and prevention. *Burns* 2006; 32:529–537.

[13] American Burn Association. Burn Incidence and Treatment in the United States: 2012 Fact Sheet. http://www.ameriburn.org/resources_factsheet.php. Accessed May 28, 2013.

[14] Brusselaers N, Monstrey S, Vogelaers D, Hoste E, Blot S. Severe burn injury in Europe: a systematic review of the incidence, etiology, morbidity, and mortality. *Critical Care* 2010, 14:R188 doi:10.1186/cc9300

[15] Peck MD. Epidemiology of burns throughout the world. Part I: Distribution and risk factors. *Burns* 2011; 37:1087-1100.

[16] Othman N, Kendrick D. Epidemiology of burn injuries in the East Mediterranean Region: a systematic review. *BMC Public Health* 2010; 10:83-93.

[17] Ahuja RB, Bhattacharya S. Burns in the developing world and burn disasters. *BMJ* 2004; 329: 447-9.

[18] World Health Organization: "The Injury Chart Book: A Graphical Overview of the Global Burden of Injuries," *Dept of Injuries and Violence Prevention + Noncommunicable Diseases and Mental Health Cluster*, Geneva, 2002.

[19] Centers for Disease Control and Prevention. Worldwide Injuries and Violence. http://www.cdc.gov/injury/global/index.html. Accessed May 25, 2013.

[20] World Health Organization (WHO). Injuries and violence: the facts. Geneva, Switzerland: WHO; 2010. http://search.yahoo.com/search;_ylt=AgtcvzZkKa8OAO7WEib10eabvZx4?p=World+Health+Organization+%28WHO%29.+Injuries+and+viole

nce%3A+the+facts&toggle=1&cop=mss&ei=UTF-8&fr=yfp-t-900. Accessed May 28,2013.

[21] Brigham PA, McLoughlin E. Burn incidence and medical care use in the United States: estimates, trends, and data sources. *J. Burn Care Rehabil.* 1996; 17:95–107.

[22] Ahuja RB, Bhattacharya S, Rai A. Changing trends of an endemic trauma. *Burns* 2009; 35:650–656.

[23] Blakeney P, Meyer W, Moore P, Broemeling L, et al. Social competence and behavioral problems of pediatric survivors of burns. *J. Burn Care Rehabil* 1993; 14:65–72.

[24] The use of epidemiological tools in conflict-affected populations: open-access educational resources for policy-makers. http://conflict.lshtm.ac.uk/page_02.htm. Accessed May 30, 2013.

[25] Younus M, Siddiqi AA, Sana Khan B, Steffey AL. Institutional and Surveillance Database use in Epidemiologic Research in Developing Countries: Revisiting Some Limitations. JPMA, March 2008. http://jpma.org.pk/full_article_text.php?article_id=1347. Accessed May 30, 2013

[26] Atiyeh B, Masellis A, Conte C.Optimizing Burn Treatment in Developing Low and Middle Income Countries with Limited Health care Resources (Part 3). *Ann. Burns Fire Disasters* 2010; 23: 13: 13-18.

[27] Keswani MH. The prevention of burning injury. *Burns* 1986; 12: 533-539.

In: Encyclopedia of Dermatology (6 Volume Set)
Editor: Meghan Pratt
ISBN: 978-1-63483-326-4

Chapter 80

CURRENT AND FUTURE DIRECTIONS OF BURN RESUSCITATION AND WOUND MANAGEMENT

Jeanne Lee, Leslie Kobayashi and Raul Coimbra
University of California San Diego, San Diego, CA, US

ABSTRACT

Burns are among the most devastating of injuries and have become an international epidemic. Fire-related injuries occur in over 1.1 per 100,000 people, and are one of the top 15 leading causes of disease globally. The populations at highest risk for burns are among the most vulnerable, including children and the elderly. Children under the age of four comprise almost 30% of the burn-injured patients worldwide.

In the United States, more than 1 million burn injuries occur every year, resulting in over 700,000 Emergency Department (ED) visits annually. Fifty percent of these occur in children, and burn injury ranks among the top ten leading causes of injury related death in children and young adults.

Burn injury can have significant long-term effects on patients. Immediate and appropriate management of burn wounds is needed to improve survival and minimize the functional impairment that often results from serious burns. Several therapies, including the use of collagenase, have been used to improve wound healing and decrease the need for surgical excision. Novel therapies including stem cells and amniotic membrane application may improve outcomes in burn patients. However, early debridement, excision and grafting are still the mainstay in the management of partial thickness to full thickness burns.

INTRODUCTION

Burns are both physically and emotionally debilitating and are a major cause of injuries both in the United States and abroad. It affects all age groups and all cultures. This injury has lifelong effects and requires a multidisciplinary approach in order to hasten recovery and optimize long term functional outcomes of the burn-injured patient.

Over the last few decades fluid management and resuscitation practices have changed minimally since the development of the Parkland formula. However, adjunctive therapies including plasma exchange and continuous renal replacement therapy have been employed to augment resuscitation efforts in patients with large burns. These practices have been associated with improvements in the preservation of renal function in these patients [1-3].

The surgical treatment of burn injuries has undergone few changes since the advent of early excision and grafting. However, several treatments have been developed which may help decrease the need for operative debridement as well as decrease the length of stay and improve recovery for the burn patient. When surgical excision is needed, new therapies including the use of amniotic membranes and stem cell therapy may lead to improved healing and long-term function for the burn patient.

Epidemiology

There are over 1 million burn injuries in the United States every year. It is one of the 10 leading causes of injury related death in children under 14 and in the elderly. Unintentional burn injury is also one of the top 20 leading causes of death in all other age groups [4]. On average, someone is injured in a fire every 30 minutes in the United States. It is a significant source of health care costs, representing $7.5 billion in dollars spent each year [5]. Over 65% of injuries occur in the home and most burns are due to fire/flame or scald injuries [6].

Burn injury is the fourth most common cause of trauma worldwide [7]. It is most prevalent in the pediatric population. In low and middle-income countries, children under 4 years old make up a third of burn victims. There is a preponderance of pediatric injuries in males. Similar to the United States, most burns in these countries also occur in the home. Worldwide, scald injuries account for up to one half of all burns followed by contact and flame burns [8-10].

Current Therapies

Resuscitation and the treatment of burn patient still typically start with the Parkland formula. Developed in 1968, this formula has been the standard for resuscitation of the burn patient. Dr. Baxter found that resuscitation in the first 24-48 hours required large amounts of fluids and calculated the average crystalloid requirements of the burn patient based on their weight and burn size. Calculated at 4ml X weight (kg) X % total body surface area burned (%TBSA), this formula gives medical providers a starting point for fluid resuscitation. The first half of the calculated amount is given in the first 8 hours from the time of the burn, with the 2nd half given in subsequent 16 hrs [11].

Since the widespread adoption of this resuscitation approach, many institutions have found that the Parkland formula underestimates initial fluid requirements [12-15]. There have been several studies examining the use of colloid resuscitation as well as adjustments to the Parkland formula to better estimate fluid replacement requirements [15, 16]. In addition, two modalities including plasma exchange and continuous renal replacement therapy have been promoted as additional adjuncts in the treatment of the burn patient.

Plasma exchange is a method that has been used to treat a multitude of inflammatory conditions including myasthenia gravis and demyelinating polyneuropathy [17, 18]. Given its therapeutic success in these inflammatory conditions, several institutions have investigated its use in the resuscitation of the patient with significant burn injury. Klein et al. examined 37 burn patients whose average TBSA was 48.6%. These patients required fluid resuscitation well in excess of the Parkland formula. Plasma exchange was initiated at an average of 17 hours from the time of injury and lasted 2.4 hours. This study was able to demonstrate a decrease in the fluid requirements and an improvement in various markers of resuscitation including urine output, base deficit, and lactate following plasma exchange [1]. Neff et al. gathered data on 40 patients who were experiencing difficult resuscitations. Difficult resuscitations were defined as patients with fluid requirements exceeding 1.2 times the Parkland Formula. Twenty-one of these patients received therapeutic plasma exchange (TPE) while 19 did not. The average TBSA was 37% vs. 27% in the group who did not receive TPE. As in the previous study, these patients also experienced an improvement in lactate and a decrease in fluid requirements after TPE [2]. However, neither of these studies was able to demonstrate a mortality benefit to TPE [1, 2], and there continues to be a lack of class I evidence in favor of TPE. While these initial results are promising, additional work needs to be performed before TPE can be formally recommended for severely burned patients.

Hemodialysis is another modality that has been utilized in complicated burn resuscitations. Renal failure is relatively rare in burn patients but has been associated with a significant increase in mortality. Hemodialysis has been demonstrated to be a safe method of treatment for renal failure [3]. In the burn patient, continuous renal replacement therapy (CRRT) has been shown to be an effective treatment of acute kidney injury [3, 19, 20]. Holm et al. found that continuous arteriovenous hemofiltration (CAVHD) was safe and effective and was well tolerated, although it did not alter the mortality rate in their group of patients. Sun et al. also demonstrated that continuous venovenous hemofiltration (CVVH) was as effective as CAVHD and had a lower incidence of vascular complications [20].

In an effort to standardize presence and severity of renal failure, two staging systems have been developed. The Acute Dialysis Quality Initiative developed the RIFLE (risk, injury, failure, loss of function, end-stage renal disease) criteria [21]. In 2007, the Acute Kidney Injury Network (AKIN) modified these criteria to further describe stages of renal failure [22]. This staging system was developed to describe and quantify the changes in serum creatinine and urine output. (Table 1) Only one criterion (creatinine or urine output) needs to be fulfilled to reach a given stage of severity. Using RIFLE and AKIN criteria, several institutions have investigated the use of CRRT in the treatment of renal failure and its influence on outcomes.

In 2008, Chung et al. analyzed the use of CRRT in severely burned military casualties with >40% TBSA. The patients were admitted to the burn unit between 2003-2007. In 2005, CRRT became available and was used to treat acute kidney injury as defined by RIFLE criteria found in patients with large burns. These patients were compared to burn patients admitted prior to 2005 who developed acute kidney injury. Both 28 day and in hospital mortality was found to be lower in the group treated with CRRT. Kaplan-Meier estimates also found a significantly higher rate of survival out to 1 year [23].

Table 1. Acute Kidney Injury Network Criteria

Stages	Serum Creatinine Criteria	Urine Output Criteria
1	Increase in serum creatinine ≥0.03 mg/dl or increase to ≥150-200% (1.5- to 2-fold) from baseline	<0.5 ml/kg/hr for >6 hours
2	Increase in serum creatinine to more than 200% to 300% (>2- to 3-fold) from baseline	<0.5 ml/kg/hr for >12 hours
3	Increase in serum creatinine to more than 300% (>3-fold) from baseline or serum creatinine of more than or equal to 4.0 mg/dl with an acute increase of at least 0.5mg/dl	<0.3 ml/kg/hr for 24 hours or anuria for 12 hours

Hemodialysis is now being considered in those patients who require volumes well in excess of that described by the Parkland Formula and exhibit evidence of renal dysfunction. Initial studies addressed the use of dialysis in the critically ill burn patient and found that CRRT was better tolerated than intermittent hemodialysis and served as a bridge until renal recovery occurred. Several studies are also advocating the early use of CRRT in these patients.

Using the AKIN criteria, Chung et al. used CRRT to treat patients with AKIN stage 3 or AKIN stage 2 with shock. These patients were compared to similar historical controls that had been treated with conventional methods including intermittent hemodialysis (IHD). CRRT was started 6 days earlier than IHD on the average. The CRRT group had a significantly lower 28-day mortality of 38% vs. 71% in the IHD group. All 29 patients treated with CRRT had return of renal function back to baseline prior to discharge vs 3 patients in the control group.

Additionally, a subgroup analysis of patients exhibiting signs of shock found a significant decrease in the type and dose of vasopressors required in patients treated with CRRT. These differences were found to be significant at both the 24 and 48-hour time points with only 24% of CRRT patients requiring vasopressors at 48 hrs vs. 94% of patients in the conventional group [24].

The timing and role of CRRT or plasmapheresis in the resuscitation of the burn patient has yet to be fully described. Further investigative work has yet to be done to identify the burn patient best suited to treatment with either or both modalities. These may yet serve to be lifesaving therapies for those patients undergoing challenging or higher volume resuscitations.

FUTURE DIRECTIONS

Improvements in burn care took a leap forward with the advent of early excision and grafting. Since the 1970's, this approach to the burn wound has improved both morbidity and mortality for the burn-injured patient. Since then, clinicians and scientists have struggled to find other advancements to improve treatment of the burn wound. Current studies have involved the use of amniotic membranes, spray cells, and stem cells to improve healing.

Amniotic membrane (AM) is the innermost layer of the fetal membranes. It is translucent and without vasculature. It is procured from donors after caesarian sections under sterile conditions. Donors are screened for HIV, hepatitis B and C, Treponema pallidum, and human transmissible spongiform encephalopathy both prior to donation and after 6 months. AM is then preserved using several methods including glycerol preservation and freeze-drying [25, 26]

Human amniotic membrane has been used for wound healing for decades. The first case series describing the use of amniotic membranes was published by the Johns Hopkins Hospital in 1910 and described its use in skin transplantation in 550 patients [27]. Other small case studies have been sporadically published over the last century [28-31]. In the last two decades, AM has been aggressively pursued as a skin substitute in the treatment of burn injuries.

Several studies have demonstrated the effectiveness of AM as a biological dressing in the treatment of superficial partial thickness or deep burns. Adly et al. treated patients with either AM or an artificial polyurethane membrane dressing either immediately or after eschar removal. Their group demonstrated improved physiology as demonstrated by electrolyte measurements as well as improved infection rates in patients treated with amniotic membranes. Forty-eight percent of patients healed within 20 days when treated with AM vs. 39% of patients treated with polyurethane membrane. Pain was also found to be significantly less in patients treated with AM [32].

Amniotic membrane has also been compared to current burn care treatments including silver sulfadiazine. A group from Sher-e-Bangla Medical College Hospital randomly assigned pediatric burn patients with partial thickness burns to treatment with either silver sulfadiazine (SSD) or AM. Patients treated with SSD underwent twice daily cleanings and dressing changes, while the group treated with AM had the dressing placed, then replaced when the integrity of the membrane was partly or fully lost. They demonstrated faster time to epithelialization as well as shorter hospital stays. These differences were statistically significant. In addition, 84% of patients who had AM applied noted painless dressing changes as opposed to 21% of patients treated with SSD [33].

In addition to aiding in primary epithelialization of burn injuries, AM has been shown to improve autograft take. Mohammadi et al. used AM in patients who presented with symmetric burns on two extremities, either upper or lower. Autograft was secured on one extremity with the standard method of skin stapling. On the other, AM was wrapped around the extremity and used to secure the skin graft. Both extremities were then examined for success of graft take after 21 days. The extremities treated with AM reached healing in 7 days vs. 14 days in the standard group. Complete graft take rates were also higher in the group treated with AM at 97% vs. 89% [34]. Current evidence shows several potential benefits for AM and support its use in the treatment of burn injuries.

As in many areas of medicine, stem cells are being actively investigated as a potential therapy in the treatment of burn wounds [35-38]. These cells contain the ability to differentiate into all cells. Mesenchymal stem cells have demonstrated great plasticity and have been found to be able to differentiate into epidermal cells. These cells have been aggressively pursued as a potential replacement for autografting in deep and full thickness burns [39]. These cells are also easily accessible from many areas of the body, including subcutaneous fat. Studies have demonstrated that lipsuctioned fat can be processed to isolate mesechymal stem cells [40, 41]. These cells are easily accessible and can potentially be donated by patients undergoing liposuction procedures.

Several animal studies have demonstrated the safety and wound healing capabilities of mesenchymal stem cells [42-44]. Researchers have found that these cells can be administered not only topically but also injected intravenously. Sasaki et al. harvested bone marrow-derived mesenchymal cells from mice and labeled them. These cells were then injected intravenously into mice that sustained full thickness skin wounds by punch biopsy. These punch biopsy sites were excised three days after injection. This group found that the wound sites had been populated by the labeled mesenchymal cells that had begun demonstrating properties of keratinocytes.

Large studies to support stem cell therapy in human burn patients is lacking. However several small case series have reported the use of mesenchymal stem cells in treating humans with burn injuries and chronic wounds [45, 46]. The first human study was reported in 2005 after a Russian female was treated with stem cells to treat extensive burns she had sustained [47]. Her wounds healed rapidly with a shorter than expected time to rehabilitation.

In the United States, there is currently a bone marrow-mesenchymal stem cell product in FDA clinical phase III trials. This product is geared towards the treatment of acute radiation syndrome and its sequellae, including cutaneous radiation syndrome [48]. Additionally, the Argentine Regulatory Agency for tissue, organ, and stem cell research and implantation (INCUCAI) gave approval for the first clinical trial to treat large burns with cadaveric bone marrow mesenchymal stem cells [38]. The first set of patients will be treated with a topical application of cells over an acellular dermal biological matrix. This study aims to demonstrate both efficacy and safety in the treatment of large and difficult burns. More work is required to find the ideal method and application of mesenchymal stem cells in the treatment of burn wounds. Current studies may provide us with better information and strategies to treat patients who may otherwise have no other coverage options.

Conclusion

The care of the burn patient is complicated. It is a long journey that starts with the initial resuscitation and treatment of the inflammatory response to the burn injury. It continues with treatment of the burn from enzymatic debridement to newer therapies involving amniotic membranes to aid not only in healing but with pain control as well. Future directions involve the continued investigation of breakthrough treatments including the use of stem cell therapy. Recent improvements in resuscitation and current studies in wound care will hopefully give physicians the tools needed to improve wound healing and long-term quality of life.

References

[1] Klein, MB; Edwards, JA; Kramer, CB; Nester, T; Heimbach, DM; Gibran, NS. The beneficial effects of plasma exchange after severe burn injury. *Journal of burn care & research: official publication of the American Burn Association*, 2009, 30, 243-8.

[2] Neff, LP; Allman, JM; Holmes, JH. The use of theraputic plasma exchange (TPE) in the setting of refractory burn shock. *Burns: journal of the International Society for Burn Injuries*, 2010, 36, 372-8.

[3] Leblanc, M; Thibeault, Y; Querin, S. Continuous haemofiltration and haemodiafiltration for acute renal failure in severely burned patients. *Burns: journal of the International Society for Burn Injuries*, 1997, 23, 160-5.

[4] 20 Leading Causes of Injury Death, United States. 2010. at http://www.cdc.gov/injury/wisqars/index.html.)

[5] Finkelstein, E; Corso, PS; Miller, TR. The incidence and economic burden of injuries in the United States. Oxford; New York: Oxford University Press; 2006.

[6] 2012 Fact Sheet. 2012. at http://www.ameriburn.org/resources_factsheet.php.)

[7] Murray, CJL; Lopez, AD. Harvard School of Public Health, World Health Organization. World Bank. The global burden of disease: a comprehensive assessment of mortality and disability from diseases, injuries, and risk factors in 1990 and projected to 2020. Cambridge, MA: Published by the Harvard School of Public Health on behalf of the World Health Organization and the World Bank; Distributed by Harvard University Press; 1996.

[8] Forjuoh, SN. Burns in low- and middle-income countries: a review of available literature on descriptive epidemiology, risk factors, treatment, and prevention. *Burns: journal of the International Society for Burn Injuries*, 2006, 32, 529-37.

[9] Iqbal, T; Saaiq, M; Ali Z. Epidemiology and outcome of burns: early experience at the country's first national burns centre. *Burns: journal of the International Society for Burn Injuries*, 2013, 39, 358-62.

[10] Duke, J; Wood, F; Semmens, J; Edgar, DW; Spilsbury, K; Rea, S. An assessment of burn injury hospitalisations of adolescents and young adults in Western Australia, 1983-2008. *Burns: journal of the International Society for Burn Injuries*, 2012, 38, 128-35.

[11] Baxter, CR; Shires, T. Physiological response to crystalloid resuscitation of severe burns. *Annals of the New York Academy of Sciences*, 1968, 150, 874-94.

[12] Saffle, JI. The phenomenon of "fluid creep" in acute burn resuscitation. *Journal of burn care & research: official publication of the American Burn Association*, 2007, 28, 382-95.

[13] Blumetti, J; Hunt, JL; Arnoldo, BD; Parks, JK; Purdue, GF. The Parkland formula under fire: is the criticism justified? *Journal of burn care & research: official publication of the American Burn Association*, 2008, 29, 180-6.

[14] White, CE; Renz, EM. Advances in surgical care: management of severe burn injury. *Critical care medicine*, 2008, 36, S318-24.

[15] Mitchell, KB; Khalil, E; Brennan, A; et al. New management strategy for fluid resuscitation: quantifying volume in the first 48 hours after burn injury. *Journal of burn care & research : official publication of the American Burn Association*, 2013, 34, 196-202.

[16] Park, SH; Hemmila, MR; Wahl, WL. Early albumin use improves mortality in difficult to resuscitate burn patients. *The journal of trauma and acute care surgery*, 2012, 73, 1294-7.

[17] Cardella, CJ. Plasma exchange--a new approach to immune modulation in rheumatic diseases. *The Journal of rheumatology*, 1979, 6, 606-9.

[18] Koo, AP. Therapeutic apheresis in autoimmune and rheumatic diseases. *Journal of clinical apheresis*, 2000, 15, 18-27.

[19] Holm, C; Horbrand, F von; Donnersmarck, GH; Muhlbauer, W. Acute renal failure in severely burned patients. *Burns: journal of the International Society for Burn Injuries*, 1999, 25, 171-8.
[20] Sun, IF; Lee, SS; Lin, SD; Lai, CS. Continuous arteriovenous hemodialysis and continuous venovenous hemofiltration in burn patients with acute renal failure. *The Kaohsiung journal of medical sciences*, 2007, 23, 344-51.
[21] Bellomo, R; Ronco, C; Kellum, JA; Mehta, RL; Palevsky, P. Acute Dialysis Quality Initiative w. Acute renal failure - definition, outcome measures, animal models, fluid therapy and information technology needs: the Second International Consensus Conference of the Acute Dialysis Quality Initiative (ADQI) Group. *Critical care*, 2004, 8, R204-12.
[22] Mehta, RL; Kellum, JA; Shah, SV; et al. Acute Kidney Injury Network: report of an initiative to improve outcomes in acute kidney injury. *Critical care*, 2007, 11, R31.
[23] Chung, KK; Juncos, LA; Wolf, SE; et al. Continuous renal replacement therapy improves survival in severely burned military casualties with acute kidney injury. *The Journal of trauma*, 2008, 64, S179-85, discussion S85-7.
[24] Chung, KK; Lundy, JB; Matson, JR; et al. Continuous venovenous hemofiltration in severely burned patients with acute kidney injury: a cohort study. *Critical care*, 2009, 13, R62.
[25] Fernandes, M; Sridhar, MS: Sangwan, VS; Rao, GN. Amniotic membrane transplantation for ocular surface reconstruction. *Cornea*, 2005, 24, 643-53.
[26] Gajiwala, K; Gajiwala, AL. Evaluation of lyophilised, gamma-irradiated amnion as a biological dressing. *Cell and tissue banking*, 2004, 5, 73-80.
[27] JD. Skin transplantation with a review of 550 cases at the Johns Hopkins Hospital. *Johns Hopkins Hosp Rep*, 1910, 15, 310.
[28] NS. Use of the fetal membranes in skin grafting. *Med Rec NY*, 1913, 83, 973.
[29] MS. The grafting of preserved amniotic membrane to burned and ulcerated skin surfaces, substituting skin grafts. *JAMA*, 1913, 60, 973.
[30] Sorsby, A; Symons, HM. Amniotic membrane grafts in caustic burns of the eye (burns of the second degree). *The British journal of ophthalmology*, 1946, 30, 337-45.
[31] Troensegaard-Hansen, E. Amniotic grafts in chronic skin ulceration. *Lancet*, 1950, 1, 859-60.
[32] Adly, OA; Moghazy, AM; Abbas, AH; Ellabban, AM; Ali, OS; Mohamed, BA. Assessment of amniotic and polyurethane membrane dressings in the treatment of burns. *Burns: journal of the International Society for Burn Injuries*, 2010, 36, 703-10.
[33] Mostaque, AK; Rahman, KB. Comparisons of the effects of biological membrane (amnion) and silver sulfadiazine in the management of burn wounds in children. *Journal of burn care & research: official publication of the American Burn Association*, 2011, 32, 200-9.
[34] Mohammadi, AA; Johari, HG; Eskandari, S. Effect of amniotic membrane on graft take in extremity burns. *Burns: journal of the International Society for Burn Injuries*, 2013, 39, 1137-41.
[35] Drago, H; Marin, GH; Sturla, F; et al. The next generation of burns treatment: intelligent films and matrix, controlled enzymatic debridement, and adult stem cells. *Transplantation proceedings*, 2010, 42, 345-9.

[36] Lootens, L; Brusselaers, N; Beele, H; Monstrey, S. Keratinocytes in the treatment of severe burn injury: an update. *International wound journal*, 2013, 10, 6-12.

[37] Leclerc, T; Thepenier, C; Jault, P; et al. Cell therapy of burns. *Cell proliferation*, 2011, 44 Suppl, 1, 48-54.

[38] Mansilla, E; Aquino, VD; Roque, G; Tau, JM; Maceira, A. Time and regeneration in burns treatment: heading into the first worldwide clinical trial with cadaveric mesenchymal stem cells. *Burns: journal of the International Society for Burn Injuries*, 2012, 38, 450-2.

[39] Burd, A; Ahmed, K; Lam, S; Ayyappan, T; Huang, L. Stem cell strategies in burns care. *Burns: journal of the International Society for Burn Injuries*, 2007, 33, 282-91.

[40] Kern, S; Eichler, H; Stoeve, J; Kluter, H; Bieback, K. Comparative analysis of mesenchymal stem cells from bone marrow, umbilical cord blood, or adipose tissue. *Stem cells*, 2006, 241, 294-301.

[41] Stanko, P; Kaiserova, K; Altanerova, V; Altaner, C. Comparison of human mesenchymal stem cells derived from dental pulp, bone marrow, adipose tissue, and umbilical cord tissue by gene expression. Biomedical papers of the Medical Faculty of the University Palacky, Olomouc, Czechoslovakia, 2013.

[42] Fang, LJ; Fu, XB; Sun, TZ; et al. [An experimental study on the differentiation of bone marrow mesenchymal stem cells into vascular endothelial cells]. *Zhonghua shao shang za zhi = Zhonghua shaoshang zazhi = Chinese journal of burns*, 2003, 19:22-4.

[43] Fu, XB; Fang, LJ; Wang, YX; Sun, TZ; Cheng, B. [Enhancing the repair quality of skin injury on porcine after autografting with the bone marrow mesenchymal stem cells]. *Zhonghua yi xue za zhi*, 2004, 84, 920-4.

[44] Sasaki, M; Abe, R; Fujita, Y; Ando, S; Inokuma, D; Shimizu, H. Mesenchymal stem cells are recruited into wounded skin and contribute to wound repair by transdifferentiation into multiple skin cell type. *Journal of immunology*, 2008, 180, 2581-7.

[45] Lataillade, JJ; Doucet, C; Bey, E; et al. New approach to radiation burn treatment by dosimetry-guided surgery combined with autologous mesenchymal stem cell therapy. *Regenerative medicine*, 2007, 2, 785-94.

[46] Wu, Y; Chen, L; Scott, PG; Tredget, EE. Mesenchymal stem cells enhance wound healing through differentiation and angiogenesis. *Stem cells*, 2007, 25, 2648-59.

[47] Rasulov, MF; Vasilchenkov, AV; Onishchenko, NA; et al. First experience of the use bone marrow mesenchymal stem cells for the treatment of a patient with deep skin burns. *Bulletin of experimental biology and medicine*, 2005, 139, 141-4.

[48] Fact Sheet; Prochymal therapy as a medical countermeasure for acute radiation syndrome. In: Osiris Therapeutics I, ed.

INDEX

#

21st century, 939, 951

A

Abraham, 517, 600
absorption spectra, 272, 274, 276, 280, 289
abuse, 353, 989, 992
academic progress, 777
academic success, 773, 777
access, xiv, 2, 66, 166, 584, 777, 797, 944
accessibility, 183, 733
accommodations, 777
accounting, 391, 484, 573, 577, 821
acellular, xiii, 1, 24, 1122, 1818
acetaldehyde, 1005, 1008
acetic acid, 163, 227, 302
acetone, 224, 424, 1005
ACF, 276
acidic, 129, 382, 913
acne, xxxiii, xxxiv, 26, 127, 131, 132, 146, 148, 401, 402, 523, 546, 558, 561, 562, 564, 569, 858, 883, 886, 899, 939
acne vulgaris, 401, 558, 858
acquired immunity, 410, 510
ACTH, xix, 83, 89, 137, 138, 193, 340, 341, 342, 359, 360, 393, 410, 441, 442, 443, 444, 445, 446, 447, 451, 991
active compound, 151, 528
active oxygen, 272
active site, 410, 448
activity level, 776
actuation, 738
acute infection, 708
acute leukemia, 587
acute lymphoblastic leukemia, 701, 714
acute renal failure, 580, 614
acute stress, 991
adalimumab, 511, 832, 833, 901, 902, 903, 906, 924, 989, 993, 1028
adaptation, xix, 175, 187, 389, 397, 400, 405, 500, 586, 659, 682, 690, 720, 728, 730, 806, 812
adaptive functioning, 786
adaptive immune response(s), 538, 934
adaptive immunity, xxii, 515, 535, 541, 552, 832, 917
adenine, 237, 696, 729
adenosine, 83, 90, 118, 128, 131, 148, 193, 256, 270, 368, 447, 874, 894, 943, 952
adenosine triphosphate, 90, 132, 447
adenovirus, 448
ADHD, 775, 780, 784
adhesion, xix, 27, 72, 73, 125, 173, 389, 405, 464, 470, 585, 621, 624, 625, 652, 657, 659, 661, 662, 668, 674, 675, 676, 677, 689, 690, 703, 707, 710, 742, 825, 830, 844, 869, 872, 876, 891, 894, 902, 942, 945, 1010, 1027
adhesive properties, 689, 993
adipocyte, 7, 904, 983
adiponectin, 948, 950, 983, 984, 989
adipose, 30, 983, 984
adipose tissue, 30, 983, 984
adjunctive therapy, 559, 561, 670, 885
adjustment, xxi, 38, 477, 489, 499, 500, 501, 513, 885
administrators, xlvi
adolescents, xxi, xxxix, xl, xlvi, 77, 324, 326, 331, 333, 346, 490, 502, 503, 564, 701, 714, 783, 786, 818, 825, 903, 904, 1032
adrenal gland(s), 171, 444, 445, 451
adrenal insufficiency, 442, 443, 446, 452
adrenocorticotropic hormone, 254, 340, 341, 342
adsorption, 189
adult stem cells, 4
adulthood, xxi, xxix, xlvii, 15, 35, 324, 326, 347, 351, 373, 445, 490, 547, 871, 983

adults, xxxv, xl, 9, 207, 326, 348, 490, 491, 496, 500, 502, 523, 547, 572, 574, 587, 589, 592, 593, 601, 608, 614, 632, 633, 653, 658, 691, 699, 701, 745, 817, 822, 825, 831, 880, 882, 886, 902, 985, 992
advancements, 70
adventitia, 301
adverse effects, xxi, xxix, xxxvii, xlix, 366, 489, 525, 530, 560, 663, 722, 738, 743, 769, 771, 816, 818, 824, 825, 831, 842, 848, 890, 893, 895, 899, 902, 941, 1000, 1001, 1020, 1021
adverse event, 712, 768, 902, 903, 906
advertisements, xlii
aerosols, 738, 740, 744, 745, 746, 748
aesthetic, xiii, xiv, xlviii, 1, 2, 24, 25, 26, 63, 64, 404, 481
aetiology, 496
affective disorder, 499
AFM, 274, 276, 285, 288, 289, 290
Africa, 179, 577
African Americans, 406, 872
agar, 168, 171, 179, 223, 224, 227, 228, 229, 230, 235, 239, 436, 589, 621, 628, 648, 679, 692, 693, 751
age spots, xv, xxxvii, 24, 83, 92, 128, 129, 402, 403
agencies, xlvi
age-related diseases, 39, 41
agglutination, 592, 708, 715
agglutination test, 592
aggregation, 19, 86, 272, 294, 295, 296, 515, 536, 540, 668, 738, 949
aggression, 509, 779, 1020
aggressive therapy, 168
aggressiveness, 539
aging population, 325
aging process, xxxiv, xxxv, 9, 13, 40
agonist, 38, 138, 340, 345, 368, 370, 391, 392, 737, 844, 860, 868, 876, 908
agranulocytosis, 696
agriculture, 143, 320
AIDS, 179, 580, 584, 608, 633, 636, 648, 651, 658, 662, 669, 673, 691, 692, 694, 699, 711, 718
airways, 737, 762
Akan, 952
alanine, xxx, 400, 643, 896, 911, 925
alanine aminotransferase, 896
albinism, xvi, 92, 93, 136, 207, 210, 216, 217, 218, 249, 251, 252, 262, 267, 268, 337, 338, 357, 390, 397, 404, 409, 410, 446
albumin, 55, 594, 689, 895, 989
alcohol consumption, xxxi, 819, 877, 898, 981, 1000, 1005
alcohol use, xxxii, 989, 999, 1005
alcoholics, 877
alcoholism, 829, 877, 895, 993
alcohols, 143
aldehydes, 116
alexithymia, xxi, 490, 497, 501, 503, 993, 994
algae, 123, 124
algorithm, 512, 558, 979
alienation, 993
alimentation, 584
alkaline phosphatase, 643, 896
allele, xvi, 191, 193, 194, 197, 198, 199, 200, 201, 202, 203, 205, 206, 207, 208, 209, 214, 347, 400, 406, 537, 835, 838
allergens, 414, 415, 424, 425, 426, 427, 428, 429, 430, 431, 432, 433, 434, 435, 436, 438, 525, 837, 838
allergic reaction, 312, 426, 435, 436, 525, 903, 931
allergic rhinitis, 436
allergy, 415, 422, 424, 427, 429, 436, 438, 560, 863
allylamines, xxvi, 717, 722, 723
aloe, 152, 314, 826
alopecia areata, xxi, xxii, 489, 490, 491, 492, 493, 494, 495, 496, 497, 498, 499, 500, 501, 502, 503, 505, 506, 508, 509, 511, 512, 513, 514, 515, 520, 521, 522, 524, 526, 528, 530, 531, 532, 533, 540, 541, 542, 543, 881
alopecia totalis, xxi, xxii, 494, 501, 505, 508, 513, 521, 522, 526, 533, 542
alopecia universalis, xxi, 505, 506, 511, 512, 513, 520, 522, 530, 542
altered peptide ligand, xxx, 911, 922, 925, 926
alternative hypothesis, 820
alters, 31, 37, 71, 139, 329, 657, 664, 828, 957, 1005
alveolar ridge, 1032
amino, xix, xlv, 3, 11, 23, 88, 116, 162, 165, 171, 174, 205, 218, 262, 308, 309, 334, 337, 340, 342, 371, 389, 400, 444, 621, 622, 625, 643, 690, 732, 873, 895, 913, 918, 921, 922, 928
amino acid(s), xix, xlv, 3, 11, 23, 88, 162, 165, 171, 174, 205, 262, 308, 309, 334, 337, 340, 342, 371, 389, 400, 621, 622, 625, 643, 732, 873, 913, 918, 921, 922
amnesia, 782
amniotic fluid, 769
amorphous polymers, 176
amphibia, 300, 303, 304
amphibians, 294, 295, 300, 458, 913
amplitude, 46, 49, 966
amputation, 636
amylase, 707
amyloidosis, 990
analgesic, 442
anatomic site, 38, 351, 584

anatomy, 27, 126, 217
ANC, 694, 696
ancestors, 443
anchoring, 15, 18
androgen, 9, 141
androgenic alopecia, 75, 500, 503
anemia, 694, 699, 884
aneurysm, 632
anger, 779
angioedema, 902
angiogenesis, xxx, 4, 453, 552, 553, 565, 820, 830, 840, 844, 848, 850, 869, 887, 891, 896, 938, 941, 946, 952, 955, 956
angiography, 478
angyogenesis, xxxi, 981
anisotropy, xxxvii, 966
ankles, 985
ankylosing spondylitis, 833, 903, 997, 1010
anorexia, 829, 849, 991
antagonism, 342, 930
antibiotic, xxiv, xxxiii, 171, 179, 585, 635, 655, 658, 697, 739, 746, 865, 939
antibody, xxiii, 165, 167, 170, 171, 356, 373, 385, 394, 395, 396, 457, 458, 460, 461, 465, 466, 571, 588, 593, 612, 703, 833, 903, 904, 906, 907, 922, 924, 934, 936, 947, 957, 1015, 1021, 1023, 1026
anti-cancer, xxxix, 727
anticoagulation, 4
antiemetics, 894
antifungal drugs, xxiv, xxv, xxvi, 165, 170, 171, 175, 176, 572, 595, 596, 598, 614, 617, 632, 646, 655, 663, 670, 677, 717, 724, 726, 727, 729, 733
antigen, xxiii, 4, 8, 251, 439, 446, 451, 510, 524, 525, 536, 538, 541, 542, 557, 571, 610, 612, 659, 693, 704, 828, 835, 837, 863, 872, 873, 901, 922, 928, 932, 934, 936, 943, 947
antigenicity, 182
antigen-presenting cell(s), 4, 439, 828, 837, 863, 943
antihistamines, 487
antihypertensive drugs, 908
anti-inflammatory agents, 1013
anti-inflammatory drugs, 891, 893, 895, 900, 991
anti-inflammatory medications, 559
antimalarials, xxix, 871, 875, 1005
antimicrobial therapy, 581, 606, 659
antinuclear antibodies, 904
antioxidant, xxxviii, xliii, xlv, 15, 25, 34, 124, 130, 150, 155, 156, 173, 180, 344, 510, 539, 670, 719, 720, 721, 724, 725, 728, 729, 733, 948, 950
antipsychotic, 177
antisense, xxx, 911, 926, 929
antisocial personality, 500
anti-TNFα, xxxii, xxxiii, 1025, 1026, 1027, 1028
antitumor, xxiii, 571, 579, 580
anus, 990
anxiety, xxi, xliii, 64, 77, 489, 499, 500, 501, 509, 514, 776, 779, 818, 853, 992, 993
aorta, 28, 768
APC(s), 918, 928
apex, 880, 913
apnea, 794, 797
apoptosis pathways, 173
apples, 130
Argentina, 574, 575, 576, 615, 619, 620, 641
arginine, 204, 527, 532, 625
aromatic compounds, 941
aromatics, 314
arousal, 994
arrest(s), 631, 781, 828, 944, 953
arrhythmia, 769
arsenic, 326, 362, 893
arterioles, 5, 553, 831, 899
arteriosclerosis, 987
arteritis, 583
artery(s), 523, 763, 768, 781, 819, 1010, 1014, 1015
arthralgia, 905, 906
arthritis, xxiv, xxxii, xli, 520, 587, 618, 630, 632, 636, 637, 651, 652, 653, 818, 840, 857, 859, 864, 872, 902, 933, 982, 985, 989, 995, 1004, 1009, 1011, 1027
arthrocentesis, 636
arthrogryposis, 795, 802
arthrogryposis multiplex congenita, 802
arthroplasty, 636, 637
arthroscopic debridement, 637
articulation, 777
artificial tanning devices, xxxix, 1265, 1266, 1281
Artisan, 561
asbestos, 327, 881
ascites, 619, 705
ascorbic acid, 53, 60, 93, 127, 128, 129, 147, 309
Asia, 575, 576, 577, 619
Asian countries, 429
asparagus, 119, 157
aspartate, 896
aspartic acid, 625
aspergillosis, 173, 174, 594, 678
asphyxia, 768, 771, 782, 784, 785
aspirate, 588
aspiration, 436, 769, 782, 783, 794, 796, 798, 801
assault, xxxv
assessment, xxxv, 57, 60, 61, 146, 158, 411, 559, 602, 604, 649, 693, 748, 755, 773, 776, 795, 796, 813, 820, 821, 897, 899, 909, 944, 963, 1006, 1014, 1019
assimilation, 167, 172, 592

assistive technology, 778
asthenia, 899
asthma, 436, 736, 737, 738, 739, 745, 746, 747, 748, 763, 838, 993
astrocytes, 516, 868
astrocytoma, 266
asymmetry, 547
asymptomatic, xxi, xxiv, 170, 171, 505, 638, 639, 655, 740, 897, 905, 989, 991
ataxia, 250, 895
atherosclerosis, xxxii, 477, 819, 844, 854, 983, 1009, 1010, 1011, 1013, 1014
atherosclerotic plaque, 982
atmosphere, xliii, 315, 331, 332
atmospheric pressure, 727
atomic force, 135, 276
atomic force microscope, 276
atoms, 48, 277
atopic dermatitis, 415, 424, 435, 436, 437, 439, 503, 506, 509, 513, 532, 563, 817, 830, 838, 851, 852, 889, 910, 917, 918, 931, 957
atopic eczema, 415, 436, 439, 930
atopy, 496, 513, 514, 530
ATP, 83, 131, 200, 362, 372, 464, 726
atrophy, xxxiv, 9, 24, 71, 257, 333, 479, 523, 526, 527, 557, 757, 774, 784, 825, 848, 886
attachment, 497, 510, 621, 741
attitudes, xxxviii, xlvi
attractant, 983
attribution, 282, 283
atypical pneumonia, 172
Austria, 575, 576, 577, 604
authorities, 593
autoantibodies, xxviii, xxxii, 711, 815, 835, 850, 1017, 1020, 1021, 1023, 1027
Autoantibodies, 711
autoantigens, 876, 921
autocrine, xx, 4, 65, 68, 71, 89, 393, 396, 409, 455, 466, 467, 837, 927, 1187, 1190
autoimmune disease(s), xxii, xxxii, 73, 377, 505, 506, 509, 514, 515, 519, 521, 530, 535, 536, 538, 699, 707, 838, 861, 876, 904, 917, 925, 936, 1010, 1015, 1017, 1020, 1023, 1025, 1026, 1028
autoimmune disorder(s), xxii, xxviii, 8, 505, 506, 510, 535, 536, 698, 815, 834, 1004
autoimmune hemolytic anemia, 990
autoimmune processes, xxi, xxxii, 489, 538, 1025, 1026
autoimmunity, 502, 513, 515, 516, 536, 542, 711, 713, 873
autonomic nervous system, 469
autopsy, 589
autosomal dominant, 250, 251, 253, 254, 255, 256, 257, 374, 914
autosomal recessive, 92, 93, 194, 203, 205, 251, 252, 255, 264
avascular, xiii, 1, 18, 24, 816, 1122, 1757
avian, 163, 457, 468, 470
avoidance, xxxix, xlii, 343, 416, 439, 497, 558
awareness, xix, xl, xliv, 32, 389, 479, 546, 564, 579, 994
axial skeleton, 985
axilla, 402
Azathioprine, 703

B

Bacillus subtilis, 668
backscattering, 276
bacteremia, 583, 594
bacteria, xvii, xxv, 61, 85, 129, 160, 164, 237, 293, 612, 635, 637, 647, 664, 665, 667, 668, 669, 681, 683, 687, 688, 689, 707, 752, 753, 757, 881
bacterial infection, 57, 579, 636, 692, 696, 697, 834, 850, 917
bacterial pathogens, 299, 588
bactericides, 424, 431
bacterium, 164
balanitis, 897
ban, xli
bandwidth, 49
Bangladesh, x, xlix
barium, 796
barriers, xxxviii, 580, 583, 584, 585, 638, 701, 742, 744
basal cell carcinoma, xvi, 72, 79, 249, 256, 269, 270, 330, 332, 351, 371, 449, 476, 484, 485, 908, 915, 927
basal lamina, 7, 44
basal layer, xxxvii, 15, 57, 86, 125, 126, 250, 253, 385, 402, 404, 414, 415, 423, 432, 446, 456, 817, 840, 841, 916, 953, 1018
base, xxxix, 14, 74, 116, 170, 207, 237, 267, 315, 328, 329, 330, 343, 344, 356, 422, 626, 657, 664, 666, 667, 679, 680, 682, 695, 795, 797, 798, 878, 879
base pair, 329, 330
base tan theory, xxxix, 1265, 1278
basement membrane, xxxvi, 3, 8, 18, 74, 77, 294, 915, 1020, 1027, 1032
basement membrane zone, 77, 1020, 1032, 1034
baths, 954
beach-day, xliii, 1445, 1452
beams, 50, 51
behavioral problems, 771, 776

behaviors, xxxviii, xxxix, xl, xlvii, 325, 355, 457, 468, 776, 779, 784, 819, 914, 961
Belgium, 600
bending, 48, 278, 280
beneficial effect, 25, 126, 176, 503, 830, 894, 938, 939
benefits, xiii, xix, xli, xlii, xliii, 26, 44, 319, 320, 333, 345, 390, 697, 748, 777, 831, 903, 909, 939, 1001, 1002
benign, xxxvii, 24, 255, 415, 474, 797, 882, 883, 1018
benzene, 327
benzyl cinnamate, xliii, 1445, 1449
benzyl salicylate, xliii, 427, 430, 431, 1254, 1445, 1449, 1454
beta blocker, 900, 1005
beverages, 554
bias, 350, 538, 561, 573
bilateral, 127, 533, 634, 798, 800, 906
bile, 300
bilirubin, 300, 895, 900
binding globulin, 141
bioassay, 733
bioavailability, 597, 743
biochemistry, 145, 157, 178, 376, 379
biological activities, 147, 170
biological markers, xxx, 613, 938, 945, 949, 950, 1431
biological processes, 67
biological samples, 718
biomarkers, xxxi, 60, 91, 594, 938, 945, 1010
biomaterials, 609, 621
biomolecules, xlv, 273, 659
biopolymer(s), xvi, 85, 87, 222, 271, 272, 274, 275, 277, 280, 282, 285, 289
biopsy, xxxii, xxxiii, 44, 57, 174, 402, 403, 588, 751, 801, 895, 896, 979, 989, 1003, 1017, 1020, 1027, 1031
bioremediation, 177
biosynthesis, xiii, xxvi, xxxvi, 87, 88, 89, 124, 132, 150, 152, 153, 161, 163, 167, 172, 175, 176, 178, 182, 185, 186, 187, 188, 215, 217, 243, 245, 250, 296, 338, 339, 360, 378, 380, 445, 597, 661, 662, 703, 717, 722, 723, 864
biotechnology, 185
bipolar disorder, 993
birds, 456, 462, 913
birefringence, 57
birth control, 402, 773
birth weight, 574, 581, 607, 609, 770, 772, 773, 780, 781, 782, 783, 785, 786, 794
births, 770
birthweight, 774, 775, 776, 785
bisphenol, 424
Blacks, 268
blastomycosis, 168, 171
blastopore, 689
bleaching, 285, 296, 376, 664
bleeding, xxiv, 93, 205, 206, 251, 655, 656, 691, 798, 820, 878, 879, 989, 1032
bleeding time, 251
blepharitis, xxiii, 545, 548, 551, 554, 555, 556, 557, 558, 559, 560, 562, 566, 568, 569, 882
blindness, 260, 588
blistering disease, xxxii, xxxiii, 8, 1017, 1031, 1032, 1042, 1048
blood circulation, 923
blood cultures, 573, 576, 586, 587, 589, 592, 598, 615, 634, 641
blood flow, xxxv, 13, 32, 55, 57, 70, 81, 526
blood monocytes, 858
blood plasma, 1004
blood pressure, 653, 885, 900
blood stream, 585
blood supply, xxvii, 18, 192, 767, 768, 780, 807
blood transfusion, 582, 583
blood transfusions, 583
blood vessels, xiv, xxxiv, 4, 13, 18, 24, 43, 54, 56, 63, 64, 296, 298, 301, 428, 736, 839, 844, 938
bloodstream, xxiv, 572, 573, 579, 585, 586, 600, 601, 602, 603, 604, 605, 606, 607, 609, 612, 613, 614, 615, 618, 619, 621, 623, 624, 628, 629, 631, 639, 640, 644, 646, 648, 649, 651, 652, 653, 660
body fat, 958
body image, 991
body mass index (BMI), 955, 983, 1002, 1010
body size, 370
body weight, 2, 360, 443, 446, 942, 1002
bonding, 288, 446
bonds, 48, 125, 126, 272
bone, xxxix, 177, 189, 366, 377, 583, 585, 607, 642, 700, 701, 832, 894, 954, 986, 988
bone form, 988
bone growth, 832
bone marrow, 177, 189, 583, 607, 700, 701, 894
bone marrow transplant, 583, 607, 700, 701
Bosnia, 521
bowel, 635, 704, 714, 986, 990, 997
bowel obstruction, 635, 990
bradycardia, 797
bradykinin, 736
brain, xxvii, 134, 167, 170, 205, 266, 444, 446, 475, 476, 477, 478, 481, 482, 487, 488, 587, 588, 632, 767, 768, 769, 770, 771, 772, 773, 774, 776, 777, 778, 780, 781, 783, 784, 786, 787
brain abnormalities, 770

brain abscess, 769
brain damage, xxvii, 475, 767, 768, 771, 787
brain functioning, 769
brain growth, 768
brain structure, 774
brain tumor, 482, 487
branching, 10, 16, 223, 240
Brazil, 63, 159, 183, 293, 574, 575, 576, 577, 578, 603, 605, 617, 619, 620, 623, 624, 631, 638, 641, 644, 646, 649, 655, 678, 717, 1017
breakdown, 447, 704, 707
breast cancer, xx, 56, 324, 473, 478, 481, 486, 488, 927, 930
breast milk, 900, 903, 906
breastfeeding, 825, 888, 895, 900, 903, 906
breathing, xxvii, 278, 761, 770, 793, 794, 797, 798, 803
breathlessness, xxvii, 761
breeding, 298, 300, 303, 840
broadband, 274, 810, 827, 890, 944, 951, 953
broad-spectrum testing, xliii, 1446, 1453
bronchial asthma, xxvi, 735, 736, 742, 745
bronchial epithelium, 838
bronchiectasis, 744
bronchiolitis, 764
bronchitis, 903, 905
bronchopulmonary dysplasia, 763, 769, 781, 785
bronchoscopy, 795
buccal mucosa, 669, 691, 757
budding, 165, 167, 168, 171, 586, 588, 661, 690
buffalo, 384
building blocks, 273, 625
Bulgaria, 435
bullous pemphigoid, viii, xiii, xxxii, xxxiii, 1017, 1018, 1020, 1022, 1023, 1025, 1026, 1027, 1028, 1029, 1045
burn, xlviii, xlix, l, 55, 56, 61, 79, 257, 325, 334, 340, 397, 479, 572, 575, 580, 893
burn-injured patients, l, 1798, 1813
by-products, xliv

C

Ca^{2+}, 167, 382, 817
cabbage, 727
cadaver, 971
caffeine, 554, 558
calcification, 819, 897
Calcineurin inhibitors, 824, 827, 858, 889
calcium, 8, 123, 333, 397, 400, 407, 742, 747, 817, 839, 841, 843, 850, 851, 852, 865, 867, 868, 875, 955
calculus, 664
caliber, 797
calibration, 55
caloric restriction, 11, 12, 13, 25, 26
calorie, xxxi, 40, 796, 999, 1000, 1002, 1005
Cambodia, 320
campaigns, xviii, 323
cancer control, xlvii, 1325, 1372, 1374, 1376, 1404, 1412, 1703, 1706, 1711, 1713, 1721
Cancer Prevention and Control, xlvii, 1325, 1640, 1651, 1703, 1736
cancer screening, xli, 346
candida, 742, 746, 750
candida albicans, 746
candidal esophagitis, 678
candidates, 400
CAP, 128
capillary, xxvii, xxx, 18, 32, 36, 75, 76, 435, 438, 707, 736, 761, 762, 830, 937, 940
capsule, xvii, 41, 163, 164, 293
carbamazepine, 875
carbohydrate(s), 172, 184, 622, 691, 696, 721, 732, 747
carbon, 131, 174, 213, 277, 939
carbon atoms, 277
carboxyl, 279, 368
carboxylic acid(s), 84, 87, 133, 148, 192, 215, 216, 255, 272, 273, 277, 370, 464, 844, 868
carcinoembryonic antigen, 8
carcinogen, xli, 127, 237, 326, 327, 343
carcinogenesis, xviii, 14, 323, 335, 341, 345, 348, 349, 350, 355, 356, 387, 828, 892, 942, 944, 953
carcinogenicity, xliv, 421, 848
carcinoma, 6, 33, 79, 355, 476, 484, 555, 558, 567, 711, 762, 876, 890, 893, 952, 953, 991
CARD15, 444
cardiac arrest, 769
cardiac failure, xxviii, 789, 822, 884
cardiac surgery, 588, 783
cardiopulmonary bypass, 781
cardiovascular disease(s), xxxii, 377, 477, 819, 830, 840, 854, 885, 958, 997, 1009, 1014, 1015
cardiovascular function, 444
cardiovascular morbidity, xxxii, 1009, 1010, 1011, 1013
cardiovascular risk, xxxi, 819, 859, 958, 981, 983, 987, 995
cardiovascular system, 768, 982
caregivers, 799
carotenoids, xxxviii, 182, 397, 405
cartilage, 464, 793
cartoon, 778
cascades, xviii, 89, 365, 392, 621, 828
case study(s), 39, 355, 774

caspases, 409
catabolism, xlviii, 163, 173, 299, 300
catalytic activity, 93, 368
cataract, 634, 646, 891
cataract extraction, 634, 646
categorization, 491
cathepsin G, 720
catheter, 573, 580, 582, 583, 584, 585, 586, 587, 599, 605, 606, 627, 631, 634, 636, 644, 653
cation, 337, 338, 357, 409, 836, 863
Caucasians, 334, 382, 536, 537, 872
causal relationship, 819
causality, 1000
causation, l, 352, 419, 427, 429, 430, 431, 435, 436, 439, 782
CBC, 435, 895, 896, 898, 900
C-C, 278
CCC, xlvii, xlviii, 1292, 1293, 1376, 1385, 1412, 1464, 1703, 1704, 1705, 1706, 1707, 1710, 1712, 1713, 1714, 1715, 1716, 1718, 1719, 1720, 1721, 1722, 1723, 1724, 1725, 1727, 1730
CD8+, 511, 520, 536, 540, 541, 557, 690, 700, 901, 924, 929, 931, 997
cDNA, 38, 204, 218, 380, 382, 443, 450, 732
CEC, 651
cell biology, 178, 212, 260, 378, 379
cell culture, xviii, 11, 65, 66, 143, 308, 378, 379, 391
cell cycle, 11, 12, 14, 22, 185, 701, 703, 828, 877, 944, 953
cell death, xxvi, 38, 61, 157, 254, 366, 597, 664, 665, 668, 718, 731, 771, 892
cell differentiation, 79, 141, 294, 396, 406, 625, 825, 875
cell division, 71, 74, 76, 621, 700, 702, 943
cell fate, 140, 378, 460, 466, 467, 470
cell line(s), 72, 74, 75, 141, 144, 156, 330, 358, 361, 367, 374, 385, 394, 487, 510, 677, 837, 918, 920
cell membranes, 121, 828
cell metabolism, xxxiv, 668
cell signaling, 621, 865, 928
cell size, 669
cell surface, 123, 173, 342, 367, 384, 527, 529, 536, 647, 661, 730, 902, 915, 946
cellular damage, xlii, xlv, 1143, 1226, 1429, 1601
cellular immunity, 707, 741, 841
cellular signaling pathway, 390
cellulitis, 905
cellulose, xxvii, 188, 242, 749, 753, 759
Central Europe, 336, 538
central nervous system (CNS), xviii, 255, 365, 609, 633, 643, 645, 769, 991, 1020
central obesity, 1003
ceramide, 91, 141, 182
cerebral blood flow, 768, 781
cerebral function, 485
cerebral hypoxia, 786
cerebral palsy, 771, 773, 780, 795
cerebrospinal fluid, 619, 633, 642, 644, 650
cerebrovascular disease, 983, 1010
chain mobility, 963, 966
chalazion, 547, 548, 549, 552, 555, 556, 558
challenges, xxvii, 85, 715, 767, 768, 774, 817, 844
channel blocker, 900
Chediak Higashi Syndrome, xv, 83
cheilitis, 656, 691, 692, 694, 696, 697, 699, 700, 701, 702, 704, 707, 709, 750, 897
chelators, xliii, 1227, 1467, 1474, 1484, 1499
chemical bonds, 48, 274
chemical degradation, 214
chemical peel, xxxiv, 25, 146, 404
chemical properties, 160, 290, 447, 452
chemical reactions, xviii, 365
chemical structures, 419, 963
chemiluminescence, 531
chemokine receptor, 931
chemokines, 552, 553, 554, 566, 836, 840, 847, 912, 915, 917, 923, 924, 928, 1004, 1010
chemotaxis, xxxiii, 525, 583, 707, 719, 942, 952
chemotherapeutic agent, 479, 487
chemotherapy, xxiii, xxiv, xxv, 73, 173, 178, 181, 183, 185, 188, 479, 481, 486, 571, 579, 580, 581, 586, 587, 607, 655, 658, 683, 688, 695, 700, 701, 702, 714
CHF, 904
chicken, xx, 361, 455, 456, 460, 462, 463, 464, 468, 469, 470, 874
chicken pox, 874
childhood, xxi, xxxii, xxxix, xlv, xlvi, xlvii, 9, 324, 333, 343, 348, 351, 477, 482, 483, 484, 485, 489, 490, 491, 496, 502, 547, 562, 563, 567, 568, 707, 715, 773, 780, 781, 784, 786, 800, 817, 823, 834, 853, 860, 1017, 1018
childhood cancer, xxxix
China, 83, 311, 426, 496, 502, 518, 540, 574, 575, 576, 620, 911, 912, 928, 930
chitin, xxvii, 165, 167, 172, 182, 185, 242, 749, 752, 753, 759
chitinase, 245, 246
Chitosan, 685
Chlamydia, 555
chloasma, 92, 146, 401, 437
chlorine, xliv
cholangitis, 587
cholecystitis, 587
cholestasis, 703, 706
cholesterol, 27, 92, 400, 408, 640, 661, 960

chondroitin sulfate, 3, 17, 559, 568
chorioretinitis, 588, 635
choroid, 206
chromatography, 151, 452, 693, 960, 979
chromatophore, xvii, 293
chromium, 326
chromosome, xx, 205, 254, 258, 262, 264, 384, 402, 443, 444, 455, 464, 510, 536, 538, 700, 838, 883, 941, 942, 985, 990
chromosome 10, 384, 510
chronic diseases, 707
chronic granulomatous disease, xxv, 688, 694, 696, 712, 713
chronic inflammatory cells, 557
chronic kidney disease, 703
chronic obstructive pulmonary disease, 737, 745, 982
chronic sun exposure, xxxviii, 1180, 1216, 1218, 1229, 1230, 1236, 1266, 1660
chymotrypsin, 726
CID, 714
cigarette smoke, 32, 878
cigarette smokers, 32
cigarette smoking, 32, 873, 878
circulation, xxvii, 32, 442, 592, 707, 762, 767, 768, 769, 784, 842, 874
cirrhosis, 582, 705, 706, 895, 989
cities, 475, 601, 605, 930
civilization, 939
classes, xxvi, xxx, xxxvi, 53, 87, 498, 527, 661, 718, 722, 724, 937, 938
classification, xxii, xlv, 31, 421, 474, 491, 505, 506, 514, 551, 552, 561, 564, 619, 645, 674, 711, 715, 770, 772, 773, 787, 800, 821, 823, 824, 868, 883, 885, 903, 909, 921
classroom, 773, 778
cleaning, 657, 680, 975
cleanup, 177
cleavage(s), 123, 199, 329, 340, 342, 360, 371, 372, 443, 926
climate, 331, 349, 352, 354, 397, 548
climate change, 349, 352
climates, 331, 578
clinical application, xxxv, 79, 661, 939
clinical assessment, 56
clinical diagnosis, 54, 693
clinical judgment, 609
clinical presentation, xxiii, xxv, 181, 486, 500, 514, 558, 572, 581, 586, 588, 598, 634, 636, 687, 688, 709, 711, 985
clinical problems, 622
clinical symptoms, xxiii, 571, 705, 820
clinical trials, xxxix, 127, 128, 132, 320, 481, 528, 599, 605, 670, 833, 884, 887, 891, 904, 926, 956, 1002, 1012
cloning, 168, 182, 261, 358, 382, 384, 442, 443, 450
closure, 57, 832
clothing, xxxviii, xlv, 331, 439, 890
clustering, xxxviii
CMC, 563, 698, 699
C-N, 278
CNS, xxvii, 446, 633, 767, 780
CO_2, 315, 797, 798
coaches, xlvi
coal, 827, 887, 890, 891, 939, 941
coal tar, 827, 887, 890, 891, 939, 941
coarctation, 768
cobalt, 326, 426
coccidioidomycosis, 168, 172, 185
cocoa, 206, 251, 252, 261
coding, xxii, 202, 361, 370, 400, 402, 411, 446, 535, 538, 539, 696, 779, 926
codon, 206, 349
coenzyme, xv, xxxii, 159, 161, 999, 1000, 1004, 1006
coffee, 98, 150, 554
cognition, 781
cognitive abilities, 768, 772
cognitive deficit(s), 774
cognitive development, 769, 770
cognitive domains, 772
cognitive dysfunction, xxvii, 767, 768
cognitive function, xxviii, 767, 771, 772, 774, 783
cognitive impairment, 770, 771, 774, 780
coherence, xiv, 43, 50, 59, 61
COI, xxviii, 805, 806, 810, 813
collaboration, xlvi, 209
college students, xxxviii, xxxix
Colombia, 574, 576, 577, 615
colon, 372, 579, 844, 990, 1019
colon cancer, 990
colonisation, 674
combination therapy, 129, 437, 598, 706, 737, 743, 832, 885, 887, 889, 891, 952, 1001
commensalism, 673, 751
commercial, xliii, xliv, xlv, 275, 331, 332, 426, 430, 560, 671, 679, 692
common signs, 548
communication, xiv, 3, 43, 63, 64, 69, 70, 72, 73, 77, 217, 650, 835
community(s), xxxix, xl, xlvi, xlvii, 575, 621, 659, 736, 739
comorbidity, 499, 501, 513, 795, 823, 853, 854, 855, 941, 982, 992, 993, 996
compatibility, 243

compensation, 372, 707
competition, xxxv, 525, 531, 925
complement, 8, 37, 165, 167, 174, 180, 182, 186, 689, 690, 719, 736, 824, 833, 943, 953, 1011
complementarity, 905, 921
complete blood count, 832
complex interactions, 449
complexity, xiv, 57, 64, 241, 449, 583, 847
compliance, xxviii, xxxiii, 560, 663, 665, 668, 737, 738, 740, 799, 805, 811, 818, 824, 830, 848, 849, 850, 886, 941
complications, xxxiii, 55, 57, 478, 524, 547, 551, 558, 583, 632, 636, 639, 641, 658, 660, 674, 701, 737, 770, 798, 800, 801, 819, 825, 831, 841, 856, 882, 895, 987, 990, 1031
composition, xiii, xiv, xvii, xxxviii, 4, 25, 41, 43, 44, 48, 49, 57, 86, 144, 177, 178, 189, 271, 281, 475, 626, 651, 668, 691, 706, 707, 890, 958, 960, 979
comprehension, 58
compression, 16, 895
compression fracture, 895
computer, 45
conception, 830
concordance, 536
condensation, 19, 665
conditioning, 548, 585, 700
conduction, 254
conference, 860
configuration, 48, 50, 413, 414
conflict, 920
confrontation, 499
congenital heart disease, 763, 768, 772, 781, 782, 783, 784, 785, 786, 787
congenital leukoderma, 250
congenital malformations, 799
congestive heart failure, 371, 769, 904
Congo, 8, 436
Congress, 320, 611
conjunctiva, xxiii, 545, 546, 547, 549, 553, 557, 559, 762, 874
conjunctivitis, xxiii, 545, 546, 548, 549, 555, 558, 562, 564, 567
connective tissue(s), xiv, xx, 3, 7, 14, 26, 30, 33, 35, 39, 43, 44, 75, 301, 455, 456, 458, 462, 463, 565, 697, 708, 816, 1122, 1132, 1150
consensus, 449, 598, 613, 739, 856, 860, 867, 900, 910, 934, 1003, 1007
conservation, xxxiv, 32
constituents, xiv, 63, 149, 150, 152, 153, 155, 314, 315, 850, 915, 1018
construction, xvi, xliv, xlv, 249, 689, 703
consumers, 126, 319, 421, 560, 1005
consumption, 605, 909, 1005, 1007
contact dermatitis, 55, 392, 414, 418, 422, 423, 424, 425, 426, 428, 429, 434, 435, 436, 437, 438, 439, 524, 526, 558, 863, 886, 890, 1018
contact time, 740
containers, 228
contaminant, xxiv, 617
contaminated sites, 177
contamination, 226, 430, 588, 592, 635, 657, 678, 679, 693
contiguity, 585
contingency, 755, 756
contour, 26
contraceptives, 883, 1000
contracture, xlviii
control group, 22, 491, 492, 497, 560, 739, 741, 772, 773, 774, 776, 926, 1004, 1010
controlled studies, 888, 902, 1011
controlled trials, 561, 1021, 1022
controversial, xxx, xxxiii, xliv, 17, 138, 218, 381, 480, 598, 693, 737, 740, 830, 831, 834, 840, 875, 883, 895, 938, 944, 946, 949, 1011
controversies, 410, 848, 858, 861, 1023, 1029
convergence, 375
cooking, 670
cooling, 226, 481, 488
cooperation, 430, 431, 541
coordination, xl, 738, 773, 777, 793
COPD, 737, 745
coping strategies, 500
copper, xxxvi, 88, 129, 130, 156, 204, 207, 216, 245, 652
cor pulmonale, 797
cornea, xxiii, 545, 546, 547, 550, 557, 559
corneal ulcer, 550, 553, 555, 561, 897
coronary angioplasty, 478
coronary artery disease, 1004
coronary heart disease, 984
correlation(s), xxi, xxxiii, 55, 56, 71, 268, 309, 490, 537, 546, 547, 553, 601, 648, 676, 703, 719, 731, 746, 758, 830, 877, 932, 934, 948, 955, 971, 977, 978
correlation coefficient, 758
corrosion, 664
cortex, 232, 236, 237, 238, 243
corticosteroid therapy, 487, 526, 714, 737, 743
corticotropin, 84, 92, 141, 450, 452, 453, 566
cortisol, 416, 742, 747, 825
cosmetic(s), xvii, xix, xxxiv, xlii, xliv, xlv, 18, 24, 25, 26, 27, 39, 41, 94, 129, 133, 143, 147, 154, 177, 189, 307, 308, 310, 311, 312, 319, 320, 345, 390, 401, 414, 426, 427, 428, 429, 430, 431, 432, 438, 449, 500, 819, 887, 890

cost, xxv, xl, xliv, 406, 579, 655, 737, 752, 824, 829, 997, 1002
cotton, xlv, 226, 435, 436, 524, 588, 753
cough, 794, 899, 906
covering, xxxvi, 424, 577, 820
cracks, 692, 699
creatine, 15
creatinine, 895, 896, 899, 900
creativity, 362
critical analysis, 1023
critical period, 351
CRM, 44, 51, 52, 53
crops, 429, 882
cross links, xxxvi, 828
croup, 740, 746, 793
crowns, 222
CRP, 948, 949, 950, 987, 988
crust, 57, 883
cryosurgery, 404
cryptococcosis, 163, 164, 178, 179, 183, 905
crystalline, 314, 523
crystals, 294
CSA, 707, 898, 899, 900
CSD, 1014
CSF, 5, 37, 65, 84, 89, 384, 633, 703, 830, 919
CT scan, 593
cultivars, 245
cultivation, 65, 75, 80, 133, 240
culture conditions, 197, 241
culture media, 169, 197, 201, 589
culture medium, 66, 171, 173, 183, 244, 419
curcumin, 25, 684, 727, 733
cure, xxix, 183, 414, 417, 422, 430, 431, 436, 437, 449, 474, 475, 598, 631, 741, 816, 847, 884, 1028
customers, xlii
cyanosis, xiii, xxvii, xxviii, 761, 762, 763, 764, 765, 767, 768, 769, 770, 776, 780, 785, 789, 790, 794, 797, 799, 805, 806, 807, 810, 812, 813, 814
Cyanosis Observation Index, xxviii, 805, 810
cyanotic, xxvii, 762, 764, 766, 767, 768, 769, 770, 772, 776, 777, 781, 785, 787
cycles, xlv, 74, 75, 479, 680, 701
cycling, 75, 80, 511, 935
cyclooxygenase, 123, 124, 864
cyclophosphamide, xxxii, 701, 702, 706, 1017, 1021, 1023
cyclosporine, xxix, xxxii, 512, 527, 532, 559, 561, 568, 702, 706, 830, 831, 847, 859, 860, 871, 883, 885, 893, 895, 898, 899, 900, 910, 924, 925, 935, 991, 993, 999, 1002, 1007
cyst, 73, 793, 794, 800
cysteine, 72, 165, 198, 199, 217, 222, 255, 334, 337, 368, 369, 842
cystic fibrosis, 173
cystine, 198
cystitis, 639
cytochrome, 176, 597, 724, 898, 900
cytochrome p450, 597
cytokine networks, 89, 918
cytology, 553, 749, 751, 752, 753, 757, 758, 759
cytomegalovirus, 510, 515, 520, 540, 583
cytometry, 553
cytoplasm, 4, 160, 171, 200, 205, 242, 296, 299, 402, 585, 659, 669, 898, 915
cytosine, 329
cytoskeleton, 22, 23, 38, 200, 253, 585, 915
cytotoxicity, 4, 146, 312, 363, 833

D

dactylitis, 872, 988, 989
daily living, xlix, 777
daily-use, xliii, 1445
damages, xiii, xlii, 2, 14, 54, 96, 584, 878
danger, 431, 476
data analysis, xiv, 43
data transfer, 45
database, 348, 641, 854
DBP, xliv
DCPC, xlvii, 1703, 1704, 1706
death rate, 346
deaths, xl, xlvi, 324, 579
debridement, l, 636, 637
debts, 493, 497
deep venous thrombosis, 990
defects, xv, xxvii, 26, 55, 83, 93, 206, 252, 326, 372, 374, 445, 480, 553, 559, 583, 587, 658, 712, 761, 765, 768, 781, 782, 784, 785, 802, 831, 835, 837, 838, 839, 863, 866
defence, 405
defense mechanisms, xv, xxvi, 160, 165, 170, 172, 658, 670, 688, 689, 690, 705, 718, 728
deficiency(s), xxviii, 13, 34, 92, 199, 207, 251, 252, 260, 261, 324, 326, 333, 337, 343, 442, 446, 452, 551, 554, 557, 582, 657, 691, 698, 703, 708, 732, 742, 805, 806, 812, 813, 814, 831, 838, 895
deficit, xlix, 12, 252, 781, 784
deformation, 45, 278
degradation, xxxv, xliv, 12, 13, 14, 15, 16, 17, 19, 20, 21, 26, 33, 70, 72, 86, 88, 91, 93, 94, 121, 127, 132, 135, 140, 144, 151, 164, 165, 174, 178, 179, 181, 197, 296, 300, 308, 349, 373, 376, 403, 408, 585, 664, 696, 708
degradation process, 70
dehydration, 15, 161, 397, 816, 823, 884
delirium, 993

dementia, 1020
demographic characteristics, 578
demyelinating disease, 905, 906
demyelination, 906
denaturation, 26
dendrites, xvii, 85, 135, 144, 192, 200, 208, 253, 307, 308, 313, 316, 318, 339, 367, 402
dendritic cell, xvii, xxix, 3, 21, 80, 307, 313, 446, 703, 815, 820, 828, 832, 837, 840, 843, 868, 878, 908, 912, 922, 930, 932, 936, 943, 947, 948, 949, 956, 991
Denmark, 423, 573, 574, 575, 576, 577, 602, 604
dental caries, 691, 715
dental plaque, 707
dentist, 755, 1032
dentures, 657, 660, 661, 663, 664, 665, 666, 667, 668, 669, 670, 671, 672, 673, 675, 678, 679, 680, 681, 682, 684, 689, 727, 743, 746
Department of Education, xlvii
dephosphorylation, 898
depolarization, 727
depolymerization, 122
deposition, 3, 4, 15, 18, 20, 26, 37, 47, 51, 58, 68, 71, 126, 167, 168, 186, 242, 288, 295, 334, 414, 737, 738, 743, 1020, 1032
deposits, xvi, 221, 523, 989
depressants, 835
depression, xxi, xli, xliii, 64, 489, 497, 499, 500, 501, 509, 526, 776, 818, 819, 821, 853, 895, 982, 992, 993
depressive symptoms, 499
deprivation, 215, 732, 769, 787
depth, xxxvi, xliv, 45, 48, 49, 50, 51, 52, 55, 207, 276, 500, 527, 960, 968, 970, 979
deregulation, 538
derivatives, 68, 87, 127, 129, 147, 150, 151, 154, 308, 371, 426, 428, 434, 438, 456, 457, 458, 460, 462, 463, 466, 467, 470, 638, 816, 867, 868
dermabrasion, 25
dermatitis, 56, 61, 414, 415, 422, 423, 424, 425, 426, 427, 428, 429, 430, 431, 432, 433, 434, 435, 436, 437, 438, 439, 479, 480, 481, 486, 487, 488, 558, 874, 880, 886, 888, 915, 918, 938, 947, 960, 1018, 1020
dermatitis herpetiformis, 1018, 1020
dermatologist, xxxiv, 401, 430, 499, 500, 522, 523, 546, 988
dermatology, xxxi, xxxviii, xlvi, 50, 59, 181, 376, 378, 382, 383, 384, 385, 386, 426, 430, 451, 453, 491, 492, 497, 499, 500, 502, 503, 532, 562, 683, 809, 853, 855, 857, 858, 859, 860, 864, 865, 959, 992, 998, 1015
dermatomyositis, 558, 1020
dermatoses, xxi, 423, 489, 526, 863, 886, 943
dermatosis, xvi, 249, 253, 257, 425, 433, 715, 1020
desiccation, xv, 160, 174, 176
desmosome, 125, 126
desorption, 592, 612
destiny, 456, 460
destruction, xiii, 2, 19, 71, 425, 479, 511, 513, 522, 660, 668, 708
detachment, 1027
detectable, xxv, 442, 592, 687, 693, 842, 941, 942
detection, xlvii, 35, 49, 52, 174, 179, 225, 242, 255, 324, 452, 592, 593, 594, 610, 612, 693, 711, 750, 754, 756, 760, 812, 847, 893
detergents, 663, 978
detonation, 486
detoxification, 15, 299, 722, 725
developed countries, l
developing countries, l
developmental change, 212
developmental disorder, 776
developmental process, xx, 455, 456
deviation, 832, 967
Dhaka Medical College Hospital (DMCH), xlix, 1775, 1776
diabetes, xxiv, xxv, xxvi, xxxi, xxxii, 55, 61, 381, 518, 519, 580, 582, 584, 655, 658, 667, 671, 672, 673, 674, 675, 676, 688, 694, 699, 703, 707, 708, 709, 715, 736, 747, 829, 858, 897, 981, 983, 984, 987, 989, 995, 997, 1000, 1003, 1004, 1007, 1009, 1010
diabetic patients, 658, 660, 671, 672, 674, 676, 715, 997
diabetic retinopathy, 55
diacylglycerol, 374
dialysis, 580, 583, 588, 635, 636, 639, 640, 641, 646, 652, 653
diaper rash, 823
diarrhea, xxiii, 585, 617, 899, 901
diet, xxiii, xxxi, 13, 40, 364, 429, 535, 691, 696, 990, 999, 1000, 1002, 1003, 1007
dietary habits, 1000
dietary interventions, xxxix, 1065, 1284
dietary supplementation, 568
differential diagnosis, 557, 757
diffraction, 287, 979
diffuse reflectance, 47, 53, 55, 60
diffusion, xxxv, 55, 614, 622, 676, 693, 771, 966, 969
diffusion-weighted imaging, 771
digestion, xv, 14, 16, 160, 624, 626
dihydroxyphenylalanine, xv, 84, 88, 159, 160, 162, 222, 296
dilation, 26, 557, 769, 770

dimerization, 161, 373
dimorphism, 639, 652, 710
diode laser, 798
diodes, 809
direct observation, 588
disability, xxix, 781, 818, 823, 853, 871, 992, 1014
disaster, 426
discharges, 573
disclosure, 926
discomfort, 523, 666, 878, 975, 1032
discontinuity, 585
discrimination, 625, 812, 993
discs, 424, 429
disease activity, 746, 876, 903, 984, 1020, 1021
disease model, 852
disease progression, 518, 559, 586, 839, 902, 996
disequilibrium, 537, 538, 863
disinfection, xxv, xliv, 474, 655, 663, 664, 665, 666, 667, 668, 669, 670, 671, 672, 678, 680, 681, 682, 684
dislocation, 585
dispersion, 127, 275, 294, 295, 296, 457, 469, 745
displacement, 45, 556, 772, 790, 792
distillation, 890
distilled water, xlv, 117, 224, 226, 315, 316, 963
distress, 478, 497, 502, 528, 560, 581, 763, 764, 768, 769, 783, 853, 903
District of Columbia, xli, xlvii
divergence, 722
diversity, 185, 252, 257, 265, 270, 305, 351, 357, 358, 381, 411, 452, 554, 605, 647, 673, 676, 715, 824
diverticulitis, 903
dizygotic, 536
dizygotic twins, 536
dizziness, 528, 830
DMCH, 1775
DMF, 842, 843, 844
DNA analysis, 539
DNA damage, xv, xviii, xxxviii, xlii, 12, 14, 83, 92, 138, 323, 329, 334, 341, 343, 344, 345, 346, 349, 350, 356, 363, 364, 366, 377, 447, 944, 953
DNA lesions, xxxviii, 349
DNA ligase, 330, 344
DNA polymerase, 330, 343, 344
DNA repair, xviii, xxxviii, xliii, 12, 13, 25, 33, 324, 326, 328, 330, 333, 341, 343, 344, 347, 349, 351, 362, 363, 364, 480, 944
DNA sequencing, 626
DNA strand breaks, xxxvii, 272
DNAs, 384
doctors, 994
dogs, 342, 361, 369, 380
dominance, 366
donors, 37, 841
dopamine, 87, 162, 165
dopaminergic, 87
dosage, 331, 446, 516, 524, 739, 743, 744, 825, 830, 885, 887, 891, 893, 894, 896, 897, 899, 902, 903, 904, 905, 906, 942, 1023, 1027
dose-response relationship, 485
dosing, 481, 894, 895, 896, 899, 902, 904, 1001, 1004
double helix, 329, 330
double-blind trial, 569, 645, 951
Down syndrome, 538, 542, 795
down-regulation, 12, 91, 92, 132, 344, 1010
drainage, 581, 637
drawing, 45
dressings, 864
Drosophila, 260
drought, 222, 242
drug action, 703
drug delivery, 59, 528, 740, 745
drug design, 345, 568
drug development, 177, 732
drug discovery, 726, 728, 733
drug interaction, 598, 662, 895, 942, 1020
drug reactions, 705, 888
drug resistance, 80, 560, 602, 605, 672, 674, 689, 693, 730
drug targets, 400, 406, 726, 857
drug therapy, 736, 737
drug treatment, 770
dry eyes, 563, 568
drying, 13, 940
duality, xxxix
duodenal ulcer, 554
DWI, 771
dyeing, xliv, 423
dyes, xliv, 415, 423, 424, 436, 438, 557, 669, 727, 752
dyslipidemia, 884, 983, 984, 989
dyspareunia, 638
dysphagia, xxviii, 789, 795
dyspnea, xxviii, 789, 790, 797, 799, 899, 905, 991

E

East Asia, 167, 407, 410
Eastern Europe, 474
eating disorders, 993, 998
E-cadherin, 67, 73, 79
ECG, 111, 254

echinocandins, xxiv, xxv, 185, 578, 579, 598, 599, 618, 622, 629, 631, 632, 639, 645, 655, 661, 662, 722
ECM, xxxv, xxxvi, 1121, 1122, 1123, 1124, 1125, 1127, 1128, 1129, 1130, 1131, 1141, 1142, 1143, 1144, 1145, 1146, 1147, 1148, 1149, 1431
ecology, 163, 178, 183
economic status, 493
ectoderm, 9, 367, 456, 457, 459, 460, 469, 470
ectopic hyperpigmentation, xx, 455, 456
ectothermic, 293, 294, 296, 299
Ecuador, 619
eczema, 838, 881, 1018
edema, 26, 46, 54, 60, 525, 551, 552, 555, 637, 736, 791, 795, 798, 884, 887, 905
edentulous patients, 657
editors, 28, 39, 995, 997
education, xxxix, xl, xlvi, xlvii, 432, 491, 500, 776, 891, 993
educational programs, xlvi
educators, xxvii, 767, 768
EEG, 477
EEG activity, 477
effluent(s), 177, 635
Egypt, 951, 956
eicosapentaenoic acid, 355
elaboration, 64
elafin, 33
elastic deformation, 45
elastosis, xiii, xxxiv, xxxv, 2, 6, 7, 10, 13, 19, 20, 23, 24, 28, 33, 36, 893, 1079, 1086, 1121, 1123, 1132, 1142, 1180, 1181, 1218, 1224, 1284
elbows, 818, 821, 876, 879, 880, 1010
elderly population, 577
electric current, 49
electric field, 48, 276
electrical conductivity, 272, 274
electrical resistance, 978
electricity, xlviii
electrolyte, 2, 597, 884
electromagnetic, 48, 50, 327, 668
electromagnetic waves, 50
electron(s), xxxi, xxxvii, 10, 17, 20, 28, 30, 46, 86, 160, 178, 182, 222, 253, 295, 436, 442, 727, 731, 959, 960, 961, 962, 975, 978
electron microscopy, 17, 436, 442
electron paramagnetic resonance, xxxi, 178, 959, 975, 978
Electron Paramagnetic Resonance, viii, 959, 960, 978, 979
electrophoresis, 625, 626
elementary school, 772
ELISA, 394, 613, 633, 693, 1020
elongation, 10, 17, 129, 820, 872
elucidation, 913
emboli, 587
embolization, 587
embryogenesis, xiii, 1, 9, 74, 75, 76, 371, 457, 468
embryology, 468
emergency, xlviii, 846, 905
Emergency Department (ED), l, 1813
emigration, 373
emission, 46, 274, 276, 277, 281, 283, 284, 285, 289, 466, 810, 891
emotional distress, xlviii
emotional health, 982
emotional problems, 786
emotional stimuli, 991
emotionality, 500
employees, xlii, 332
EMS, 1014
emulsions, xliii
encephalopathy, 770, 782, 783, 784, 785, 786
encoding, xix, 38, 74, 92, 165, 186, 205, 265, 372, 374, 380, 389, 447, 464, 510, 625, 728, 838, 935
endocrine, 23, 367, 387, 713, 736, 991
endocrine disorders, 736
endocrinology, 387, 450, 452
endogenous mechanisms, 585
endonuclease, 344, 625
endorphins, 333
endoscopy, 766, 795, 796, 801
endothelial cells, xviii, 67, 73, 148, 365, 366, 382, 411, 703, 705, 820, 837, 840, 842, 843, 844, 845, 847, 848, 849, 850, 894, 941, 943, 945, 948, 952
endothelial dysfunction, 819, 982, 983
endothelium, 382, 830, 866
endotoxins, 585
endotracheal intubation, 572, 583
energy, xxviii, xxxvi, xlv, 14, 26, 37, 41, 44, 46, 48, 49, 51, 52, 53, 85, 121, 131, 177, 272, 274, 280, 281, 282, 283, 284, 285, 289, 327, 329, 330, 334, 442, 450, 666, 667, 668, 682, 690, 700, 805, 809, 810, 813, 892, 962, 1002, 1007
energy efficiency, xxviii, 805
England, 179, 185, 354, 575, 576, 1018
enlargement, xxxvi, 251, 879
enthesitis, 872, 989
entrapment, 664
environmental change, xlvi, xlvii
environmental conditions, 164, 169, 170, 301
environmental control, 709
environmental factors, xxii, xxix, xxxv, 193, 250, 257, 334, 351, 506, 535, 540, 548, 815, 820, 834, 835, 871, 872
environmental influences, 9

environmental stimuli, 838
environmental stress(s), xv, 160, 168, 175, 960
enzymatic activity, 170, 339, 390
enzyme immunoassay, 592
enzyme induction, 138
enzyme inhibitors, 900
enzyme-linked immunosorbent assay, 610, 1020
eosinophilia, 901
eosinophils, 1020
epidemic, xlv, l, 55, 474, 656
epidemiologic, l, 330, 653, 660, 819, 822, 856
epidemiology, xiii, xxiii, xlix, l, 32, 178, 324, 346, 348, 351, 352, 355, 449, 484, 502, 540, 572, 589, 600, 601, 603, 604, 605, 606, 607, 609, 615, 627, 641, 649, 650, 651, 653, 674, 712, 718, 733, 907, 929
epidermal melanocytes, xvi, 135, 137, 141, 152, 153, 191, 192, 193, 197, 199, 205, 208, 209, 210, 211, 212, 213, 214, 217, 264, 308, 338, 339, 345, 377, 378, 387, 408, 410, 467, 468
epidermolysis bullosa, 74, 77, 1020
epiglottis, 790, 791, 792, 797, 798, 802
epilepsy, 771
epinephrine, 170, 176
episcleritis, 551, 552, 556, 559, 990
episodic memory, 774
epithelia, xxx, 207, 624, 911, 913, 929, 930, 935, 936
epithelial cells, xxx, 65, 67, 72, 74, 93, 253, 553, 624, 643, 659, 661, 668, 670, 674, 675, 676, 684, 689, 741, 742, 747, 751, 752, 753, 760, 844, 868, 911, 913
epithelial-mesenchymal interactions, xiv, 63, 65, 66, 72, 74, 76, 80, 1187
epithelium, xxxiii, 2, 57, 72, 80, 206, 273, 373, 511, 555, 557, 562, 624, 644, 650, 657, 689, 690, 700, 701, 705, 710, 741, 760, 795, 1031
epitopes, 922, 923, 925, 928, 934
EPR, xxxi, 178, 959, 960, 961, 962, 963, 964, 965, 966, 967, 968, 969, 970, 971, 972, 973, 974, 975, 976, 977, 978, 979, 980
Epstein-Barr virus, 581
equipment, xxiv, 332, 475, 477, 617, 814
erosion, 549, 555, 823
erysipelas, 903, 906
erythema multiforme, 738
erythema nodosum, 990
erythematous papules, 879
erythrocyte sedimentation rate, 882, 884, 987
erythrocytes, 721
erythrodermic psoriasis, xxix, 822, 823, 846, 856, 871, 882, 883, 896
esophageal cancer, 713
esophageal varices, 705
ESR, 160, 171, 727, 882, 960, 979, 987, 988
ESR spectroscopy, 171
ester, 96, 113, 131, 154, 623, 869
estrogen, xxxiv, 12, 13, 202, 217
etanercept, 511, 832, 860, 901, 903, 904, 906, 924, 934, 989, 993, 1028
ethanol, 118, 123, 132, 156, 224, 227, 228, 315, 424, 527, 532, 1005
ethnic background, xxxiii
ethnic groups, xxix, 537, 547, 871
ethnicity, 346, 997
etiology, xxii, xxix, 218, 403, 490, 503, 521, 522, 536, 538, 539, 577, 588, 631, 642, 660, 672, 765, 799, 815, 819, 820, 832, 834, 842, 845, 847, 873, 1003, 1005, 1029
eukaryotic, xxvi, 173, 717, 722, 725
eukaryotic cell, 173, 725
Europe, xxiv, xxxii, l, 325, 347, 382, 547, 573, 574, 575, 576, 577, 578, 593, 601, 602, 618, 619, 620, 817, 872, 900, 902, 1009, 1018
European Commission, 94
European market, 738
evaporation, xiv, 63, 65, 551
evolution, xiii, 1, 72, 354, 356, 357, 361, 377, 407, 409, 410, 449, 450, 453, 469, 474, 514, 586, 607, 794, 878, 879, 955, 984, 985, 986, 989
examinations, 750, 751, 752, 754, 755, 757, 758, 759
excimer lasers, 892
excision, l, 14, 326, 330, 343, 344, 347, 362, 800
excitation, 46, 47, 51, 52, 53, 59, 276, 281, 282, 283, 284, 285, 289
excretion, 64, 132, 426
execution, 795
executive function(s), xxviii, 767, 770, 774, 775
executive functioning, xxviii, 767, 774, 775
exercise(s), xxxv, 27, 777, 806, 807, 830, 897
exertion, 798
exocytosis, 87, 263
exons, 205
expertise, 559
exploitation, xxvi, 718, 927, 928
extensor, 821, 879, 880, 1010
external environment, xxxv, 44, 64
externalizing behavior, 776
extracellular matrix, xxxvi, 3, 4, 5, 11, 14, 17, 20, 23, 25, 26, 32, 64, 67, 69, 71, 72, 73, 187, 467, 553, 621, 689, 1081, 1084, 1089, 1122, 1126, 1136, 1141, 1142, 1154, 1155, 1217, 1227, 1228, 1472, 1477, 1763, 1766
Extracellular matrix (ECM) proteins, xxxv, 1121
extraction, 133, 160, 310, 315, 319, 762

extracts, xvii, xxxviii, 96, 106, 119, 125, 129, 133, 143, 144, 146, 147, 151, 153, 155, 156, 157, 171, 177, 204, 307, 310, 314, 315, 316, 317, 318, 319, 320
extraversion, 776
extrusion, 721

F

FAA, 227
facial palsy, 633
Factor XIIIa, 8
failure to thrive, xxviii, 789, 794, 795, 797
fairness, xvii, 307, 308, 309, 310, 339
faith, xxxix, xl
false negative, 755
false positive, 693
families, xxxix, xl, xlvi, 255, 267, 296, 301, 358, 359, 493, 495, 514, 541, 542, 625, 818
family history, 326, 402, 492, 494, 496, 502, 514, 530, 536, 547, 818, 821, 874, 988
family members, xix, xlvi, 441, 985
family physician, 783
fascia, 986
fasting, 1003
fat, 9, 23, 44, 71, 360, 443, 446, 451, 452, 523, 528, 594, 890, 897, 967, 984
fatty acids, xxxii, 9, 121, 131, 144, 559, 569, 664, 960, 999, 1004, 1007
fauna, 415, 436, 437
FDR, 403
fear, 499, 848
feces, xxiii, 617, 618
feelings, xliii, 992, 993, 994
fermentation, 129, 418, 419, 527, 592, 690
ferritin, 564
fetal distress, 785
fetus, xxvii, 767, 831, 893, 903
fever, 586, 587, 588, 598, 633, 635, 822, 882, 884, 990, 991
fiber(s), xiii, xiv, xxxvi, xliv, xlv, 1, 3, 4, 6, 7, 8, 9, 10, 13, 15, 16, 17, 18, 19, 20, 21, 22, 24, 26, 27, 28, 35, 36, 37, 43, 44, 47, 48, 51, 53, 54, 55, 56, 64, 71, 295, 511, 753
fibrils, xiii, 1, 16, 18, 86, 192, 204, 509, 1082, 1084, 1123, 1130, 1132
fibrin, 67, 650
fibrinogen, 8, 621, 689
fibroblast growth factor, 65, 68, 210, 211, 254, 467, 480, 487
fibroblast proliferation, 26, 65, 70
fibrocytes, 4, 29, 30
fibromyalgia, xli, 993
fibrosis, 77, 205, 206, 478, 555, 762, 858, 895, 989
fibrous tissue, 56, 479
fidelity, 809
filament, xxx, 253, 296, 809, 911, 934
filiform, 129, 692, 882
films, 683, 994
filters, xxxviii, xliv, 594
filtration, 60, 224, 225, 896
financial, 301, 490, 493, 495, 498
financial support, 301
fine tuning, 538
fingerprints, 24, 449
Finland, 574, 576, 602, 620
first aid, 1783, 1786, 1811
first degree relative, 540, 819
first generation, 669
fish, xx, 294, 295, 300, 361, 366, 419, 455, 458, 460, 468, 469, 559, 1007
fish oil, 559, 1007
fishing, 422
fistulas, 583, 1028
fitness, 331, 366
fixation, 397, 719
flame, xlix
flavonoids, 150, 151, 152
flavor, 155
flavour, 315
flexibility, 44, 64, 460, 466, 659, 885
flight, 592, 612
floaters, 588, 634
flora, 569, 676, 688, 690, 691, 707, 838, 865
fluctuations, 47
fluid, 54, 60, 71, 526, 553, 562, 565, 619, 635, 642, 653, 663, 769, 884, 1026
fluorescence, xiv, xlv, 43, 46, 47, 49, 51, 52, 53, 54, 56, 59, 60, 61, 243, 273, 276, 281, 285, 289, 465, 466, 592, 594, 611, 749, 753, 754, 759
fluorescent tube, xxviii, 805, 809, 810, 813
fluorescent whitening agents, xliv, 1541, 1574, 1593
fluorophores, 46, 47, 52
fluoroquinolones, 893
fluoxetine, 875
foams, 885, 886
folate, 397, 829, 849, 895
folic acid, 691, 701, 829, 893, 894
follicle(s), xxi, xxii, 18, 44, 74, 75, 76, 80, 416, 477, 479, 480, 487, 505, 506, 510, 511, 520, 523, 529, 537, 879
follicle stimulating hormone, 416
folliculitis, 523, 525, 886, 889, 890, 895
food, 25, 300, 426, 429, 443, 446, 487, 493, 585, 586, 682, 893, 942

Food and Drug Administration (FDA), xlii, xliii, 127, 353, 669, 826, 830, 832, 833, 889, 900, 901, 903, 924
food habits, 493
food intake, 443, 446
force, 35, 46, 244, 277, 558, 907
Ford, 385, 853
formaldehyde, 227, 327, 423
formula, 157, 887
foundations, 468
FOV, 757, 758
fragile site, xxxi, 959
fragility, 23, 24, 74, 438, 897
fragments, 193, 625, 949, 966
frameshift mutation, 200, 205, 263, 444, 451
France, 43, 267, 429, 453, 577, 590, 592, 594, 638, 642, 751, 797, 1007, 1018, 1022
fraternities, xxxviii, 1265, 1267, 1278
free radicals, xxvi, 12, 14, 15, 131, 133, 160, 296, 328, 329, 344, 480, 525, 669, 718, 728, 878, 961, 963
freedom, 960, 968
freezing, 176
friction, xlix, 434, 657, 663, 876, 886, 993
fruits, 126, 149
FTIR, 274, 277, 279
fucoxanthin, 123, 124, 145
functional analysis, 539, 929
functional changes, 31
functional food, 155
funding, xlvii, 481
funds, xlvii
fungal arthritis, 637
fungal cell, xxvi, xxvii, 164, 165, 167, 172, 222, 582, 597, 598, 621, 662, 665, 689, 690, 717, 719, 720, 721, 722, 724, 725, 726, 733, 741, 749, 752, 753
fungal disease, xx, xxvi, 176, 473, 474, 613, 636, 717, 722, 724
fungal metabolite, 693
fusion, 186, 207, 251, 262, 527, 833, 901, 903, 924, 1026
FWA, xliv, xlv, 1541, 1545, 1568, 1571, 1572, 1573, 1575, 1576, 1578, 1580, 1581, 1582, 1583, 1584, 1586, 1592, 1593, 1595, 1596, 1597

G

gallbladder, 1019
gallium, 48
gametogenesis, 384
gamma radiation, 939
gamma rays, 486
ganglion, 457
gastritis, 554
gastroesophageal reflux, xxviii, 789, 791, 795, 801, 982
gastrointestinal tract, 443, 446, 583, 584, 585, 595, 660, 661, 701, 704, 718, 898
GDP, 255
GEF, 552
gel, 70, 79, 148, 395, 529, 533, 559, 626, 670, 677, 679, 693, 741, 826, 888, 1001
gene expression, xxvi, xxxvi, 5, 12, 33, 38, 90, 91, 139, 141, 144, 156, 184, 340, 344, 363, 375, 391, 392, 402, 409, 447, 448, 516, 586, 650, 710, 717, 728, 730, 732, 863, 866, 878, 947, 1012
gene mutations, xv, 83, 266, 268, 442, 696, 929, 1245
gene promoter, 91
gene silencing, 510, 520
gene therapy, 25, 532
general anesthesia, 703, 796
general practitioner, 490
genetic background, 193, 194, 212, 359, 538, 539
genetic defect, 837, 839
genetic disease, 264
genetic disorders, 264, 696, 795
genetic factors, xxi, 192, 480, 489, 509, 536, 538, 835
genetic information, 689
genetic load, 536
genetic marker, 536
genetic predisposition, 402, 541, 707, 983
genetic risk, xviii, xxiii, 323, 535, 539, 540, 1314, 1315
genetics, xiii, xxi, xxxiv, 133, 142, 184, 185, 188, 209, 210, 351, 357, 361, 376, 380, 381, 382, 383, 386, 387, 390, 411, 450, 451, 452, 453, 489, 515, 540, 543, 644, 839, 852, 862, 863, 934, 995
genital warts, 529
genitals, 880, 884, 942
genome, xxii, xlv, 11, 12, 330, 344, 351, 397, 400, 402, 408, 411, 505, 506, 509, 513, 515, 518, 520, 536, 537, 538, 542, 855, 861, 862, 864
genomic instability, 328, 344, 364
genomic stability, 13, 341, 343, 363
genomics, xix, 32, 356, 389, 397, 407, 730
genotype, 267, 268, 358, 359, 513, 584, 875, 953
genotyping, 627, 644, 652
genus, 111, 154, 167, 172, 173, 175, 303, 572, 576, 645, 665, 718, 729
genus Candida, 172, 572, 576, 645, 729
geographic tongue, 694, 882
geometry, xxxvii, 276
Georgia, 767, 815, 999
germ cells, 372

Germany, 45, 264, 346, 386, 575, 576, 577, 653, 753, 826, 842, 848, 868, 1002, 1018, 1022
germination, 243, 621
germline mutations, 267
gestation, 9, 202, 769, 784, 898
gestational age, 782, 786, 794
gestational diabetes, 768
ginger, 124, 125
gingivae, 882
gingival, 692, 700, 711, 735, 1032
gingivitis, xxxiii, 679, 897, 1031, 1032
ginseng, 25, 41, 95, 149
gland, xxiii, xxxv, 6, 29, 30, 445, 446, 451, 467, 545, 548, 549, 555, 556, 557, 558, 560, 564, 566, 567, 568, 569, 914
glaucoma, 67, 78, 635, 886
glaucoma surgery, 78
glia, 456, 460, 466, 469
glial cells, 5, 140, 367, 444, 462, 466, 471
globalization, 178
glomerulonephritis, 702
glossitis, 656, 691, 692, 699, 704, 706, 707, 735, 750, 882
glucocorticoid(s), 406, 442, 445, 446, 512, 700, 702, 705, 706, 708, 712, 714, 747, 825, 850, 925, 935
glucocorticoid receptor, 825, 850
gluconeogenesis, 445, 451
glucose, xxiv, 55, 61, 99, 108, 111, 131, 160, 445, 594, 617, 621, 636, 648, 658, 696, 707, 724, 742, 747, 898, 984, 1003
glucose tolerance, 984
glucoside, 101, 110, 129, 147
glue, 125, 963
glutamate, 198, 971
glutamic acid, 537
glutamine, 204, 315, 625
glutathione, 255, 470, 722, 728, 843, 868
glycerol, 175
glycine, 160
glycogen, 8, 67, 84, 91, 188, 696, 712
glycol, 123, 319, 329, 356
glycolysis, 161, 622
glycoproteins, 3, 44, 86, 121, 536, 625
glycosaminoglycans, xxxvi, 3, 4, 21, 37, 71, 126
glycoside, 127, 314
glycosylation, 93, 674
glyoxylate cycle, 721
goblet cells, 553, 559
gonads, 296, 301
governments, xl
grading, 55, 552, 557, 564
grain size, 287
grants, 449, 468, 1013, 1014
granules, xvi, 4, 10, 71, 182, 206, 222, 224, 249, 250, 251, 253, 255, 257, 294, 295, 300, 690, 719, 720
granulomas, 169, 897
graph, 45, 48, 777
grass(d), 222, 246
gravity, xxxiv, 46, 435
gray matter, 783
Greece, 562, 642
Griscelli Syndrome, xv, 83
growth arrest, 622, 727
growth rate, 224, 229, 230, 240, 241
GTPases, 263, 466, 470
guanine, 14, 237, 246, 329, 703
guidance, xiii, 55, 61
guidelines, xlvi, xlvii, 407, 593, 598, 599, 609, 610, 629, 648, 650, 677, 798, 831, 852, 856, 857, 859, 867, 868, 884, 885, 891, 895, 900, 909, 910, 933, 1002, 1006, 1022, 1023
guilt, xliii
Guinea, 603, 610, 615, 861, 866
guttate psoriasis, xxix, 823, 827, 834, 838, 846, 856, 871, 872, 873, 880, 883, 892, 896, 932

H

H&E, 6, 8, 22
H. pylori, 554
habitat(s), 169, 376, 718
HaCaT cells, 79, 394, 395, 837, 918, 919
haemoglobin, xix, 389
hair depigmentation, xv, 83, 373
hair loss, xxi, xxii, 477, 478, 479, 480, 481, 486, 487, 489, 490, 493, 494, 495, 496, 498, 499, 500, 501, 503, 506, 507, 521, 522, 523, 526, 530, 531, 535, 536, 540, 822
hairless, 210, 213, 216, 350, 971
half-life, 842, 898, 1000
halitosis, 656
halogen, 48, 557, 809
handwriting, 775, 778
haplotypes, 537, 538, 542
harbors, 953
hardness, 664, 665, 667, 680, 682
harmonization, 693
harmony, 70
harvesting, 133
hazards, xliv, 353, 476
HBV, 581
head and neck cancer, 481, 487
head trauma, 588
headache, 528, 588, 597, 598, 633, 830, 897, 899, 902, 905, 906

healing, xiv, 18, 24, 26, 56, 57, 61, 63, 67, 68, 69, 211, 701, 915
health care, xxiv, xl, xlviii, 584, 617, 818, 998, 1032
health care costs, xl
health care system, 818
health effects, xiii, 250, 334
health problems, 333
health risks, xli, 333, 353
health services, xlvi, xlvii
health status, 474, 715
hearing loss, 250
heart attack, 1010
heart disease, xxxii, 55, 366, 762, 763, 764, 783, 784, 785, 787, 818, 982, 983, 1004, 1009
heart failure, 762, 763, 986
heart valves, 572, 587
heat shock protein, xxxvi, 26, 42, 586
heavy metals, xv, 85, 160
height, 287, 288
Helicobacter pylori, 554, 566
hemangioma, 793
hematology, 581
hematopoietic stem cells, 299, 696
heme, 40
heme oxygenase, 40
hemidesmosome, xxxii, 1017, 1020
hemiplegia, 773
hemisphere, 619
hemodialysis, 579, 580, 582, 620
hemoglobin, xxvii, 55, 300, 709, 761, 762, 949, 950
hemorrhage, 435, 436, 588, 632, 770
hepatitis, 597, 830, 832, 834, 835, 859, 895, 897, 900, 905, 907, 989
hepatitis a, 832, 905
hepatitis b, 859
hepatitis b surface antigen, 859
hepatitis b virus, 859
hepatocellular carcinoma, 989
hepatocytes, 5, 844, 989
hepatotoxic drugs, 989
hepatotoxicity, 598, 830, 894, 895, 897
herbal medicine, 143, 212, 320
herbicide, 176
heredity, 381, 383
heritability, 539, 821
Hermenksky Pudluk Syndrome, xv, 83
heroin, 581, 636, 643
heroin addicts, 636, 643
herpes, 714, 874, 889, 891, 905, 906
herpes simplex, 714, 889, 891
herpes zoster, 874, 905, 906
heterogeneity, 30, 289, 350, 537, 542, 625, 626, 627, 639, 646, 823, 872
heterotopic ossification, xlviii, 1739, 1746, 1750, 1767, 1770, 1772, 1773, 1774
heterozygote, 449
Hibiscus mutabilis, 311
HIES, 697, 698, 699
high school, 490, 779
hippocampus, 771, 774
Hispanics, 334, 352
histamine, 4, 54, 480, 487, 736, 796, 830
histidine, 625
histogenesis, 4
histological examination, xxvii, 658, 749, 750
histological improvement, xxx, 911
histology, 27, 40, 51, 404, 851, 878
histone, 206
histoplasmosis, 168, 170, 834, 905
historical data, 478
history, xxx, xxxix, xliii, xlvi, xlvii, 330, 343, 348, 361, 402, 426, 432, 485, 497, 502, 598, 633, 772, 773, 774, 777, 795, 821, 831, 883, 891, 893, 895, 896, 899, 902, 904, 907, 908, 937, 938, 939, 941, 942, 951, 988, 1010
HIV, xxiv, xxix, 172, 179, 185, 572, 579, 580, 607, 620, 623, 633, 640, 645, 647, 655, 658, 660, 661, 662, 670, 672, 673, 675, 676, 678, 684, 691, 735, 742, 744, 747, 850, 871, 873, 897, 902
HIV/AIDS, 179
HLA, xxii, xxx, 510, 511, 516, 518, 535, 536, 537, 538, 539, 541, 542, 553, 704, 705, 821, 835, 838, 850, 872, 878, 880, 883, 911, 922, 934, 984, 985, 986, 996, 997
HLA antigens, 541, 996
HLA-B27, 984, 986, 997
homeostasis, xiv, 2, 4, 9, 22, 25, 29, 63, 64, 65, 68, 70, 78, 442, 529, 708, 722, 817, 825, 839, 841, 844, 852, 904, 991
homes, 415, 436
homework, 498, 777, 779
homocysteine, 893
homogeneity, 49, 523
Hong Kong, 430
hordeolum, 547, 548, 552, 555, 556, 558
Hormesis, xxxviii, 25, 39, 40, 1216
hormonal control, 138, 294, 452
horses, 170
hospitalization, 581, 583, 584, 586, 1021
hotels, xlix
House, ix, xli, 376, 439, 1014
house dust, 415, 436, 437, 439
House of Representatives, ix
HPV, 889
hue, 397, 762, 807
human body, xiv, 5, 43, 63, 64, 72, 400, 670

human brain, 136, 180
human development, 356, 378, 784
human genome, 402, 411
human health, xlii, xliv, 163, 352
human immunodeficiency virus, 572, 647, 672, 676, 736, 860, 873
human leukocyte antigen, 516, 821, 835
human neutrophils, 183, 531, 721, 732
human subjects, 710, 760, 842
humidity, 77, 406
humoral immunity, 634, 697
Hungary, 620, 645
Hunter, 266, 353, 362, 382, 662, 676, 680
hunting, 80
hyaline, 168, 170, 172, 175, 223, 224, 234, 235, 236, 238, 243
hybrid, 208
hybridization, 373
hydrocortisone, 437, 523, 531, 738, 885
hydrogen, xvii, xxvi, 15, 171, 227, 243, 271, 272, 275, 296, 300, 328, 344, 510, 717, 720, 724, 729, 927
hydrogen peroxide, xvii, xxvi, 15, 171, 227, 243, 271, 272, 275, 300, 328, 344, 510, 717, 720, 724, 729, 927
hydrolysis, 129, 150, 624, 843
hydroperoxides, 510
hydrophobicity, 160, 621, 660, 661, 675, 676
hydroquinone, 84, 131, 148, 309, 310, 421, 437
hydroxide, 300
hydroxyacids, 126
hydroxyl, xxvi, 165, 300, 309, 328, 717, 727
hydroxyl groups, 165
hygiene, xxiii, xxv, 545, 559, 560, 595, 655, 657, 661, 663, 672, 673, 678, 679, 691, 899, 1032
hyperactivity, 775, 776, 781, 784, 913
hyperalimentation, 618, 634
hypercalcemia, 887
hypercholesterolemia, 899, 983
hyperemia, 549, 552, 555, 558, 560
hyperglycemia, 446, 707, 708
hyperinsulinemia, 446
hyperkalemia, 900
hyperlipidemia, xxxi, 706, 832, 897, 981, 1000, 1010
hyperparathyroidism, 484
hyperplasia, xxxvii, 18, 387, 414, 476, 527, 551, 656, 836, 839, 878, 899, 902, 938, 946
hyperproliferative inflammatory disease, xxviii, 815
hyperpyrexia, 585
hypersensitivity, 416, 435, 555, 557, 902, 905, 940
hypertelorism, 254
hypertension, xxxi, 371, 382, 525, 793, 831, 860, 884, 899, 900, 981, 983, 989, 993, 1000, 1003, 1004, 1010
hypertrichosis, 475, 483, 523, 526, 527, 899
hypertrophic cardiomyopathy, 265
hypertrophy, xxxiv
hyperuricemia, 899
hypnosis, 499
hypodermis, xiv, 5, 63, 71, 816
hypoglycemia, 696
hypoparathyroidism, 699, 883
hypoplasia, 803
hypothalamus, 295, 443
hypothermia, 884
hypothesis, xvii, xxix, 215, 271, 274, 393, 397, 448, 522, 528, 622, 815, 819, 820, 832, 839, 843, 950, 982, 1003
hypothyroidism, 699
hypoxemia, 769
hypoxia, 25, 300, 768, 769, 770, 771, 780, 781, 782, 793, 794
hysteresis, 272

I

ibuprofen, 1005
ICAM, 553, 703, 848, 902, 952
Iceland, 574, 575, 576, 602
ideal, 2, 319, 426, 808, 824
identical twins, 540
identity, 589
idiopathic, 127, 520, 555, 706, 897
idiosyncratic, 893
IFN, xxx, 522, 526, 527, 529, 690, 703, 721, 830, 832, 835, 843, 875, 876, 911, 914, 917, 918, 919, 920, 921, 922, 923, 924, 925, 926, 927, 928, 929, 931, 932, 935, 936, 943, 946, 947, 949, 951, 955, 957, 1005
IFN-β, 919
IL-17, xxx, 74, 79, 80, 552, 554, 582, 690, 711, 713, 832, 872, 911, 917, 918, 919, 920, 921, 923, 924, 925, 927, 928, 932, 934, 935, 947, 949, 950, 955, 957, 1015
IL-8, 5, 65, 73, 78, 703, 836, 837, 838, 940, 946, 947, 949, 950, 955, 1004
ileum, 636
illiteracy, l
illumination, 48, 557, 813
image(s), xxxv, 49, 50, 51, 52, 54, 58, 59, 228, 275, 276, 277, 288, 289, 466, 639, 753, 985
image analysis, 58, 59
imbalances, 401
immersion, 664, 665, 679, 680, 942

immobilization, 57
immune defense, 165, 552, 582
immune disorders, 857
immune function, 13, 326, 405, 914
immune reaction, xix, 389, 938
immune regulation, 520
immune response, xxix, xxxii, 165, 167, 177, 499, 529, 538, 582, 622, 658, 688, 690, 702, 708, 736, 815, 843, 847, 863, 876, 930, 932, 991, 993, 1005, 1025, 1028
immune system, xxx, xli, 14, 67, 78, 163, 167, 347, 443, 510, 552, 553, 582, 583, 584, 607, 670, 690, 691, 700, 703, 706, 736, 832, 834, 837, 844, 850, 889, 894, 907, 911, 947, 984, 1000, 1020, 1026, 1027
immune system cells, 167
immune-mediated disorder, xxviii, 815, 817, 821, 835, 845, 982
immunity, xxv, xxix, 178, 179, 180, 181, 182, 183, 184, 185, 186, 187, 188, 347, 366, 442, 446, 510, 538, 552, 565, 582, 583, 657, 687, 690, 701, 703, 713, 742, 816
immunization, 176, 180
immunocompetent cells, 690, 924
immunocompromised, xxiii, xxiv, xxv, 24, 173, 174, 571, 572, 583, 613, 643, 655, 656, 658, 660, 662, 675, 687, 709, 711, 714
immunodeficiency(s), xxv, 572, 580, 581, 582, 687, 688, 691, 692, 693, 694, 695, 696, 697, 699, 700, 705, 712, 873, 900
immunofluorescence, xxxii, xxxiii, 8, 437, 457, 458, 461, 557, 693, 1017, 1020, 1027, 1031, 1032
immunogenetics, 856, 929
immunogenicity, 903
immunoglobulin, 84, 90, 372, 510, 623, 638, 701, 703, 706, 708, 833, 901, 905, 1021
immunoglobulin superfamily, 510
immunoglobulins, 8, 426, 582, 594
immunohistochemistry, 8, 27
immunomodulation, 825, 848, 850, 927
immunomodulator, 927
immunomodulatory, xxii, xxx, 521, 522, 527, 528, 876, 896, 917, 926, 938, 939, 940, 943
immunomodulatory agent, 527
immunoreactivity, 17, 20
immunostimulatory, 917, 936
immunosuppression, xxv, xlii, 13, 14, 333, 526, 688, 691, 694, 700, 701, 703, 714, 742, 849, 877, 892, 895, 897, 898, 900, 902, 951, 1000, 1090, 1245, 1260, 1429, 1430, 1433, 1470, 1478, 1479, 1481
immunosuppressive agent, 525, 526, 532, 898, 902
immunosuppressive drugs, 658, 703, 830
immunosuppressive therapies, 326
immunosuppressive treatment, xxxiii, 702, 703, 705, 706, 740, 1031, 1040
immunotherapy, xxii, xxv, 512, 521, 524, 525, 530, 531, 565, 656, 666, 670, 681, 713
impaired wound healing, xxxvi, 1122, 1141
impairments, 771, 774, 777, 975
impetigo, 705, 882
implants, 645
imports, 430
improvements, xliii, 58, 436, 439, 524, 728, 902, 942, 947, 950, 1003
impulsive, 774, 993
impulsivity, 779
impurities, 421, 424
in situ hybridization, 592, 611
in utero, 769, 900
inattention, 768, 775, 779
income, l, 993
incubation period, 589, 634
incubation time, 466
indentation, 45, 46
independence, 285
India, 307, 311, 313, 314, 315, 319, 389, 404, 409, 426, 496, 502
Indians, 827
indirect effect, 173, 175, 328, 891
indium, 48
individual sweat glands, xxxv, 1099, 1108
indolent, 588
inducer, 868
industrialized countries, 989
industry(d), xvii, xlii, xliii, xliv, xlv, xlix, 143, 307, 310, 320, 332, 423, 424, 425, 426, 430, 431, 432, 621, 738
INF, xxxi, 705, 876, 898, 949, 950, 981, 990, 993
infancy, 783, 786, 801
infant mortality, 769
infants, xxviii, 574, 607, 608, 609, 643, 691, 694, 718, 769, 770, 771, 772, 777, 780, 781, 782, 784, 785, 789, 790, 793, 794, 795, 797, 798, 799, 801, 802, 886
infarction, 983, 1010
infected hair, xx, 473, 474
infectious conjunctivitis, 558
inflammasome, 393, 407
inflammatory bowel disease, xxxi, xxxii, 93, 444, 934, 981, 982, 990, 997, 1009
inflammatory cell migration, 836
inflammatory cells, 3, 11, 68, 69, 73, 366, 402, 511, 557, 829, 832, 837, 838, 887, 917, 926, 943, 952
inflammatory disease, xxviii, xxix, xxxi, xxxii, 65, 406, 557, 815, 834, 836, 853, 863, 871, 872, 903, 981, 983, 990, 1009, 1010, 1014, 1026

inflammatory mediators, 14, 553, 838, 841, 847, 848, 983
inflammatory responses, 188, 444
infliximab, 511, 581, 833, 847, 856, 901, 905, 906, 907, 924, 993, 1028, 1029
informed consent, 963
infrared spectroscopy, 58, 979
infundibulum, 74, 913
ingestion, 169, 426, 427, 898, 942, 1028
ingredients, xvii, 47, 94, 95, 307, 309, 310, 319, 429, 430, 431, 888
inguinal, 880, 887
inhaler, 737, 738, 743, 745, 747, 748
inheritance, 251, 256, 264, 339
inherited disorder, 250, 254
inhibitor, xxxvi, 5, 66, 81, 84, 85, 90, 121, 122, 130, 140, 147, 149, 150, 151, 153, 154, 155, 156, 176, 181, 197, 203, 309, 310, 345, 391, 527, 623, 678, 724, 732, 796, 830, 833, 843, 868, 875, 876, 925, 933, 956, 983
initiation, 26, 79, 349, 368, 600, 624, 632, 636, 656, 820, 825, 829, 831, 835, 839, 840, 847, 885, 902, 904, 905, 915, 952
injections, 445, 523, 917
injury(s), xv, xxxii, xl, xlii, xlviii, xlix, l, 55, 69, 77, 79, 83, 334, 337, 343, 401, 476, 477, 479, 481, 485, 486, 487, 488, 529, 566, 657, 664, 705, 763, 769, 770, 771, 773, 776, 780, 782, 783, 784, 786, 837, 838, 876, 902, 915, 944, 1017, 1019, 1020
injury mechanisms, l
innate immune response, xxix, 815
innate immunity, 342, 564, 690, 836, 862, 865
inner ear, 366, 372, 374, 377, 386
inoculation, 166, 182, 223, 226, 234, 236, 243, 244, 245, 253, 587, 636, 741
inoculum, 226, 227, 581, 585
inorganic products, xxxviii, 1245
inositol, 130, 314, 405, 875
INS, 706, 707, 708
insects, xxiii, 150, 617, 619
insecurity, 500
insertion, 205, 238, 239, 240, 241, 242, 267, 344, 400, 468
insomnia, 982
institutions, 475
insulation, 44
insulin, 71, 193, 370, 401, 446, 467, 673, 674, 707, 708, 819, 884, 983, 984, 989, 995
insulin resistance, 401, 707, 708, 819, 884, 983, 984, 989, 995
insulin sensitivity, 984
insulin signaling, 984
integration, 272, 276, 582
integrin(s), 78, 464, 467, 1005
integrity, xxxvi, 35, 71, 178, 253, 326, 366, 583, 595, 623, 638, 664, 668, 682, 708, 724, 835, 837, 838, 865, 913
integument, xx, xxiii, 217, 455, 460, 463, 617, 619
intellect, xxviii, 767
intellectual disabilities, 768
intelligence, 782, 783
intensive acute sun exposure, xxxviii, 1216, 1236
intensive care unit, 575, 603, 606, 607, 608, 630, 631, 641, 642, 643, 649, 653
intentional/non accidental burn, 1779
intercellular adhesion molecule, 848
interface, 43, 66
interference, 50, 93, 121, 165, 242, 345, 663, 752, 925, 928
interferon(s) (IFN), xxxi, 522, 525, 542, 552, 582, 708, 733, 830, 832, 872, 873, 912, 929, 930, 934, 935, 936, 940, 950, 951, 953, 958, 981
interferon gamma, 830, 930, 951
interferon-γ, 522, 873
interleukin-17, 932, 934, 935, 947, 957, 1015
interleukin-8, 355
internalization, 167
internalizing, 776
interstitial lung disease, xxxii, 1025, 1026
intertrigo, 880
intervention, xx, xxxvii, 39, 40, 391, 400, 407, 447, 473, 479, 481, 500, 552, 636, 703, 776, 777, 779, 780, 795, 827, 855, 905, 939
interventional radiology, xxi, 473, 486
intestinal obstruction, 585, 608
intestinal tract, 639
intestine, xx, 455, 585, 842
intima, 1010, 1014
intoxication, 301
intracellular calcium, 123, 843, 844, 874
intracranial pressure, 633
intraocular, 559, 634, 646, 990
intraocular pressure, 559
intravenously, 635, 639, 905
intron, 206, 261, 406
intronic region, xxii, 535
inversion, 208
invertebrates, 293, 296
involution, 479
iodine, xlii, 474, 1028
ion channels, 725
ionising radiation, 482
ionization, 592, 612
ionizing radiation, 177, 189, 193, 477, 479, 482, 484, 485, 486, 487, 488, 893, 939
ions, 214, 300, 597, 661, 724, 817

Iowa, 601
IPPD, 434
IQ scores, 772
Iran, 713
iris, 67
iritis, 551, 552, 555, 556, 559
iron, xliii, 136, 170, 193, 299, 300, 350, 584, 624, 657, 690, 691, 724, 733
irradiation, xxx, 13, 25, 33, 38, 85, 123, 212, 409, 474, 475, 476, 477, 479, 480, 483, 484, 485, 488, 666, 667, 668, 669, 671, 679, 681, 682, 683, 684, 827, 828, 863, 937, 938, 940, 942, 944, 951, 956
irrigation, 18, 634, 636, 639
irritability, 768, 776, 779
IRS, 74
ischaemic heart disease, xxxii, 1009, 1010
ischemia, 12, 13, 770, 771, 780, 782, 786
Islam, 517
isolation, 64, 65, 151, 171, 280, 526, 572, 584, 586, 589, 599, 604, 611, 619, 623, 631, 637, 649, 751, 880, 992
isomerization, xliv, 14
isomers, xliv, 951
Israel, 174, 187, 476, 576, 609, 620
issues, xxvii, xliii, 60, 242, 352, 492, 498, 738, 767, 768, 769, 770, 772, 777, 780, 806, 819, 820, 831, 833, 848, 849, 860, 890
Italy, 271, 535, 576, 602, 608, 620, 642, 789, 1025

J

Japan, 143, 191, 249, 311, 413, 418, 423, 424, 425, 426, 430, 431, 455, 505, 526, 574, 594, 644, 752, 753, 959, 963, 998
jaundice, 705, 770
joint contracture, xlviii, 1739, 1746, 1750, 1768
joint damage, 986
joint deformities, xlix, 1789, 1792
joint destruction, 985
joints, xxviii, xlix, l, 572, 621, 636, 640, 815, 817, 819, 823, 845, 982, 985, 988, 989, 1010
Jordan, 258, 360, 566, 639
jurisdiction, xlvii, xlviii
juvenile rheumatoid arthritis, 833, 903

K

K^+, 597
karyotype, 625, 640
KBr, 276, 279
Keinbock-Adamson technique, xx, 473
keratin, xxxvii, 23, 51, 67, 72, 126, 253, 263, 383, 409, 839, 840, 866, 873, 902, 912, 913, 918, 922, 929, 930, 931, 932, 933, 934, 935, 936, 970, 971
Keratin 17, viii, xxx, 911, 912, 913, 914, 915, 916, 929, 930, 931, 932, 934, 935, 936
keratoconjunctivitis, 555, 557, 558, 562, 564, 567
keratosis, 24, 382, 415, 699
kidney(s), xxv, xxxiii, 39, 55, 205, 296, 298, 300, 301, 583, 585, 587, 597, 636, 652, 661, 663, 688, 694, 695, 702, 703, 704, 712, 714, 720, 890, 894, 904
kidney recipients, xxv, 688, 694, 695, 703, 704
kidney transplantation, 712
kill, 168, 186, 245, 690, 696, 710, 719, 721
killer cells, 690
kinase activity, 15, 210, 373
kindergarten, 495, 498
kinetics, 94, 136, 210
knee arthroplasty, 640, 653
knees, 250, 818, 821, 876, 879, 880, 985, 1010
Korea, 41, 185, 311, 426, 496, 502
Kurd, 853, 854
Kuwait, 496, 502, 639, 735

L

labeling, xliii, 53, 174, 458, 462, 465, 466, 890
laboratory studies, xxxix, 896, 898, 907
laboratory tests, 539, 556, 895
lack of confidence, 993
lactation, 826, 827, 828, 890, 893
lactic acid, 126, 128, 132, 149, 696
lactoferrin, 690, 701, 721, 948, 949
lakes, 882, 883
lamella, 960
laminar, 226
Langerhans cells, 2, 4, 67, 439, 524, 525, 529, 828, 844, 849, 891, 941, 943
language development, 784
language impairment, 773
languages, 500
larvae, 457
laryngomalacia, xxviii, 789, 790, 793, 794, 795, 796, 797, 798, 799, 800, 801, 802, 803
laryngoscope, 797, 798
laryngoscopy, 795, 796
laryngotracheobronchitis, 740
larynx, 790, 795, 797, 799
lasers, xxxiv, xxxvii, 50
latency, 77, 325, 326, 339, 476, 875, 1026
Latin America, xxiv, 171, 575, 577, 618, 619, 647
laxity, xxxvii, 15, 1122, 1215, 1218, 1763
LBA, 223, 224, 225, 228, 229, 240

LDL, 948, 950
leakage, 597, 661
lean body mass, 451
learning, xxvii, 767, 768, 770, 771, 773, 774, 776, 778, 782, 785
learning disabilities, 771, 782, 785
learning task, 774
LED, xxviii, 669, 670, 684, 805, 806, 810, 811, 813, 814
left hemisphere, 777
legislation, 354
legs, 404, 415, 433, 478, 884, 906
leisure, 992
lens, 51, 634, 646
lentigo, xv, 83, 85, 128, 130, 131, 372, 383, 415, 421
Leopard syndrome, 254, 264, 401
leptin, 983
leptomeninges, xv, 83
lesional keratinocytes, xxix, 815
leucine, 90, 139, 338, 625
leucocyte, 872, 957, 1010
leukemia, 84, 89, 144, 215, 254, 467, 584, 701, 713, 919, 1019
leukocyte function antigen, 902
leukocytes, 14, 67, 176, 589, 633, 839, 896, 938, 948, 957, 958
leukocytosis, 635, 884
leukopenia, 884, 896, 903
leukoplakia, 673, 691, 705, 711
leukotrienes, 4, 84, 123, 875
LFA, 641, 833, 901, 902
LGE, 692
liberation, 340
lichen, 154, 426, 497, 558, 738, 740, 746, 836, 881, 1018
lichen planus, 426, 497, 558, 738, 740, 746, 836, 881, 1018
life cycle, 164, 167, 169, 991
life expectancy, 11, 21, 983
life quality, 992
lifestyle changes, xxxv
lifestyle differences, xxxv, 1099
lifetime, xiii, xlv, xlvi, 1, 39, 74, 324, 325, 326, 330, 333, 334, 348, 496, 502, 506, 536, 658, 828, 852
ligament, 28, 798, 897
ligand, 210, 217, 250, 258, 264, 338, 339, 340, 366, 368, 369, 370, 371, 374, 384, 385, 386, 392, 409, 448, 464, 467, 520, 582, 625, 703, 825, 1004
light emitting diode, xxviii, 805, 810
light scattering, 52
light-emitting diodes, 669
lignans, 154
linear model, 225, 403
linoleic acid, 121, 132, 148
lip balms, xliii, 1445, 1452
lipases, xxiv, 586, 618, 620, 622, 624, 689
lipid metabolism, xix, 389
lipid peroxidation, xxxvii, 543, 828, 939
lipid peroxides, 34
lipids, xxxviii, 32, 48, 58, 126, 328, 329, 405, 622, 624, 640, 885, 900, 960, 961, 967, 968, 969, 970, 971, 973, 975, 978, 979, 1002
liposomes, 33, 528
liquid chromatography, 214
liquids, 1032
lithium, xxix, 49, 871, 874, 875
liver damage, 705, 895, 990
liver disease, 694, 695, 705, 712, 715, 893, 895, 909, 989, 997, 1008
liver enzymes, 445, 598, 898, 900, 989
liver failure, 705, 904, 905
liver function tests, 426, 832, 895, 907
liver spots, 148
liver transplant, 608, 714
liver transplantation, 608
local conditions, 23, 656
local mobility, 967
local order, 966
localization, 16, 217, 245, 378, 457, 471, 480, 515, 649, 841, 851, 867, 992
loci, xxii, 133, 194, 197, 203, 209, 213, 217, 254, 256, 257, 269, 359, 370, 374, 397, 406, 447, 515, 516, 518, 519, 535, 536, 537, 538, 539, 540, 820, 835, 836, 838, 850, 861, 862, 863
longevity, 13, 31, 71, 811
longitudinal study, 662, 958
long-term memory, 774
low birthweight, 774, 775, 776, 781, 782
low temperatures, 300
low-density lipoprotein, 948, 950
low-grade inflammation, 984
LTB4, 948
LTC, 123
lubricants, 559
lumen, 339, 580, 793
lung disease, 93, 763, 770, 794
Luo, 154, 356, 393, 409, 950
lupus, xxxii, xli, 3, 561, 566, 746, 893, 903, 906, 1010, 1011, 1020, 1025, 1026
lupus erythematosus, 3, 566, 893, 1020
luteinizing hormone, 416
lying, 9, 480, 796
lymph, 5, 60, 171, 525, 585, 705, 741, 884, 912
lymph node, 171, 585, 741, 912
lymphadenopathy, 525, 884
lymphangiogenesis, 552

lymphangitis, 170
lymphatic system, 54, 585
lymphedema, 60
lymphocytes, 5, 414, 425, 426, 435, 446, 511, 531, 557, 582, 633, 658, 690, 703, 705, 736, 828, 829, 830, 837, 843, 844, 866, 877, 886, 891, 901, 943, 947, 951, 952, 991, 1021, 1027
lymphoid, 84, 90, 861, 894, 921
lymphoid tissue, 894, 921
lymphoma, 533, 584, 819, 834, 849, 850, 855, 902, 903, 905, 906, 991, 1026, 1029
lysine, 625
lysis, 690
lysozyme, 20, 28

M

mAb, 956
machinery, 263
macromolecules, 12, 14, 289, 327, 328, 329, 341, 961
macrophage inflammatory protein, 931
macrophages, 3, 15, 44, 164, 165, 167, 169, 173, 179, 181, 182, 186, 252, 303, 444, 450, 529, 690, 705, 707, 719, 720, 721, 724, 733, 736, 820, 828, 829, 830, 832, 837, 878, 943, 945, 948, 984
macroscopic symptoms, xvi, 221
magnesium, 128, 129, 147, 900
magnetic field(s), xxxi, 959, 961, 962, 973, 975
magnetic resonance, 771, 784, 960, 979, 980
magnetic resonance imaging, 771, 784
magnitude, l, 273, 807
major depressive disorder, 499
major histocompatibility complex, 516, 518, 838
major issues, 820
majority, xxx, xxxviii, xli, xliii, xlvii, 65, 66, 299, 301, 328, 339, 402, 426, 523, 561, 577, 770, 806, 824, 831, 841, 885, 904, 938, 1010, 1021
malaise, 822, 829, 849, 991
Malaysia, 307, 311, 406, 578
MALDI, 592
malignancy(s), xiii, xviii, xxxi, xxxiii, xxxix, 1, 93, 323, 324, 330, 333, 343, 352, 484, 587, 603, 613, 614, 651, 714, 831, 833, 834, 861, 900, 902, 903, 906, 907, 942, 956, 981, 982, 1019, 1045, 1046, 1047, 1048, 1049, 1050, 1283, 1411, 1461
malignant cells, 515
malignant melanoma, xvi, 33, 249, 256, 257, 347, 348, 349, 352, 354, 356, 357, 942, 952
malignant neoplasms, xxxvii, 1049, 1215, 1430
malignant tumors, 8, 255, 944
malnutrition, 579, 582, 583, 700, 705, 706
malocclusion, 682
malondialdehyde, 1053, 1483
maltose, xxiii, 617, 618
mammal, 172
mammalian cells, 177, 181, 662
mammalian skin, xviii, 92, 138, 341, 360, 365, 366, 1191
mammals, 136, 168, 211, 294, 356, 366, 378, 380, 444, 456, 458, 522, 726, 913
manipulation, 345, 385, 820, 841
mannitol, 693
mantle, 232, 235
Manual Therapy (MT), xi, xlix, 1789, 1794, 1800, 1801
manufacturing, 309, 423, 671
mapping, 55, 58, 456, 516
marine environment, xxiii, 617, 619
marketing, xliii, 41
marrow, 607
MAS, 769
masking, 295
mass, 6, 46, 224, 241, 446, 451, 452, 475, 479, 592, 612, 693, 886
mass spectrometry, 452, 612, 693
mast cells, 3, 4, 8, 20, 21, 29, 33, 44, 372, 384, 487, 565, 830, 943
materials, xlvii, xlviii, 26, 49, 53, 150, 155, 286, 423, 424, 430, 595, 644, 664, 666, 667, 680, 727, 779
matrix metalloproteinase, xxxviii, 5, 11, 12, 13, 15, 16, 17, 21, 25, 36, 70, 471, 553
matter, 56, 599, 769, 771, 847, 944
maturation process, 367
MCP, 1004
MCP-1, 1004
MDA, 1521
measurement(s), xvii, xviii, xxviii, xlv, 46, 47, 48, 54, 55, 56, 58, 61, 223, 228, 229, 239, 271, 274, 275, 276, 285, 286, 305, 308, 320, 391, 405, 421, 805, 806, 807, 810, 814, 884, 900, 955, 961, 974, 976
mechanical properties, 45, 46, 57, 666, 667
mechanical ventilation, 580, 631, 803
meconium, 769, 782, 783
media, 49, 162, 164, 170, 223, 224, 225, 228, 229, 238, 239, 240, 241, 391, 394, 396, 621, 624, 650, 724, 742, 747, 1010, 1014
median, 87, 560, 579, 593, 634, 637, 656, 691, 704, 706, 735, 750, 798, 818, 901, 904, 906, 940
mediation, 4, 65, 76, 837
medical care, xlviii, xlix, 579
medical history, 484, 772, 780, 896
medical science, 319
medication, xxxiii, 414, 416, 558, 691, 705, 706, 744, 777, 829, 830, 867, 869, 874, 889, 907, 1005

medicine, 2, 26, 180, 385, 451, 452, 759, 802, 997
Mediterranean, 336, 348, 401, 474, 577, 578
Mediterranean countries, 577, 578
medulla, 445, 457
medulloblastoma, 701
meiosis, 384
MEK, 118, 119, 375
melanin granules, xvi, 249, 250, 253, 255, 257, 294, 300, 1199, 1231
melanoblasts, xvi, xx, 145, 191, 193, 197, 199, 200, 201, 202, 203, 204, 205, 206, 208, 210, 211, 212, 213, 214, 216, 249, 250, 367, 371, 373, 378, 396, 408, 455, 456, 457, 458, 460, 461, 462, 463, 466, 468, 469, 470
melanocortin-1 receptor (MC1R), xviii, 137, 197, 323, 358, 359, 360, 405, 450, 453, 1460
melanocyte protein tyrosinase, xxxvii, 1179
melanocyte stimulating hormone, 83, 89, 135, 149, 254, 268, 337, 339, 341, 379, 380, 381, 453
melanophore(s), 294, 295, 457, 458, 459, 460, 466, 468, 469, 471
Melatonin, x, xliii, 295, 302, 1467, 1485, 1487, 1488, 1489, 1490, 1491, 1499, 1500, 1501, 1502, 1503, 1504
mellitus, xxxii, 536, 580, 582, 584, 672, 673, 674, 675, 676, 699, 715, 736, 747, 885, 897, 984, 989, 1000, 1004, 1009
melting, 559
membrane permeability, 597, 661
membranes, xxxiii, 122, 188, 296, 301, 594, 623, 640, 720, 960, 966, 978, 979, 1031
memory, xxviii, 272, 767, 771, 774, 778, 858, 901
memory function, 774
menadione, 724
meninges, 296, 587
meningioma, 476, 482, 484
meningismus, 588
meningitis, xxiv, 179, 572, 587, 588, 618, 630, 632, 633, 643, 644, 646, 651, 697
meningomyelocele, 898
menopause, 31
mental disorder, 476
mental health, 490
mental retardation, 250, 795
mental state, 994
merchandise, 425
mercury, 424, 810, 939
MES, 678
mesenchymal stem cells, 5, 30, 74, 1767, 1773, 1774, 1818, 1821
mesenchyme, 72, 75, 76, 78, 81, 456
mesoderm, 4, 9, 470
messengers, 825
meta-analysis, 353, 516, 519, 605, 613, 652, 715, 783, 865, 909, 995, 1001, 1004, 1005, 1007
Metabolic, 715, 983, 1003
metabolic disorder(s), 429, 705, 983
metabolic dysfunction, 583
metabolic pathways, 161, 722
metabolic syndrome, xxxii, 451, 819, 854, 855, 884, 982, 989, 998, 999, 1000, 1003, 1006, 1007
metabolism, xiii, xxvi, xxxvi, 1, 11, 12, 21, 31, 37, 70, 71, 132, 178, 333, 379, 400, 403, 405, 419, 450, 452, 584, 622, 659, 664, 717, 725, 784, 839, 841, 850, 865, 875, 895, 898
metabolite profiles, xlii, 1429, 1431
metabolites, 72, 173, 182, 218, 411, 690, 868, 1005
metabolized, 598, 720, 875, 890, 900, 1000
metabolomics, xlii, 1429, 1431, 1432, 1433, 1438, 1439, 1440, 1441, 1442, 1443
metal ion(s), 116, 222
metalloproteinase, 32, 553
metals, 87, 326, 414, 425
metaphor, 779
metastasis, 264
methanol, 117, 154, 155
methemoglobinemia, 764, 766
methodology, xlii
methotrexate, xxix, xxxii, 512, 528, 701, 728, 822, 829, 847, 858, 859, 861, 871, 884, 892, 893, 894, 895, 896, 903, 905, 910, 924, 945, 983, 990, 991, 993, 1011, 1017, 1021
methylation, 27
methylene blue, 436, 648, 669, 670, 683, 684, 685, 752
Mexico, 171, 423, 574, 576, 600, 619
MHC, 251, 510, 515, 518, 541, 703, 835, 838
Miami, 365
miconazole, xxv, xxvi, 188, 630, 638, 655, 661, 667, 718, 731, 741
microarray technology, 38
microbial cells, xxv, 656, 668
microbial community(s), 621, 727
microbial survival, xv, 159
microbiota, 580, 582, 584, 586, 595
microcephaly, 795
microcrystalline, 738
microemulsion, 898
microenvironments, 720, 932
micrometer, 51, 223
micronucleus, 941
microorganism(s), 172, 174, 243, 308, 342, 554, 556, 573, 585, 621, 624, 656, 657, 659, 660, 664, 666, 667, 668, 682, 684, 693, 707, 718, 719, 747, 873
microRNA, 403, 980

microscope, xviii, xxxvii, 51, 59, 223, 227, 228, 275, 276, 308, 316, 692, 751, 752, 753, 757
microscopy, xiv, xxxvi, 28, 43, 48, 51, 53, 55, 56, 57, 59, 60, 61, 135, 172, 243, 295, 557, 566, 567, 669, 753, 754, 757, 759
microspectroscopy, xiv, 43, 979
microstructure(s), 51, 55, 56
microtome, 227
microwave radiation, 682
microwaves, 667, 668, 961
middle ear infection, 652
Middle East, 402, 620
migration routes, 457
migratory properties, 71
minors, 354
miscarriages, 770
misuse, 877, 908
mitochondria, 51, 202, 203, 300, 445, 719, 731, 826, 857
mitochondrial DNA, 12, 32, 397, 406
mitogen(s), xx, 39, 70, 84, 91, 141, 208, 254, 267, 387, 392, 408, 455, 464, 525, 703, 729, 875, 878, 919, 951, 952
mitosis, xxx, 363, 524, 701, 722, 937, 940
mitral valve, 587
mixing, 762
MMP, xxxiii, xxxvi, 70, 71, 79, 81, 553, 565, 1031, 1032
MMP-2, xxxvi, 71
MMP-9, 553
MMPs, xxxvi, 70, 71
mobilisations with movement (MWM), xlix, 1789, 1794, 1797
model system, 137, 142, 157, 262, 357, 391
models, xvi, xxiii, 55, 65, 66, 73, 76, 79, 94, 163, 165, 205, 216, 249, 250, 257, 273, 481, 535, 623, 643, 670, 720, 741, 746, 771, 820, 839, 840, 848, 850, 852, 855, 861, 866, 915, 940, 984, 1004
modifications, xxxi, 53, 71, 328, 374, 510, 708, 794, 891, 939, 948, 999, 1002
modifier gene, 256
moisture, xliv, 65, 222, 240, 826, 849
moisture content, xliv, 65
moisturizers, xliii, 126, 826, 827, 1445, 1452
mold(s), 227, 295, 726
mole, 324, 961
molecular biology, 35, 136, 693
molecular mass, 622
molecular mimicry, 861
molecular orbital, 274
molecular oxygen, 727
molecular structure, xv, 48, 159
molecular weight, xv, 11, 17, 159, 160
monoclonal antibody, 184, 468, 469, 728, 730, 833, 902, 905, 907, 924, 932, 947, 957, 1012, 1013, 1015
monocyte chemoattractant protein, 1004
monolayer, 9, 143
monomeric units, xvii, 271, 282, 284
monomers, xvii, 271, 272, 274, 277, 279, 282, 285, 289, 913
monozygotic twins, 997
Montenegro, x
Moon, 149, 151, 321, 406
morbidity, xxi, xxiii, xxxii, xlvii, xlviii, l, 489, 547, 571, 583, 586, 633, 635, 660, 722, 740, 770, 782, 819, 821, 882, 884, 895, 998, 999, 1011
morphine, 333
morphogenesis, 31, 74, 75, 76, 78, 80, 134, 175, 625, 659, 709, 710
mortality rate, l, 85, 324, 579, 583, 609, 635, 660
morula, 202
mosaic, xix, 389, 404, 446
Moses, ix
motif, 90, 91, 207, 372, 921
motivation, 779
motor skills, 773, 777, 778
motor task, 773
MRI, 771, 989
mRNA(s), xxx, 34, 38, 90, 92, 93, 100, 102, 105, 109, 112, 113, 117, 119, 126, 136, 145, 152, 153, 206, 214, 217, 262, 360, 392, 395, 402, 403, 406, 411, 448, 480, 525, 566, 911, 918, 919, 926, 947, 949, 1005
MTI, 447
mucin, 8, 664, 760
mucoid, 167
mucosa, xxiv, xxv, xxxii, 580, 585, 655, 656, 657, 658, 660, 663, 664, 668, 669, 673, 674, 691, 694, 695, 712, 721, 741, 743, 755, 797, 874, 1017, 1019, 1032
mucous membrane(s), xxv, xxvii, xxxiii, 74, 555, 558, 567, 688, 690, 691, 693, 694, 698, 701, 704, 707, 712, 761, 764, 882, 897, 1019, 1020, 1031, 1032
mucus, xxvii, 547, 637, 761, 762
multilayered structure, 816
multiple sclerosis, xxii, 505, 509, 510, 516, 517, 518, 867, 868, 906, 1020
multiples, 663
multiplication, 37, 80, 661
multipotent, 4, 5, 29, 367, 726
multivariate analysis, 55, 580, 632
murmur, 764
muscle mass, 896
muscle strength, 778

muscles, 37, 446
musculoskeletal, 250, 897, 899
musculoskeletal complaints, 897
music, 362
mutagen, 237, 245
mutagenesis, xxxviii, 85, 237, 325, 326, 328, 329, 334, 341, 343, 344, 349, 350, 830
MWM, xlix, 1790, 1794, 1795, 1796, 1797, 1800
myalgia, 897, 905
mycelium, 166, 174, 226, 232, 233, 235, 240, 241, 246, 759
mycobacterial infection, 834
mycology, 178
Mycophenolate mofetil, xxxii, 703, 1017
mycosis fungoides, 529, 954
myeloid cells, 518
myelosuppression, 701
myocardial infarction, 854, 885, 983, 993, 1010, 1011, 1014, 1015
myocarditis, 587
myofibroblasts, 67, 69, 78, 79
myosin, 87, 200, 215, 218, 252, 262, 296

N

NaCl, 223, 224
nail beds, xxviii, xxx, 764, 805, 806, 807, 911, 913
nail changes, xxix, 509, 522, 823, 871, 874
naming, 812
nanometers, 275, 288
nanoparticles, xliv, xlv, 177, 189, 670, 685
nares, 803
nasopharynx, 795
National Academy of Sciences, 29, 33, 34, 37, 179, 188, 377, 379, 380, 381, 382, 383, 385, 387, 451, 453, 730, 731, 732
National Comprehensive Cancer Control Program, xlvii, 1376, 1385, 1412, 1703, 1736
National Health and Nutrition Examination Survey, 513
National Institutes of Health, 324
natural compound, 670, 725
natural disaster, l
natural disasters, l
natural killer cell, 93, 251, 525, 901, 940, 943, 951
nausea, 524, 597, 663, 829, 893, 894, 897, 899, 905, 942
NCCCP, xlvii, 1376, 1385, 1703, 1736
neck tumors, xx, 473
necrosis, xxxi, 29, 125, 243, 300, 514, 520, 588, 860, 876, 950, 955, 956, 981, 1025
negative effects, 222
negativity, 876
nematic liquid crystals, 979
neon, 811
neonates, xxiii, 445, 571, 573, 574, 577, 580, 587, 588, 592, 607, 609, 614, 633, 639, 651, 652, 763, 769, 770, 780, 784, 785, 787, 795
neovascularization, 57
nephritic syndrome, 715
nephritis, 702
nephrotic syndrome, xxv, xxvi, 688, 695, 706, 714
nephrotoxic drugs, 900
nerve, 18, 44, 65, 67, 84, 89, 254, 378, 411, 456, 457, 800, 872
nerve fibers, 44
nerve growth factor, 65, 84, 89, 254, 411, 872
nervous system, 368, 484
Netherlands, 40, 41
neural crest, xviii, xx, 74, 86, 140, 191, 215, 216, 250, 299, 338, 365, 367, 378, 383, 385, 386, 446, 455, 456, 457, 458, 459, 460, 461, 462, 463, 467, 468, 469, 470, 471
neuroblastoma, 266
neuroblasts, 469
neuroendocrine cells, 9
neuroimaging, 784
neurokinin, 487
neuroleptics, 893, 942
neurological disease, 769, 1020
neuromotor, 784
neurons, 87, 263, 366, 367, 378, 456, 460, 468
neuropathy, 55
neuropeptides, 443, 540, 872
neuropsychology, 785
neuroscience, 782
neurosurgery, 588, 609
neurotoxicity, 597
neurotransmitters, 991
neutral, 342, 391, 836, 913
neutropenia, xxv, 572, 574, 579, 580, 581, 582, 583, 584, 586, 587, 612, 639, 688, 694, 696, 700, 701, 731
neutrophils, 78, 168, 174, 251, 531, 565, 580, 583, 633, 634, 658, 690, 720, 721, 724, 726, 728, 732, 820, 823, 836, 839, 848, 872, 940, 942, 946, 948, 952, 956, 957, 1011
nevus, 404, 409, 421, 426
New England, 33, 451, 781, 783, 851, 853, 859
New South Wales, 805
New Zealand, xxviii, 325, 805, 814
next generation, xxvi, 431, 717, 724
NH_2, 340
niacin, xxxvi, 122, 309
niacinamide, 122, 123, 143, 144, 318, 320
niche market, xliv

nickel, 426, 428
nicotinamide, xxxvi, 122, 696, 729
nicotine, 993
nicotinic acid, 309, 868, 869
NIR, 44, 47, 48, 53, 54, 55, 57
NIR spectra, 48, 54
nitric oxide, 15, 34, 84, 89, 137, 167, 171, 182, 333, 720, 726, 825, 947, 949, 958
nitric oxide synthase, 15, 34, 720, 947, 949, 958
nitrogen, 163, 165, 181, 222, 272, 720, 896, 962, 967, 970, 976, 1004
nitrosamines, 692
nitroxide, 480, 962, 963, 964, 965, 966, 967, 968, 969
nitroxide radicals, 964
NK cells, 538, 543, 705
NMR, 960, 961
nodes, 585
nodules, 255, 299, 429, 551, 698, 985, 1018
non-enzymatic antioxidants, 722
nonirritant, 430
non-polar, 3
nonsense mutation, 259
norepinephrine, 165
normal aging, 31, 78
normal children, 567
normal development, 903
North America, xxiv, 58, 133, 184, 361, 483, 486, 532, 618, 619, 620, 817
Norway, 331, 352, 574, 602, 872
notochord, 460, 461, 462, 464
Nrf2, 344, 363
NSAIDs, 875, 989
nuchal rigidity, 588
nuclear magnetic resonance, 37, 597, 960
nuclear membrane, 669
nuclear receptors, 121, 344
nuclei, 51, 414, 820
nucleic acid, xxiii, 571, 592, 611, 703, 828, 829
nucleic acid synthesis, 829
nucleotides, 328, 329, 343, 344, 611
nucleus, 87, 127, 200, 339, 368, 376, 825, 898, 920, 962
nuisance, 897
null, 370, 371, 382, 446, 453, 915, 932
nurses, xlvi
nursing, 886
nutrient(s), xxiv, 44, 64, 144, 165, 169, 240, 241, 243, 246, 366, 617, 624, 664, 689, 822
nutrition, xxiv, xxxi, 243, 480, 572, 577, 582, 583, 584, 585, 595, 618, 621, 632, 651, 653, 769, 770, 999, 1004
nutritional deficiencies, 536, 736
nutritional status, xvii, 293
nystagmus, 92

O

OAS, 993
obesity, xxxi, 370, 380, 381, 442, 444, 446, 448, 451, 452, 819, 855, 884, 897, 981, 982, 983, 984, 985, 989, 995, 1000, 1003
obsessive-compulsive disorder, 499
obstacles, 671
obstruction, xxviii, 549, 581, 763, 789, 793, 794, 795, 798, 800
obstructive sleep apnea, 803
occipital regions, 881
occlusion, 70, 657, 850, 886, 888, 889
occupational risks, 351
occupational therapy, 776
Oceania, 574, 575, 576
oil, xlii, 427, 430, 649, 986, 987
olanzapine, 875
old age, 1023
older adults, xxxv, 572, 1099, 1100, 1103, 1104, 1105, 1106, 1107, 1108, 1109, 1110, 1111, 1112, 1116, 1309, 1326, 1768
oleic acid, 121, 434
oligomeric structures, xvii, 271
oligomers, 272, 274, 286, 532
olive oil, 155
omega-3, xxxii, 355, 559, 568, 999, 1004, 1007
online advertising, xli, xlii
onycholysis, 881, 893, 975, 987, 988
onychomycosis, xxiv, 174, 618, 630, 634, 642, 647, 650
open angle glaucoma, 874
open heart surgery, 784
operations, 495, 776
ophiasis inversus, xxi, 505, 506, 508
ophiasis type, xxi, 505
ophthalmologist, 554, 556, 559, 635
opioids, 566
opportunism, 185
opportunities, xl, xlvi, 331, 353
optical density, xvii, 53, 225, 230, 271, 276, 280
optical microscopy, xiv, 43
optical properties, 289, 897
oral antibiotic(s), xxxiii, 560
oral cavity, xxvi, 476, 611, 620, 633, 656, 657, 658, 660, 665, 669, 673, 678, 695, 697, 710, 711, 712, 714, 718, 735, 739, 740, 743, 746, 751, 759, 1032
oral diseases, 755
oral health, 712, 715, 744
oral lesion, 657, 712

oral surgeon, 755
orbit, 46
organelle(s), xvii, 51, 86, 87, 93, 133, 134, 135, 142, 160, 192, 206, 216, 218, 251, 260, 261, 263, 272, 293, 295, 308, 357, 367, 381, 397, 400, 405, 410, 447
organic compounds, xliv
organic products, xxxviii, 1245
organic solvents, 160, 624
organism, xiv, xlii, 4, 63, 72, 94, 163, 164, 169, 187, 296, 301, 368, 554, 586, 588, 619, 620, 630, 659, 718, 721, 728
organize, 779
oropharyngeal, xxiv, 633, 655, 658, 673, 678, 737, 738, 739, 740, 742, 743, 744, 745, 747
oropharyngeal region, 737, 742
osmolytes, xliii, 187, 1467, 1474, 1484
ossification, xlviii, 988
osteomalacia, 333
osteomyelitis, 572, 587, 609, 645
osteopathy, 895
osteoporosis, xli, 333, 895, 897
otitis externa, 646
otorrhea, 646
outpatient(s), 431, 639, 826, 827, 890, 996
ovarian cancer, 371
overlap, xxii, 3, 257, 270, 480, 519, 535, 538, 720, 751, 770, 878, 883
overproduction, 19, 92, 872
overweight, 446, 903
ovulation, 895
ox, 762, 768
oxidation, xvi, xviii, xxxvii, 14, 88, 136, 163, 165, 172, 176, 192, 214, 271, 272, 275, 308, 316, 367, 369, 380, 719, 1005
oxidative agents, 721
oxidative damage, 12, 13, 32, 34, 119, 328, 329, 344, 350, 377, 724, 728, 733, 878
oxygen, xxv, xxvi, xxvii, xxxvii, 14, 15, 34, 72, 165, 181, 272, 328, 329, 443, 480, 656, 668, 696, 707, 717, 725, 726, 729, 762, 763, 767, 768, 769, 770, 780, 787, 794, 806, 807, 808, 828
oxygen consumption, 443, 726
oyster, 879
ozone, 14, 327, 328, 331, 332, 352, 738
ozone layer, 14, 738

P

p16INK4A, 326
p53, 12, 14, 33, 91, 92, 141, 147, 330, 340, 341, 344, 346, 350, 351, 355, 359, 944, 953
pain, xxi, xlix, 333, 490, 523, 547, 555, 566, 587, 597, 634, 635, 755, 757, 878, 895, 899, 901, 912, 989, 1032
pairing, 328, 330
Pakistan, 311
palate, 691, 757, 762, 1032
palliate, 24
palliative, 478, 481, 488
palmoplantar pustulosis, 872, 883, 896
palpitations, 526
PAN, 430, 432
pancreas, 446, 579, 585
pancreatitis, 579, 581, 583
pannus formation, 550
papillary dermis, xiii, 1, 6, 7, 10, 13, 16, 17, 18, 19, 20, 26, 820, 872, 1122, 1123, 1167, 1237
papulosquamous plaques, xxix, 871
paracoccidioidomycosis, 168, 171, 184
paracrine, xx, 4, 65, 68, 70, 71, 73, 77, 79, 89, 92, 137, 145, 211, 214, 253, 383, 385, 393, 408, 448, 455, 466, 467, 837, 1182, 1186, 1190, 1193, 1228
paradigm shift, 391
parallel, xxxvi, 7, 9, 44, 50, 51, 68, 69, 286, 295, 400, 409, 460, 659, 964, 965, 967, 968, 976
paralysis, 793, 794
parasite, xvi, 221, 223, 244, 742, 747
parasites, 244, 299
parathyroid, 476, 484
parenchyma, 13, 300
parents, xxvii, 237, 475, 490, 494, 495, 498, 536, 767, 768, 775, 777, 779, 799
paronychia, 897
parotid, 476, 1019
participants, 54, 772, 773, 774, 775
pathogens, xiv, xxvi, 63, 64, 133, 163, 175, 176, 177, 178, 572, 576, 578, 582, 584, 589, 601, 603, 612, 622, 647, 656, 658, 670, 688, 690, 693, 710, 717, 718, 721, 722, 724, 726, 731
pathologic diagnosis, 567
pathology, xxxvii, 30, 385, 386, 410, 566, 711, 768, 770, 772, 782, 786, 809, 852, 866
pathophysiological, 565
pathophysiology, xlviii, 56, 357, 393, 486, 552, 564, 565, 795, 819, 820, 855, 997
pattern recognition, 421, 719
PBMC, 949, 950
PCR, 197, 205, 395, 589, 592, 611, 612, 626, 627, 653
PDT, 668, 669, 670
pediatric burn, xlix, 1740, 1762, 1768, 1769, 1772, 1775, 1776, 1777, 1782, 1784, 1797, 1817
pediatric erythema dyschromicum perstans, xvi, 249

pediatrics, xlvi, 781, 782, 783, 784, 1295, 1298, 1465, 1619
pellagra, 939
pelvis, 587
pemphigoid, xiii, xxxii, xxxiii, 555, 558, 567, 1017, 1018, 1019, 1020, 1022, 1023, 1025, 1026, 1027, 1028, 1029, 1031, 1032, 1041, 1042, 1043, 1044, 1045, 1046, 1047, 1048, 1049, 1050
pemphigus, xxxii, 558, 738, 1022, 1025, 1026, 1027, 1028, 1029
penetrance, 339
penicillin, 669, 875
perforation, 550, 582, 585, 588, 635, 636, 651, 990
perfusion, 764, 770, 1010, 1014
pericardium, 587
perinatal, xxvii, 767, 768, 771, 772, 780, 782, 783, 784
periodontal, 715
periodontal disease, 715
peripheral blood, xxvii, 21, 30, 37, 565, 701, 761, 831, 840, 873, 921, 946, 947, 950, 956
peripheral blood mononuclear cell, 873, 947, 950, 956
peripheral nervous system, 367
peripheral neuropathy, 250
peripheral vascular disease, xxxii, 1009, 1010, 1015
peritoneal cavity, 585, 588, 636
peritoneum, 295, 296, 298, 587
peritonitis, xxiv, 572, 579, 581, 584, 588, 618, 619, 630, 635, 636, 639, 640, 641, 644, 646, 652, 653, 905
permeability, 77, 167, 175, 246, 597, 657, 668, 736, 817, 841, 851, 991
permeation, xliv, 960, 972, 973
permit, xvii, xxviii, xlii, 25, 271, 466, 659, 805
pernicious anemia, xxii, 505, 509
peroxide, 15
peroxynitrite, 720
persistent asthma, 745
personal communication, 242, 245
personal history, 479, 988
personal problems, 490, 497
personal relations, 992
personal relationship, 992
personality, xxi, 476, 489, 490, 497, 776, 783, 877
personality characteristics, xxi, 489, 497
personality disorder, 476
personality traits, xxi, 489
pertussis, 843
petechiae, 656
pH, 8, 47, 81, 125, 126, 128, 132, 146, 160, 169, 202, 216, 222, 252, 262, 382, 527, 657, 664, 690, 691, 701, 707, 742, 796, 801, 826, 849
pH monitoring, 801
phage, 922, 936
phagocyte, 299, 690, 720
phagocytic cells, 171, 173, 557
phagocytosis, xvii, 86, 87, 121, 122, 134, 144, 165, 167, 168, 169, 171, 173, 183, 184, 252, 253, 263, 293, 299, 367, 583, 585, 674, 690, 703, 707, 719, 720, 721
phalanx, 883
pharmaceutical(s), xix, xliv, xlv, 58, 94, 186, 188, 390, 738, 745, 842, 844
pharmacokinetics, 568, 643, 850, 904
pharmacological treatment, 796
pharmacology, 360, 437, 532, 745, 851, 868
pharmacotherapy, 702
pharyngitis, 822, 902
pharynx, 740, 796, 880
phenol, 95, 96, 97, 98, 99, 100, 101, 102, 103, 104, 105, 106, 107, 108, 109, 110, 111, 112, 113, 114, 115, 116, 117, 118, 119, 120
phenolic compounds, 125, 127, 164, 165, 168, 170, 171, 172
phenylalanine, 174, 280, 296, 309, 625
phenytoin, 898
Philadelphia, 27, 28, 35, 37, 799, 932
phosphate, 91, 128, 129, 140, 147, 161, 309, 315, 316, 344, 559, 663, 696, 730, 738
phosphatidylcholine, 979
phospholipids, 123, 527, 532, 664, 979
phosphorylation, 11, 21, 37, 91, 207, 363, 373, 375, 376, 391, 447, 730, 919, 925, 927
photobleaching, 51, 52, 53
photocarcinogensis, xxxviii, 1245
photochemotherapy (PUVA), xxii, xxx, 512, 521, 522, 531, 853, 858, 893, 909, 933, 937, 938, 939, 941, 951, 952, 953, 954, 955, 957, 1397
photoconductivity, 272, 274
photodermatoses, xxxviii, 942, 1245, 1473, 1493
photodynamic therapy, xxv, 26, 40, 656, 666, 681, 683, 684, 685
photographs, 421, 812
photolysis, xliv
photon, xiv, xlii, 43, 46, 48, 51, 52, 53, 54, 55, 56, 59, 61, 828, 1221, 1429, 1472, 1475
photons, 13, 46, 48, 51, 52, 327, 329
photophobia, xxiii, 92, 255, 257, 545, 547, 555, 556
photoproducts, xxxvii, 14, 328, 329, 343, 349, 366, 377, 1215, 1224, 1232, 1234, 1462, 1463, 1603, 1613
photosensitivity, 405, 552, 560, 897, 941
photosensitizing, xxv, 328, 524, 656, 892, 893, 1150, 1227, 1238, 1602
photosynthesis, 366

phototoxicity, 53, 683, 892, 942
physical activity, xxxv, 855
physical environment, xlvii
physical properties, 272, 275, 680
physical therapy, xlviii
physicians, 477, 827, 895, 907
physicochemical characteristics, 664
physicochemical properties, 176, 961
physics, 189, 737
physiological factors, xvii, 293
physiology, 23, 27, 65, 126, 137, 144, 342, 379, 448, 526, 866, 984
physiopathology, 636
PI3K, 72, 79, 118, 186, 914, 927
PI3K/AKT, 72, 79, 927
pigment cells, xvii, xx, 138, 140, 188, 216, 293, 294, 296, 386, 452, 455, 456, 457, 458, 468, 471
pigmentary changes, xxxvii, 343, 1087, 1123, 1208, 1215
pigs, 125, 361, 373, 608
pilot study, 350, 481, 488, 955
pineal gland, 302
pipeline, 677
pituitary gland, 89, 192, 341
placebo, 421, 529, 607, 745, 833, 888, 889, 903, 904, 910, 956, 1015
placenta, 446, 780
placental abruption, 771
plants, xvi, xvii, xliv, 94, 126, 130, 133, 143, 149, 151, 155, 221, 222, 226, 228, 232, 233, 235, 236, 242, 243, 244, 245, 272, 307, 310, 313, 315, 320, 321, 366, 892
plasma levels, 946, 956, 984
plasma membrane, 72, 122, 165, 198, 200, 207, 597, 625, 676, 726, 732, 843
plasminogen, 131, 956, 983
plasticity, 74, 75, 140, 460, 462, 470
plastics, 619, 621
platelet count, 832, 907
platelets, 251, 260, 825
Plato, 351
playing, 467, 471, 623, 778, 820, 835, 848
pleasure, 319
pleura, xx, 455, 458, 463
plexus, 3, 5, 7, 19, 298, 309, 457, 946
plutonium, 327
PM, 185, 407, 410, 453, 482, 484, 487, 517, 518, 519, 603, 680, 682, 951
PNA, 434, 592
pneumocystis carinii, 905
pneumonia, xxvii, 171, 174, 697, 761, 764, 765, 798, 903, 905
pneumothorax, 762, 769
point mutation, 199, 200, 215, 217, 358, 381, 450, 944
poison, 366
Poland, 620, 687
polar, 11, 23, 331, 333, 640
polarity, 914
polarizability, 48
polarization, 57, 843, 868, 913
policy, xlvii, xlviii, l, 353
policy issues, xlviii
policy makers, l
pollutants, xxxv, 85
pollution, 548
polyamine(s), 154, 829, 894
polycarbonate, 743
polycythemia, 763, 769
polydactyly, 469
polyenes, xxv, 629, 640, 655, 661, 662, 722
polymer, 87, 160, 242, 296, 334, 424, 680
polymerase, 12, 32, 197, 246, 626
polymerase chain reaction, 197, 246, 626
polymerization, xv, 66, 88, 129, 159, 160, 163, 173, 176, 285, 300, 338
polymers, xv, 49, 159, 160, 163, 173, 274
polymorphism(s), 268, 338, 339, 340, 343, 357, 382, 406, 407, 409, 411, 412, 451, 453, 510, 518, 536, 538, 542, 626, 627, 630, 878, 985
polypeptide, 340, 342, 443, 527
polyphenols, xxxviii, 25, 94, 95, 96, 97, 98, 99, 100, 101, 102, 103, 104, 105, 106, 107, 108, 109, 110, 111, 112, 113, 114, 115, 116, 117, 118, 119, 120, 153
polysaccharide(s), xxvii, 163, 594, 662, 679, 689, 749, 752, 753, 759
polystyrene, 238
polyunsaturated fat, 300
polyunsaturated fatty acids, 300
POMC, vi, xix, xx, 84, 89, 91, 137, 138, 340, 341, 342, 359, 360, 368, 377, 379, 393, 395, 402, 409, 410, 441, 442, 443, 444, 445, 446, 447, 448, 449, 450, 451, 452, 1232
pons, 87
population group, 739
porosity, xliv, 165, 667, 682
porphyria, 893
portability, 737
portraits, 546
Portugal, 473, 474, 476, 482, 483, 620, 937
positive correlation, 759, 946
positive feedback, 66, 912, 923, 924, 927, 928
positron, 854
positron emission tomography, 854

post-inflammatory hyperpigmentation, xv, 83, 85, 123, 126, 128, 129, 402, 1052, 1181
postpolymerization, 680
post-transcriptional regulation, 402
post-transplant, 704
potassium, 130, 227, 397, 407, 900
potato, 223, 227
potential benefits, 222, 831
poverty, l
PPP, 424, 425
precancer, 760
precipitation, 874
precursor cells, 74, 86, 145, 339, 373
predation, 366, 376
predators, 169
prednisone, 1021
pregnancy, 31, 402, 416, 493, 497, 718, 825, 826, 827, 828, 830, 831, 849, 857, 859, 882, 886, 888, 889, 890, 892, 893, 895, 897, 898, 900, 902, 903, 942, 958
premature death, 72, 372
premature infant, 643, 653, 783
prematurity, xxvii, 574, 767, 770, 784, 785, 794
preparation, 49, 136, 281, 301, 468, 661, 692, 747, 887, 888, 890
preschool, 782, 783, 787
preschool children, 782
prescription drugs, 738
preservation, 481, 598
preservative, 559
preterm infants, 583, 785, 786
prevention, xiii, xix, xxxix, xl, xli, xliii, xlvi, xlvii, l, 37, 39, 123, 143, 349, 352, 353, 354, 363, 366, 377, 413, 480, 481, 486, 488, 595, 603, 614, 660, 667, 702, 709, 758, 849, 1002, 1004
primary function, 65, 68
primary hyperparathyroidism, 484
primary pulmonary hypertension, 762
primate, 865
priming, 531
principal component analysis, 54, 60
principles, xiv, xliv, 43, 44, 45, 58, 59, 81, 155, 274, 960, 997
private practice, xxxiv
probability, 769, 905
probands, 536
probe, 45, 46, 47, 48, 49, 626, 801, 960, 961, 962, 963, 964, 965, 966, 967, 968, 969, 970, 971, 972, 973, 975, 976, 977, 978
professional development, xlvi, xlvii
professionals, xlvi, 627
progenitor cell(s), 4, 5, 21, 25, 38, 41, 74, 75, 76, 696
progesterone, 217, 402, 414, 415, 416, 417
prognosis, xxiii, xxxiii, 347, 508, 514, 522, 571, 594, 604, 639, 822, 856, 877, 880, 1031
progressive multifocal leukoencephalopathy, 902
pro-inflammatory, xxx, xxxiii, 70, 71, 165, 333, 409, 552, 553, 554, 701, 705, 707, 825, 836, 837, 838, 840, 843, 847, 887, 938, 940, 944, 945, 946, 951, 983, 984, 1004, 1005
project, 302, 397, 402, 411, 427, 429, 430, 481
prokaryotes, 366
prolactin, 416
prolapse, 790
proline, 23, 625, 643
promoter, 90, 91, 139, 140, 370, 371, 376, 386, 387, 411, 447, 518, 825, 839, 840, 866, 918, 919, 920, 927, 933
pro-opiomelanocortin (POMC), 84, 89, 148, 341, 442, 449, 452, 453
propagation, 656
prophylactic, 593, 607, 661, 740, 744
prophylaxis, xliii, 572, 574, 581, 583, 587, 589, 594, 597, 607, 683, 744, 748
propylene, 319
prostaglandin, 67, 124, 145, 254, 355, 488, 528, 703, 837, 864
prostaglandins, 4, 131, 137, 333, 392, 480, 875
prostheses, 663, 666, 678, 679, 689, 727
prosthesis, 636, 637, 656, 666, 668, 682
prosthetic device, xxiv, 617, 619, 656, 669
protease inhibitors, 623
proteases, xxiv, xxxviii, 14, 121, 393, 553, 565, 618, 620, 649, 674, 689, 690, 719, 948, 1004, 1142, 1143, 1215, 1223
proteasome, 26, 42, 91, 121, 143, 144
protected areas, 36
protection, xiii, xiv, xv, xviii, xxxviii, xxxix, xl, xlii, xliii, xliv, xlv, xlvi, 63, 64, 159, 171, 175, 177, 189, 323, 324, 334, 345, 348, 355, 358, 366, 377, 387, 397, 453, 480, 481, 582, 607, 659, 664, 670, 726, 797, 891, 942, 943
protective role, xxxix, 17, 85, 243, 244, 838
protein components, 278, 280, 281
protein kinase C, 67, 84, 89, 120, 201
protein kinases, 387, 408
protein oxidation, xxxviii
protein structure, 54
protein synthesis, 625, 722, 726, 825, 914, 927, 931
proteinase, 67, 134, 144, 622, 623, 638, 639, 642, 646, 650, 660, 676
proteinuria, 706
proteoglycans, xxxvi, 11, 17
proteolysis, 624
proteolytic enzyme, 17, 160, 689

proteome, 378, 447
proto-oncogene, 22, 257, 258, 384, 411
pruritus, 423, 434, 525, 547, 555, 822, 849, 878, 884, 887, 891, 893, 903, 940, 1018
PSA, 995
pseudogene, 623
Pseudomonas aeruginosa, 594, 650, 668
pseudotumor cerebri, 899
psoriatic arthritis, xxix, xxxi, 510, 518, 818, 823, 832, 833, 835, 840, 852, 853, 855, 856, 857, 858, 859, 861, 862, 864, 871, 872, 881, 885, 898, 902, 903, 907, 909, 910, 917, 925, 933, 952, 981, 983, 995, 996, 1001, 1014
psychiatric disorder(s), 499, 501, 503, 506, 509, 782, 993, 998, 1020
psychiatric illness, 477
psychiatric morbidity, xxii, 505, 991
psychiatrist, 499
psychiatry, 503
psychological aspects, xliii, 1457, 1459
psychological development, 785
psychological distress, 401, 908
psychological stress, 496, 536, 877, 975, 991
psychological well-being, xlix, 499, 503
psychosis, 476
psychosocial factors, 770, 991
psychosocial functioning, 776
psychosocial stigmatization, xxix, 871
psychosomatic, xxi, 489, 490, 497, 499, 501, 503, 853, 908, 998
psychotic symptoms, 895
psychotropic drugs, 875
puberty, 9, 475, 530
public education, xviii, 323
public health, xxxix, xl, xlvi, 325, 352, 356, 601, 648, 658
publishing, 606, 607
Puerto Rico, 261, 618
pulmonary artery, 793
pulmonary edema, 762, 764
pulmonary embolism, 762, 1010
pulmonary hypertension, 764, 769, 794
pulse oximeters, xxviii, 805
pumps, 662, 852
purification, 119, 133, 143, 272, 280, 287
purines, 894
purpura, 433, 434, 439, 886
pus, 760, 882, 883
pustular psoriasis, xxix, 823, 832, 846, 856, 871, 874, 875, 876, 878, 882, 883, 896, 898, 905, 990, 1001, 1002, 1026, 1029
pustules, xxix, 551, 823, 846, 871, 878, 882, 883, 1052, 1053
PUVA, xxx, 350, 512, 524, 530, 822, 827, 828, 829, 831, 849, 850, 887, 890, 891, 892, 893, 896, 897, 900, 937, 938, 939, 941, 942, 943, 944, 945, 946, 947, 948, 949, 950, 952, 953, 954, 956, 957, 958, 1001
pyelonephritis, 587, 903, 905
pyoderma gangrenosum, 990
pyogenic, 564, 897
pyrimidine, 14, 237, 246, 329, 349, 350, 366, 377, 524, 828, 941, 944, 953

Q

qualitative research, 79
quantification, 47, 61, 225, 242, 356, 406, 566, 651, 807
quantified data, xxxv, 1093
quantum state, 961, 962
quartz, 49, 276, 809
Queensland, 604
quercetin, 108, 153, 310
questioning, 874
questionnaire, xxxiv, xxxviii, 490, 499, 500, 503, 540, 884, 987, 992, 993, 994
quinone(s), 88, 127, 129, 165, 277, 296

R

Rab, 87, 263, 650
race, 327, 334, 335, 346, 402, 794
radiation damage, 14, 19
radiation therapy, xx, 189, 473, 478, 480, 481, 482, 484, 485, 486, 957, 1020
radiation treatment, xx, 174, 473, 477, 479, 480, 485, 487
radical formation, xlii
radicals, xxvi, xxxviii, xliv, 12, 15, 31, 182, 300, 717, 727, 729
radio, xx, 473, 475, 682
radiodermitis, xx, 473, 476, 477, 480
radiography, 635
radiotherapy, xliii, 54, 56, 478, 479, 480, 481, 485, 486, 487, 488, 581
radius, 277
radon, 327
Raman spectra, 48, 49, 54, 275, 277, 278
Raman spectroscopy, 48, 49, 54, 55, 58, 60
RAS, xvi, 249, 254, 255, 264, 266, 373, 375, 694, 704
rash, 587, 598, 823, 1018
rate of change, 812
rating scale, 490, 502

RBC, 949
reaction rate, 316
reactions, xliv, 55, 88, 133, 161, 163, 167, 200, 225, 328, 333, 334, 380, 424, 428, 436, 480, 487, 520, 822, 876, 888, 893, 902, 903, 904, 905, 906, 938
reactive oxygen, xxvi, xxxiii, xxxv, xlii, xlv, 14, 15, 34, 84, 85, 171, 173, 328, 349, 364, 392, 669, 690, 717, 730, 731, 733, 828, 878, 944, 1004, 1005
Reactive Oxygen Species, xxxvii, 1215, 1222, 1493
reactivity, 200, 416, 497, 876, 933, 948, 950
reading, 205, 728, 775, 777, 779
reagents, 1002
real time, 55, 76
reality, 486
reasoning, 772
recall, 774
reception, 64
recessive allele, 198, 199, 202
recidivism, 497, 500
recognition, xxviii, xxxiii, 122, 167, 171, 330, 343, 344, 362, 410, 516, 536, 582, 607, 659, 805, 810, 812, 814, 950, 1031
recombinant DNA, 527, 832, 901
recombination, 285, 363, 371, 446, 627, 644
recommendations, xxviii, xxxiv, xxxix, xlii, xlvi, xlviii, 552, 593, 594, 598, 599, 612, 613, 632, 638, 767, 777, 803, 810, 990, 1006
reconstruction, 50
recovery, xxxix, xlix, 34, 38, 57, 65, 171, 582, 595, 633, 850, 1001
recreational, 325, 331, 333, 334, 337, 773
rectum, 301
recurrence, 474, 491, 497, 527, 536, 537, 560, 659, 662, 670, 678, 822, 830, 874, 879, 891, 912
recycling, 299, 300
red blood cells, 624, 949
red shift, 283
redshift, 282
reflectance spectra, 53
reflectivity, 51
refractive indices, 51
regenerate, 25
regeneration, xiv, 25, 29, 64, 74, 75, 76, 77, 78, 80, 760
regenerative medicine, 25
regions of the world, 823
Registry, 513, 540
regression, xxxviii, 16, 55, 74, 75, 225, 230, 511, 758, 1007
regression equation, 758
regression line, 230
regrowth, xx, 473, 475, 478, 479, 480, 481, 511, 522, 523, 524, 525, 527, 528, 529, 530, 531, 679
regulations, 919
regulator gene, 699, 730
regulatory changes, 409
rehabilitation, xlvii, 818
rejection, 702, 830, 831
relapses, 845, 879, 904, 920
relatives, 499, 536, 539, 813, 872, 992
relaxation, 272, 979
relevance, 79, 343, 377, 630, 710, 757, 932
reliability, 755, 786
relief, 404, 638, 825, 827
remediation, 775
remission, xxix, xlv, 530, 817, 821, 822, 871, 888, 892, 938, 941, 945, 948, 950, 952, 954, 984, 1002, 1007, 1027
renaissance, 546
renal cell carcinoma, 1019
renal dysfunction, 900
renal failure, 631
renin, 360
repair, xiv, xxxviii, 14, 25, 26, 29, 31, 33, 37, 39, 41, 57, 63, 65, 67, 68, 70, 72, 77, 78, 324, 330, 343, 344, 345, 347, 349, 362, 363, 364, 552, 769, 774, 781, 782, 785, 851
repair mechanisms, xxxviii, 25, 324, 349, 552, 1153, 1216, 1223, 1225, 1236, 1248, 1260, 1431, 1496, 1498
repetitions, 223, 230
replication, xxx, 11, 22, 23, 328, 363, 828, 894, 938, 941
repression, 12, 720
repressor, 733
reproduction, 165, 170, 175, 397, 597
requirement(s), 209, 243, 262, 377, 383, 468, 770, 778, 810, 813, 814
researchers, xiv, xxxv, 2, 55, 73, 164, 240, 244, 626, 740, 768, 771, 772, 773, 774, 775, 912, 918
resection, 636, 637, 797, 798
residue(s), xxx, 11, 14, 23, 91, 122, 199, 237, 344, 360, 371, 373, 410, 748, 911, 922, 925
resilience, xxxiv, 46
resins, 663, 665, 667, 680, 682
resolution, xxx, 49, 51, 53, 57, 59, 158, 275, 538, 558, 560, 586, 598, 637, 794, 800, 891, 896, 913, 938, 940, 946, 947, 979, 1027, 1028
resorcinol, 95
resources, xlvii, xlviii, 658
respiration, 726, 732, 769, 793, 794
respiratory distress syndrome, 769, 785
responsiveness, xxiv, 35, 184, 467, 524, 618, 825, 863, 955

restaurants, xlix
restoration, 4, 38, 41, 741
restriction enzyme, 626
restriction fragment length polymorphis, 626
restrictions, xxxiii, 378, 498, 737
resveratrol, 138, 386
retardation, 831, 832
reticulum, 11, 21, 26, 86, 88, 136, 367, 715
retinal detachment, 635
retinol, 127, 146
retrovirus, 380
rheumatic diseases, 829, 861
rheumatoid arthritis, 510, 518, 519, 528, 533, 609, 829, 833, 838, 859, 865, 903, 985, 987, 1010, 1011, 1015, 1020, 1026
rheumatoid factor, 693, 818, 872, 985, 987, 988, 1011
rheumatologist, 988
rhinitis, 899
rhinophyma, 546, 548
rhizome, 314
Rhizopus, 726
rhythm, 764
ribosomal RNA, 653
ribosome(s), 88, 622
rickets, 333
rings, 279, 699
ringworm, 175, 474, 483, 484
rituximab, 702, 1023
RNA(s), xxx, 202, 256, 257, 270, 328, 329, 330, 344, 349, 368, 381, 385, 395, 402, 405, 412, 626, 722, 723, 726, 911, 930, 937, 940, 943
RNAi, xxx, 911, 929
rodents, 11, 13, 26, 180
rods, 693
Romania, 489, 490, 492
room temperature, 224, 226, 275, 276, 277, 278, 279, 280, 281, 282, 283, 284, 286, 316
root(s), xvi, 41, 74, 116, 122, 123, 124, 150, 151, 152, 153, 154, 155, 175, 221, 222, 223, 226, 227, 228, 232, 234, 235, 236, 237, 238, 239, 243, 244, 245, 246, 247, 314, 315, 457, 511, 523, 840, 913
root rot, xvi, 221, 222, 245, 246
rosacea, xiii, xxiii, 545, 546, 547, 548, 549, 550, 551, 552, 553, 554, 556, 557, 558, 559, 560, 561, 562, 563, 564, 565, 566, 567, 568, 569, 886
rotations, 48
roughness, xxxvii, 132, 664, 665, 679, 680
Rouleau, 406
routes, 456, 458, 460, 462, 467, 721
routines, 778, 926, 928
rubber(s), 415, 425, 434, 436, 439
rubella, 768
rubrics, 779
rules, xliii, 776, 962
Russia, 620

S

sadness, 776
saliva, 657, 661, 663, 689, 690, 701, 742, 747, 751, 758, 760
salivary gland, 713
salmon, 1009
salts, xlv, 474, 726, 733, 842, 1005
saponin, 145
Sarajevo, 521
SAS, 225, 226
saturation, xxvii, 391, 767, 768, 780, 794, 806, 807, 808
Saudi Arabia, 955
scaling, 525, 552, 555, 556, 822, 826, 879, 881, 883, 884
Scandinavia, 331
scanning electron microscopy, 30, 675
scar tissue, 56, 474
scatter, 51, 275
scattering, xvii, 48, 49, 51, 53, 271, 274
SCF, 85, 123, 258, 390, 393, 395, 1182, 1183, 1184, 1187, 1189, 1194
schizophrenia, 477, 485
school, xiii, xlii, xlvi, xlvii, xlviii, 474, 490, 491, 493, 495, 498, 671, 772, 773, 775, 778, 780, 781, 782, 783, 784, 785, 787, 992
school grounds, xlvii, 1352, 1372, 1631, 1652, 1653, 1657, 1663, 1664, 1665, 1667, 1670, 1671, 1672, 1673, 1675, 1676, 1689, 1690, 1691, 1692, 1693, 1694, 1695, 1696
school performance, 787
School-based Education, 1734
science, xxxix, xlix, 189, 272, 319, 353, 409, 526, 786
scientific investigations, 390
scleroderma, 46
sclerosis, 519
scope, xli, 477, 1002
scrotum, 890
SCT, 613
SDS, 913
SDS-PAGE, 913
seasonal change(s), 294
seborrheic dermatitis, 881
sebum, 44
second generation, 46, 1000
secrete, 4, 68, 69, 173, 177, 192, 366, 392, 582, 622, 689, 690, 921, 924

security, 499, 939, 989
seed, 124, 125, 222, 226
seeding, 224, 587
segregation, 239, 385, 469
selective serotonin reuptake inhibitor, 993
selectivity, 917
selenium, 1000, 1004, 1007
self esteem, 319
self-assessment, 487
self-awareness, 500
self-efficacy, 777
self-esteem, xli, 64, 333, 500, 776, 777, 991, 992
self-image, xxi, 489, 499
self-regulation, 770, 777
self-tanning creams, xxxviii, 1265
semantic memory, 786
semiconductors, 272, 274
senescence, xxxvi, 38, 40, 42, 53, 72, 387, 580
sensation(s), xiv, xxiii, xxiv, 63, 64, 545, 547, 553, 555, 556, 655, 656, 691, 793, 889, 994, 1032
senses, 319
sensing, 621, 622, 644, 647, 649, 817, 841, 851
sensitivity, xxiv, xxvii, xxxv, xxxviii, 256, 282, 283, 284, 333, 334, 335, 339, 343, 345, 371, 486, 551, 553, 588, 589, 592, 593, 617, 693, 724, 749, 755, 756, 759, 848, 961, 987, 989, 1005
sensitization, xxvi, 421, 422, 426, 431, 524, 525, 718, 838
sensor, 77
sensorineural hearing loss, 250
sensors, 144
sepsis, 579, 588, 638, 646, 649
septic arthritis, 619, 903
septic shock, 583, 764
sequencing, 330, 626, 627, 653, 773
serine, 91, 121, 217, 443, 565, 934
serology, 537
serotonin, 101, 726
serum, 55, 61, 131, 193, 210, 211, 212, 213, 315, 415, 417, 419, 426, 436, 589, 591, 592, 593, 594, 634, 689, 711, 740, 833, 842, 895, 896, 897, 899, 900, 927, 944, 946, 948, 955, 958, 979, 997, 1001, 1002, 1003, 1020, 1023, 1026
serum albumin, 55, 61, 193, 896, 979, 1023
services, 578, 609, 775, 777, 779
severe muscle catabolism, xlviii, 1739
sex, 13, 31, 34, 35, 59, 92, 141, 201, 210, 401, 475, 497, 648, 697, 885, 1003, 1010
sex hormones, 92
sexual problems, 493
sexual reproduction, 640
shade, xlvii, 768
shape, xvi, 17, 86, 135, 160, 167, 171, 172, 206, 218, 221, 240, 275, 277, 294, 295, 721, 846, 879, 964, 968, 975
shear, 663, 664
sheep, 28, 41
shock, 25, 26, 42, 585, 905
short supply, 243
shortage, 708, 954
shortness of breath, xxvii, 761
showing, xv, xvi, xxi, xxxix, xlii, 12, 18, 20, 26, 48, 54, 55, 64, 66, 249, 295, 297, 299, 324, 400, 414, 457, 458, 463, 467, 481, 505, 506, 511, 538, 546, 548, 588, 619, 623, 630, 637, 639, 659, 670, 679, 751, 754, 775, 776, 807, 1028
shrink scars, xlix, 1789, 1792
Si_3N_4, 277
sibling, 498
siblings, 536
signal transduction, 38, 89, 91, 137, 373, 405, 408, 538, 624, 625, 928, 934, 935, 1005
signalling, 140, 157, 186, 361, 383, 385, 866, 868, 878, 901, 943
signals, xviii, 4, 27, 53, 64, 72, 74, 76, 91, 160, 218, 323, 338, 366, 392, 467, 468, 518, 642, 817, 837, 866, 919, 948, 961, 965, 968, 1012
silicon, 48, 272, 424
silver, 8, 135, 203, 209, 210, 215, 218, 245, 381, 419, 589, 884
simulation(s), xxxi, 55, 959, 961, 966, 967, 968, 970, 971, 978
Singapore, 496, 501, 502, 514, 761
single chain, 972
single-nucleotide polymorphism, xxii, 406, 535
siRNA, xxx, 391, 392, 397, 407, 911, 919, 926
skeletal muscle, 21, 23, 121, 144, 205
skeleton, 152, 456, 460, 476
skimming, 779
Skin Cancer Prevention/, 1731, 1732
Skin Cancer Risk Factors, 1734
skin cancer risks, xlvi
skin diseases, xxxii, xxxiii, 59, 174, 403, 490, 502, 527, 532, 817, 820, 830, 837, 838, 844, 877, 927, 932, 934, 975, 991, 1021, 1025, 1026, 1028
skin lightening formulations, xvii, 307
skin permeation, xliv, 1523, 1524, 1525, 1528, 1529, 1530, 1532, 1533, 1534, 1536, 1537, 1538
SLE, 510, 518, 519, 740
sleep apnea, 797
Slovakia, 642
small intestine, 842
smoking, xiii, xxxi, xxxiv, 2, 13, 31, 32, 657, 673, 855, 878, 883, 981, 990, 993, 1004, 1010
smooth muscle, 5, 7, 38, 67, 78, 79, 382, 525

smooth muscle cells, 5
SNAP, 22
snoring, 794
SNP, xix, 389, 397, 400, 518, 539
sociability, 776
social behavior, xliii, 776
social class, 354
social competence, 776
social context, 294
social costs, 818
social environment, xlvi
social interaction, 773
social life, 500
social phobia, xxi, 489, 499
social relations, xxi, 489, 499
social support, 497, 499
social withdrawal, 818
socialization, 991
society, 500, 818
Socrates, 291
sodium, 129, 144, 193, 226, 316, 397, 406, 407, 663, 664, 665, 666, 667, 678, 679, 680, 702, 738, 836, 971
software, 225, 226, 276, 395
solar ultraviolet (UV) radiation, xxxvi, xlv, xlvi, 1141, 1545, 1571, 1572, 1602, 1651
solid tumors, 577, 584, 701
solidification, 228
solubility, 10, 127, 275, 424
solution, xxvii, xxviii, 126, 129, 225, 227, 230, 242, 276, 282, 283, 284, 285, 288, 289, 299, 426, 523, 524, 568, 584, 634, 661, 663, 664, 665, 680, 681, 738, 749, 752, 805, 806, 886, 906, 963, 970, 971, 972, 973, 976
solvents, 255, 310, 319
somatic mutations, 351
sororities, xxxviii, 1265, 1267, 1278
South Africa, 127, 154, 620, 744
South America, 171, 303, 619, 620
South Asia, xix, 389, 397
Southeast Asia, 172
Southern blot, 626
Spain, 1, 573, 574, 575, 576, 577, 590, 592, 594, 602, 604, 606, 608, 615, 620, 639, 643, 861, 907, 981, 994, 997
spasticity, 250
special education, 775
specialisation, 410
specialists, xlvi
specialization, 260
spectroscopy, xiv, xvii, 37, 43, 46, 47, 53, 55, 58, 60, 178, 271, 273, 274, 784, 960, 961
speech, 498, 773, 776, 777, 801
spelling, 775
spending, xxxviii
SPF capping, xliii, 1446, 1453
spin, 160, 727, 960, 961, 962, 963, 964, 965, 966, 967, 970, 971, 975, 979
spin labels, 963
spindle, 67
spine, 793
spleen, 205, 296, 299, 300, 443, 446, 585, 587
splinting, xlix
spondyloarthropathy, 823
sponge, 176, 594
spontaneous abortion, 830
spontaneous recovery, 508
sporotrichosis, 168, 169, 170, 183
Spring, ix
spring break, xxxviii, 1265, 1267, 1268, 1269, 1270, 1271, 1272, 1274, 1275, 1276, 1277, 1278, 1399
sprue, 639
sputum, 757
squamous cell, xvi, 6, 14, 33, 72, 80, 81, 249, 256, 268, 330, 332, 333, 351, 353, 359, 449, 475, 484, 692, 711, 829, 831, 902, 942, 944, 952, 953, 1001
squamous cell carcinoma, xvi, 6, 14, 33, 72, 81, 249, 256, 268, 330, 332, 333, 351, 359, 449, 476, 692, 711, 829, 831, 942, 944, 953, 1001
stab-and-roll biopsy, xxxiii, 1031, 1033, 1042
stability, 93, 421, 557, 564, 624, 665, 666, 667, 682, 811, 896
stabilization, xxvii, 215, 330, 338, 376, 558, 574, 761, 765
standard deviation, 226, 491, 772, 775, 776, 948
standard error, 55, 231, 232
standardization, 133, 592
staphylococci, 558, 573
starvation, 170, 721, 732
state(s), xxx, xl, xli, xlv, xlvi, xlvii, xlviii, 45, 46, 52, 56, 70, 168, 245, 285, 355, 378, 402, 447, 460, 475, 478, 499, 503, 649, 674, 701, 721, 722, 747, 762, 806, 837, 861, 876, 915, 917, 921, 922, 931, 937, 940, 948, 956, 962, 998
statistics, 225, 346, 347, 770
steel, 89, 217, 384, 385, 467, 470
stele, 222, 223, 232, 234, 235, 236, 237, 238, 242, 243, 244
stem cell factor (SCF), xxxvii, 145, 211, 384, 385, 386, 406, 1179, 1182, 1193
stem cells, l, 4, 5, 21, 23, 25, 29, 37, 38, 74, 76, 214, 479, 511, 701
stenosis, 254, 793, 794, 795, 798, 802
sterile, xxiv, 225, 226, 227, 374, 588, 589, 618, 619, 754, 823, 846, 882, 883
steroid inhaler, 736, 739, 743

steroids, xxiii, xxvi, 92, 114, 480, 523, 532, 545, 635, 735, 736, 737, 738, 739, 740, 741, 742, 743, 744, 745, 746, 824, 882, 883, 885, 886, 1001, 1002, 1006, 1021
sterols, 314
stigmatized, 998
stimulant, 123, 124, 777
stimulation, 9, 35, 68, 69, 92, 145, 205, 343, 344, 345, 375, 379, 383, 384, 405, 444, 446, 553, 747, 797, 921, 924
stimulus, 294, 393, 847, 876
stock, 204, 208, 211, 225, 970, 971, 973
stomatitis, 656, 657, 660, 668, 670, 671, 672, 673, 674, 675, 676, 677, 678, 679, 681, 683, 692, 735, 750, 895
storage, 44, 133, 260, 261, 299, 682, 712
stratification, 580, 816
strenuous exercise, xxxv, 1099, 1100, 1638
streptococci, 873, 875, 921, 922, 935
stress factors, 927, 992
stress response, xxvi, 40, 41, 180, 662, 718, 720, 721, 722, 724, 728, 730, 877
stressful events, xxi, xxiii, 489, 490, 492, 495, 496, 497, 498, 500, 503, 535
stressful life events, 497, 499, 873
stressors, xxi, xlv, 25, 174, 489, 720, 877
stretching, 48, 277, 279, 960
striae, 825, 886
stridor, xxviii, 789, 790, 793, 794, 799, 801, 802, 803
stroke, 55, 819, 854, 958, 983, 1010, 1014
stroma, xvii, 293, 296, 301, 557
stromal cells, 73
structural changes, 34
structural protein, 86, 90, 447, 913
structuring, xxxvi
style, 810
subacute, 421
sub-clinical levels, xxxv, 1121, 1125
subcutaneous injection, 894, 906
subcutaneous tissue, xxxiv, 5, 7, 9, 71, 816
subepithelial fibrosis, 555
subgroups, 376, 626
submucosa, 585
substance abuse, 877
substance use, 499
substitutes, 77
substitution(s), xxx, 194, 199, 211, 213, 217, 237, 911, 922, 925
substrate(s), 44, 94, 127, 132, 136, 164, 165, 170, 172, 177, 180, 210, 255, 267, 275, 276, 277, 288, 289, 410, 621
success rate, 529, 798, 834
succession, 51, 757
sucrose, 223, 409
sugar beet, 126
sugarcane, 126
suicidal ideation, 992, 993
sulfate, 5, 17, 836, 971
sulfonamide, 171, 528
sulfur, 87, 334, 337, 509
sulphur, 272, 474
Sun, ix, x, xxxviii, xxxix, xliii, xlv, xlvii, xlviii, 10, 11, 15, 18, 21, 59, 78, 79, 331, 348, 350, 352, 355, 378, 402, 415, 441, 515, 518, 727, 733, 864, 929
sun-sensitivity, xxxviii, 1265, 1267, 1659
supervision, 886, 894
supplementation, xxxii, xxxviii, xxxix, 559, 830, 999, 1004, 1006, 1007
suppliers, 129, 169
suppression, xxxv, xxxviii, 12, 70, 123, 144, 145, 163, 318, 320, 326, 437, 528, 736, 741, 794, 797, 825, 848, 863, 894, 947, 957, 1002
surface area, 816, 821, 824, 829, 848, 849, 884, 887, 942, 992
surface hardness, 666
surface structure, 679
surfactant(s), 260, 960, 961, 971, 978
surgical intervention, xxxiii, 769, 794, 795, 797, 1031
surgical technique, 798
surgical techniques, 798
surveillance, xl, xlviii, 325, 326, 348, 573, 577, 600, 601, 602, 603, 604, 605, 608, 610, 615, 619, 626, 639, 641, 644, 646, 648, 653, 660, 730, 934
survival rate, 367, 584, 770
survivors, xxxix, 478, 587, 772
suspensions, 208, 666, 667, 668, 740
suture, 579, 797
sweat, xiv, xxx, xxxv, 5, 44, 63, 217, 816, 911, 913, 914
sweating response, xxxv, 1099, 1108, 1109, 1110, 1111, 1117, 1118, 1119, 1120
Sweden, 576, 577, 615, 1002
swelling, xxiv, 16, 54, 655, 656, 903, 986
Switzerland, 1022
symmetry, 53, 966, 969
symptomatic treatment, 826
synaptic vesicles, 252, 260
synergistic effect, 319, 386
synovial fluid, 642
synovitis, 872, 883, 996
synthetic polymers, 689
syphilis, 415, 939
systemic immune response, 527

systemic lupus erythematosus, xxii, xxxii, 505, 509, 510, 511, 518, 519, 558, 740, 891, 1020, 1025, 1026
systolic blood pressure, 1003

T

T cell receptor, 516, 873, 936
T lymphocytes, xxv, 251, 252, 511, 525, 526, 527, 541, 688, 694, 872, 878, 891, 892, 901, 921, 931, 990
T regulatory cells, 542, 708
tachycardia, 526, 884
tachypnea, 769
Taiwan, 83, 150, 311, 426, 441, 501, 575, 576, 578, 605, 615, 620, 641, 713, 800
tandem repeats, 873
tanners, xli, xliii, 353, 1275, 1279, 1280, 1321, 1325, 1326, 1330, 1337, 1344, 1348, 1349, 1362, 1363, 1415, 1417, 1418, 1426, 1457, 1461, 1465
tanning attitudes, xxxviii, 1265, 1267, 1269, 1280, 1281, 1348
tanning beds, xxxviii, xli, 332, 333, 1265, 1266, 1274, 1275, 1277, 1278, 1302, 1319, 1338, 1341, 1342, 1347, 1363, 1375, 1380, 1381, 1393, 1394, 1415, 1417, 1418, 1419, 1420, 1423, 1461, 1621, 1624, 1626, 1708, 1733
tanning behaviors, xl, 1276, 1277, 1279, 1305, 1331, 1345, 1346, 1347, 1357, 1362, 1363, 1367
tanning salons, xli, xlii, xliii, 327, 332, 345, 1275, 1337, 1338, 1340, 1341, 1349, 1363, 1368, 1377, 1411, 1415, 1416, 1417, 1420, 1421, 1422, 1423, 1424, 1425, 1426, 1457
tannins, 314
tar, 827, 884, 890, 891
TBA, 948, 949, 950
T-cell mediated autoimmune mechanism, xxi, 505, 506
T-cell receptor, 922, 929
TCR, xxx, 911, 921, 934
teachers, xlvi, 498, 779
tear shaped papules, xxix, 871
technical support, xlvii
techniques, xiii, xvii, xxvii, xliv, xlix, 1, 8, 26, 55, 172, 271, 273, 274, 285, 290, 330, 480, 527, 567, 592, 593, 610, 613, 625, 627, 711, 739, 749, 751, 752, 797, 798
technology(s), xxviii, 41, 51, 61, 567, 737, 738, 805, 806, 807, 810, 811, 832, 840, 901
teenage girls, xli, xlii
teeth, 663, 665, 666, 667, 669, 680, 682, 697, 779, 798
telangiectasia(s), xiii, xxxiv, xxxvii, 2, 13, 19, 24, 343, 549, 551, 552, 554, 555, 556, 886, 1213
telomere, 11, 31
TEM, 285, 442, 448, 450
temperature, xv, xvii, 2, 47, 160, 169, 176, 181, 182, 222, 225, 293, 719, 779, 808, 809, 811, 816, 961, 971, 979
tendon(s), 819, 986
tensile strength, xxxvii
tension, xxxvi, 35, 762, 993
teratogen, 895
terminals, 44
termination codon, 206
terpenes, 971
territorial, xl
territory, xlvii, xlviii
test scores, 565
testicle, 295, 301
testing, xxxiii, xxxv, xliii, 46, 241, 403, 414, 424, 427, 428, 429, 430, 436, 439, 563, 592, 600, 605, 612, 628, 633, 641, 642, 643, 650, 653, 675, 676, 692, 693, 720, 728, 732, 898, 907, 940, 1031, 1032
testosterone, 376
tetracyclines, xxiii, 545, 569, 893, 897, 899
textbook(s), 430, 757, 779
textiles, xliv, xlv, 423, 424, 425, 435
texture, xxxiv, 132
TGF, xxxvi, 65, 67, 68, 69, 77, 85, 91, 141, 703, 836, 875, 926, 1005
Th cells, 923
Thailand, 311, 496, 502
thalamus, 771
theatre, 813
T-helper cell, 736, 830, 831, 887
therapeutic agents, 88, 531, 874, 950
therapeutic approaches, xxiii, xxxiv, 501, 530, 572, 839
therapeutic effect(s), 147, 176, 894
therapeutic goal, 526, 842
therapeutic ointments, xx, 473, 474
therapeutic targets, 73
therapeutic use, 867
therapeutics, 449, 528
therapist, xlix
thermal heat, xlviii, 1739
thermoregulation, xiv, xxxv, 63, 64
thiazide, 900
thiazide diuretics, 900
thinning, xxii, xxxvi, 11, 16, 126, 343, 505, 549, 550
thoughts, 818, 821
three-dimensional confocal microscopy, xxxvi, 1157
three-dimensional model, 75

threonine, 400
thrombin, 144
thrombocytopenia, 903, 1020
thrombophlebitis, 583, 587, 598
thrombosis, 523, 588, 840, 867
thromboxanes, 123
thrush, 653, 697, 699, 735
thulium, 798
thymine, xlv, 329, 350, 356
thymoma, 691, 699, 711
thymus, 296, 510, 538, 953
thyroid, xxii, 476, 482, 483, 484, 505, 536
thyroid cancer, 476, 482
thyroiditis, 510, 518, 1020
tibia, 895
TID, 796
time constraints, 827
time periods, 897
time-frame, 244
TIMP, xxxvi, 81
TIMP-1, xxxvi
TIMP-2, xxxvi
tin, 227, 411
tincture, 474
tinea capitis, xx, 473, 474, 475, 476, 477, 478, 482, 483, 484, 485, 881
tinea corporis, 494
tinea pedis, 494
tissue engineering, 29, 79
TLR2, 553, 565
TLR4, 553
TLR9, 933
TNF-alpha, xxxi, 382, 701, 953, 954, 955, 981, 983, 984, 989, 990, 993, 1000, 1028
TNF-α, xxxv, 85, 123, 124, 125, 526, 528, 690, 703, 707, 736, 832, 833, 836, 837, 844, 847, 876, 902, 903, 905, 906, 907, 915, 923, 924, 945, 946, 947, 949, 950, 980, 1002, 1026
tobacco, 32, 554, 657, 819
tobacco smoke, 32
tobacco smoking, 32, 657, 819
tones, 334, 401, 809
tonsils, 880, 908, 921
tooth, 663, 715
toothbrushing, 678, 680
topical agents, xxix, xxx, 437, 662, 722, 723, 824, 871, 885, 886, 937, 938, 1257
topical anesthetic, 523, 795
topical applications, xxxvi, 226, 480, 1142, 1148
torsion, 45, 46
torture, xlix
total parenteral nutrition, 579, 580, 631
toxic effect, 127, 669, 903, 906
toxic metals, 87
toxicity, xxvi, 94, 421, 480, 481, 486, 528, 661, 663, 717, 722, 827, 829, 849, 859, 884, 889, 893, 894, 895, 896, 899, 939
toxin, 689, 843
TPA, 85, 124, 125
trachea, 793, 796
trafficking, 4, 86, 87, 122, 134, 135, 136, 142, 203, 210, 218, 251, 260, 261, 262, 553, 902, 932
training, 500, 799
traits, xviii, 173, 209, 301, 348, 365, 400, 407, 469, 497, 710
transaminases, 597, 884, 894, 897, 905
transcription factors, xxvi, 12, 22, 90, 91, 139, 140, 341, 374, 510, 717, 828, 896, 927, 943, 979
transcripts, 216, 402, 465, 951
transducer, 49, 85, 90, 209, 379
transduction, 27, 81, 371, 384, 919
transfection, 92
transferrin, 689
transformation(s), xxvi, 5, 67, 69, 73, 75, 166, 185, 237, 272, 364, 474, 525, 692, 735, 932
transforming growth factor, xxxvi, 65, 79, 80, 85, 836, 875, 887, 931, 936
transition metal, 961
transition mutation, 330
translation, 390, 403, 926
translocation, xvi, 134, 249, 253, 257, 263, 585, 586, 608, 688, 843, 868, 898, 931
translocation of melanosomes, xvi, 249
transmission, xlv, 17, 30, 295, 585, 897
transmission electron microscopy, 17
transplant, 24, 39, 73, 326, 574, 577, 578, 583, 607, 608, 636, 652, 677, 702, 704, 712, 713, 714, 715, 759, 830, 831
transplant recipients, 39, 326, 574, 577, 578, 583, 607, 608, 704, 713, 714, 715, 759
transplantation, xxiii, xxiv, 77, 571, 581, 583, 607, 614, 655, 658, 672, 681, 703, 704, 714, 715, 898, 905, 926
transport, 87, 133, 134, 135, 136, 198, 200, 202, 205, 210, 214, 218, 222, 252, 260, 296, 357, 405, 625, 664, 836
transportation, 252, 447
transverse section, 236, 237, 238, 457
transversion mutation, 329
trauma, 54, 56, 479, 491, 495, 575, 583, 657, 763, 780, 834, 837, 847, 873, 876, 877, 883, 948, 992
traumatic events, 502
traumatic experiences, 496
treatment methods, 677, 679
tremor, 899

trial, 127, 129, 132, 148, 149, 353, 418, 421, 439, 488, 529, 559, 560, 561, 593, 598, 599, 607, 670, 671, 681, 745, 746, 781, 854, 906, 910, 954, 956, 1002, 1003, 1007
triazoles, xxv, 595, 655, 661
tribal organization, xlvii, 1376, 1703
tricarboxylic acid, 197, 214
trichotillomania, 501
tricuspid valve, 587
triggers, xxxii, 41, 89, 123, 135, 141, 254, 390, 487, 540, 551, 554, 558, 730, 731, 733, 779, 834, 875, 877, 878, 1005, 1025, 1028
triglycerides, 594, 897, 899, 989, 1003
tropism, 587
trypsin, 85, 121, 122, 726, 732
tryptophan, 281
tuberculosis, 757, 830, 832, 834, 895, 900, 905, 906, 907
tumor cells, 72, 73, 927
tumor development, 72
tumor growth, 565, 915, 930
tumor invasion, 71, 72, 73
tumor necrosis factor, xxxii, xxxv, 38, 85, 123, 137, 355, 450, 520, 522, 525, 528, 529, 690, 736, 832, 833, 840, 850, 872, 912, 940, 950, 958, 983, 1007, 1015, 1025, 1028, 1029
tumor progression, xv, 64, 264
tumorigenesis, 23, 866
tumours, 354, 953
tungsten, 48, 809
turgor, 188, 239, 240, 244, 246
Turkey, 502, 541, 576, 604, 620
turnover, 125, 131, 148, 366, 722, 820, 872
twins, 381, 453, 515, 540
twist, 543
tympanic membrane, 637
type 1 diabetes, 510, 518, 519, 520, 536
type 2 diabetes, 671, 672, 885, 984
tyrosine hydroxylase, 129

U

ubiquitin, 91, 121, 143, 144, 369, 836
ulcer, 759
ulcerative colitis, xxii, 505, 509, 510, 1010
ultrasonography, xiv, 43, 50
ultrasound, 49, 50, 53, 55, 59, 81
ultrastructure, 17, 448
ultraviolet irradiation, xxxv, 9, 13, 33, 409
umbilical cord, xxvii, 767, 768, 780
underlying mechanisms, 728
underproduction, 92
uniform, 70, 232, 236, 245, 993
United Kingdom, 127, 620, 745, 842
United States, ix, xxxii, xxxix, xl, xliii, xlvi, l, 29, 33, 34, 37, 179, 188, 324, 325, 332, 334, 346, 352, 354, 377, 379, 380, 381, 382, 383, 385, 387, 451, 453, 475, 547, 601, 603, 619, 671, 818, 851, 902, 997, 1002, 1009
unstable patients, 598
upper respiratory infection, 902
upper respiratory tract, 882, 903, 905, 906
upstream regulator, xix, 389, 915
urban, 997
urban population, 997
urea, 896
urethritis, 897
uric acid, 884, 900
urinalysis, 900
urinary tract, xxiv, 583, 584, 585, 618, 630, 757, 903
urinary tract infection, xxiv, 583, 618, 630, 757
urine, 55, 416, 638, 694, 760, 842, 868
urticaria, 436, 501, 525, 902, 903
USA, xxxviii, l, 127, 131, 134, 139, 144, 159, 171, 210, 216, 217, 221, 223, 225, 226, 259, 260, 405, 407, 411, 469, 475, 566, 573, 574, 575, 576, 577, 592, 593, 594, 612, 730, 731, 732, 738, 824, 827, 872, 1031
UV absorbers, xliv, xlv, 1541, 1571, 1573, 1574, 1592, 1593, 1610
UV DNA damage, xviii, 323, 344
UV irradiation, xv, 14, 85, 89, 92, 123, 128, 141, 160, 174, 222, 354, 393, 418, 827, 927, 939, 960
UV light, xv, 83, 160, 164, 175, 179, 328, 333, 353, 891, 893, 943
UV penetration, xviii, 323
UV protective clothes, xxxviii, 1216, 1236
UV spectrum, 328
UVA irradiation, xxx, 15, 418, 892, 938, 941, 942, 943, 944
UVB irradiation, xxx, 125, 410, 937, 938, 940, 946, 951
uveitis, 986, 990, 996, 998
UV-irradiation, 554
UV-mediated carcinogenesis, xviii, 323
UV-radiation, 349, 354

V

vaccinations, 832, 907, 910
vacuole, 585
vacuum, 45, 224, 225
vagina, 584, 637, 718, 897
vaginitis, 611, 619, 642
vagus, 87
vagus nerve, 87

Valencia, 134, 135, 136, 139, 142, 144, 210, 218, 361, 386, 452
validation, 319, 592, 728, 741
valuation, 784
valve, 587, 647, 738, 986
variables, 305, 479, 632, 745, 770, 776
variations, xx, xxxviii, 49, 51, 53, 59, 73, 344, 368, 370, 390, 397, 401, 441, 463, 624, 630, 812, 838, 855, 861, 873
varieties, 170, 246, 332, 883
vascular bundle, 236, 237, 238
vascular diseases, 859, 1015
vascular endothelial growth factor (VEGF), 552, 848, 859, 896, 946, 950, 955, 956
vascular occlusion, 222
vascular system, 301
vascularization, 18, 550, 553, 557, 946
vasculature, 56, 552, 554, 840, 844
vasculitis, xxxii, 511, 588, 1025, 1026
vasoconstriction, xxvii, 13, 761, 763, 824, 857, 885
vasodilation, 555, 900
vasodilator, 267
VCAM, 703, 952
vector, 55
vegetable oil, 434
vegetables, 122
VEGF, 5, 552, 848, 850, 946, 947, 949, 950, 955, 956
VEGFR, 946
vehicles, xxxiii, 421
vein, 464
velocity, 55
Venezuela, 619
ventilation, 582, 770, 797, 798, 803
ventricle, 771
venules, 5, 553
Vermeer, 39, 268, 359, 450, 453
vertebrates, xx, 293, 294, 295, 296, 299, 443, 455, 456, 462, 467
vesicle, 261
vessels, xiv, 3, 5, 18, 43, 44, 56, 65, 67, 296, 397, 436, 547, 552, 769, 881
vibration, 49, 668
Vickers hardness, 682
viral infection, 700, 703, 704, 705, 883, 889, 915
virus infection, 581, 714
viruses, 215, 581, 669, 697
viscera, 572
viscosity, 44
vision, xxiii, xxviii, 390, 545, 547, 552, 555, 556, 634, 757, 805, 806, 812, 813, 814, 991
visual acuity, 92, 205, 255, 257, 635
visualization, 51, 242, 752
vitamin A, xxxii, 309, 831, 898, 999, 1001
vitamin B3, xxxvi, 122, 309
vitamin C, 147, 309, 417, 426, 691
vitamin D, xxxii, xxxix, 333, 352, 354, 366, 377, 397, 481, 486, 824, 825, 850, 886, 887, 890, 892, 925, 935, 957, 999, 1001, 1002, 1005, 1006
vitamin D deficiency, xxxix
vitamin E, xxxii, 999, 1000, 1004
vitamins, xxxii, 999, 1000
vitiligo, xix, xxii, 77, 389, 404, 497, 498, 503, 505, 509, 510, 514, 515, 536, 699, 827, 858, 954
vomiting, 633, 893, 897, 899, 942
vulgaris stratum corneum, xxxi, 959, 975, 980
vulnerability, 497, 499, 877
vulva, 637

W

walking, 777, 823
war, 572, 575, 578, 939
warts, 39
washing procedures, 748
Washington, 27, 332, 475, 603, 610
waste, xxiv, 617, 707
water permeability, 978
waterproof, xliii, 1339, 1446, 1453, 1454, 1639
watershed, 771
wavelengths, 46, 49, 281, 294, 328, 330, 447, 809, 890, 891
weakness, xxvii, 24, 333, 426, 761, 772, 773
wear, 331, 530, 657, 664, 680, 992
wearing apparel, 426, 438
web, 397, 793
websites, xlii
Wechsler Intelligence Scale, 774, 786
weight loss, xli, 664, 794, 1002
welfare, 474
well-being, xlix, 64, 331, 844
West Indies, 314
Western blot, 633
wheezing, 764, 793
white blood cells, 736
white hair, xx, 208, 255, 473, 478
white matter, 771, 782, 783
wild type, xx, 167, 168, 169, 174, 175, 194, 198, 199, 224, 228, 229, 243, 244, 455, 464, 480
Wisconsin, 304
withdrawal, 353, 776, 822, 876, 882, 883, 897, 902, 1001, 1028
Wnt signaling, 66, 91
wood, 153
workers, xxiv, 419, 423, 584, 617, 618, 620, 626, 648, 652, 740, 939, 1010, 1032

working memory, 774, 786
World Health Organization (WHO), xli, 55, 327, 674, 768, 787
World War I, 429, 433
worldwide, xxix, xl, l, 166, 172, 397, 406, 475, 478, 572, 577, 658, 670, 817, 842, 844, 871, 912, 1007
wound healing, xiv, xxxvi, l, 18, 23, 24, 26, 29, 37, 40, 57, 61, 63, 65, 68, 69, 78, 80, 81, 393, 403, 836, 839, 914, 915
wrists, 881, 985
writing process, 779

X

X chromosome, 207
xenografts, 33, 375, 386
xenon, 529, 533
xeroderma pigmentosum, 324, 326, 347, 351, 362, 891, 893
xerostomia, 657, 673, 705
X-irradiation, 477
X-ray diffraction, xvii, 271, 286, 960
x-rays, 327, 485
XRD, 274, 276, 286, 290
xylem, 234

Y

Yale University, 304, 561
yang, 361
yield, xiv, 43, 67, 169, 171, 172, 176, 212, 213, 214, 272, 274, 341, 342, 407, 750, 1001
yin, 361
yolk, 461
young adults, xl, l, 324, 326, 331, 346, 347, 522, 712, 780, 1032
young people, xli, xlvii, xlviii, 17, 990

Z

zinc, 685, 890
zinc oxide, 890